Guides to the Evaluation of Permanent Impairment

Alan L. Engelberg, M.D., M.P.H.
Editor

Third Edition

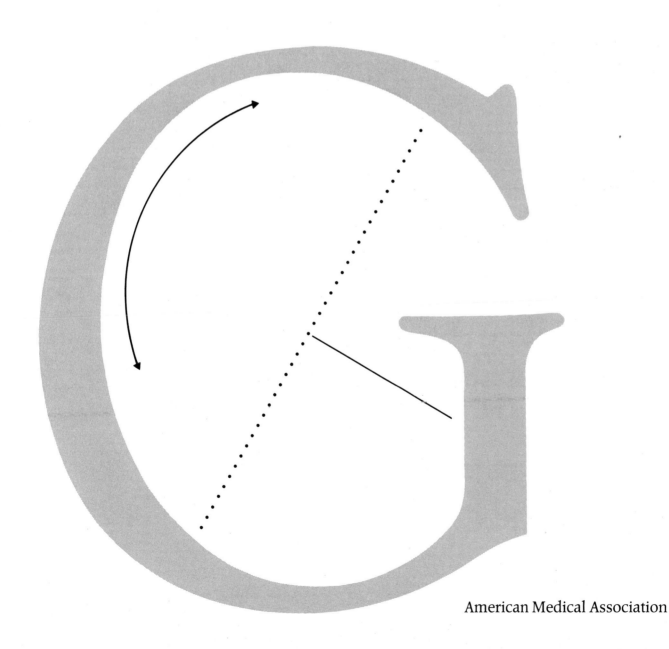

American Medical Association

American Medical Association

Copyright © 1988, 1984, 1977, 1971 by the
American Medical Association
All rights reserved
First Printing March 1984
Second Printing November 1984
Third Printing March 1985
Fourth Printing November 1985
Fifth Printing November 1986
Third Edition—First Printing November 1988
ISBN: 0-89970-338-0

Additional copies may be purchased from:
Order Department OP-254/8
American Medical Association
P.O. Box 10946
Chicago, Illinois 60610

Comments or Inquiries to:
Department of Public Health
American Medical Association
535 North Dearborn Street
Chicago, Illinois 60610

HEA: 88-389:15M: 11/88

Table of Contents

List of Tables
and Figures

Foreword to Third Edition

Thirteen years elapsed between the publishing of the first and second editions of the *Guides to the Evaluation of Permanent Impairment.* The third edition is published only four years after the second, yet this new edition is substantially revised. A number of trends account for this: first, the clinical knowledge about impairment, and how it is evaluated and rated, has developed rapidly in the 1980's. Major studies have appeared in the medical literature, and have been commissioned by authoritative national organizations. Second, the growth of interest in impairment by nearly all medical specialties has been truly remarkable. Conferences in this subject, which used to attract only a die-hard few, are now over-subscribed. And finally, the expanded use of the *Guides* has enlarged the pool of practitioners who provide comments and suggestions for improvements. The numerous letters the American Medical Association has received since 1984 provided us with a major impetus to review and revise the *Guides* as quickly as we did.

In this edition the reader will note substantial changes. The Preface of the 2nd edition, which provided the philosophical underpinning for the *Guides,* is expanded into two chapters. The emphasis on thorough report-writing and better use of the patient's past medical records in the impairment evaluation process is strengthened. The message that the *Guides* provides a system for *evaluating,* and not just rating impairment, is made clearer. To assist in the evaluation process, each chapter is divided into numbered sections, or protocols, the evaluative processes of which can be referenced by the physician in his or her report.

The chapter on the Extremities, Spine, and Pelvis is altered considerably from the 2nd edition. The evaluation of the upper extremity is revised in accordance with the methods adopted by the International Federation of Societies of Surgery of the Hand. The evaluation of the spine uses inclinometers, rather than goniometers, for the measurement of range of motion, a technique that provides more accurate, reproducible results. An expanded list of specific acquired spine disorders provides ratings to combine with the ratings for limited range of motion. To reduce the need for cross-referencing, for both the upper and lower extremities, guidance for evaluating peripheral nerve and vascular impairments are placed next to the respective sections on range of motion impairments.

The chapter on Mental and Behavioral Disorders relies upon a review of the "Listings of Mental Impairments" of the Social Security Administration, which was published in 1985. Four broad areas are defined in the evaluation process: limitation on activities of daily living; social functioning; concentration, persistence, and pace; and adaptation to stressful situations, such as work.

Other chapters with major revisions include Respiratory (in accordance with new guidelines from the American Thoracic Society), Visual (discussion of new technologies and inclusions of a binocular grid for visual field testing), Digestive (evaluation of abdominal wall and inguinal hernias), and Skin (nail disorders).

An issue of great concern to many users of the *Guides* is chronic pain. In recent years the Institute of Medicine and the Social Security Administration have conducted major reviews of chronic pain and its implications for impairment and disability. Both studies conclude that chronic pain should be attended to in a more thorough and systematic fashion in clinical practice, but that it is undesirable at this time to add chronic pain as an impairment listing under Social Security. Similarly, in this edition of the *Guides* we include an appendix that summarizes the biopsychosocial issues involved in chronic pain that make it difficult to address chronic pain in a standardized impairment evaluation system.

Finally, the *Guides* continue to espouse the philosophy that all impairments affect the whole person, and therefore, all impairment ratings should be combined to be expressed as impairment of the whole person. This is done with the aid of the familiar "Combined Values Chart."

Since the 3rd edition of the *Guides* builds upon the work of the many consultants who assisted AMA in revising the 2nd edition, we would again like to acknowledge their contribution to the furthering of our knowledge of impairment evaluation. AMA also thanks the following consultants whose efforts are largely responsible for the preparation of this new edition.

Consultants

Robert G. Addison, M.D.,
Rehabilitation Institute of Chicago, Chicago, IL

Sidney J. Blair, M.D.,
Loyola University, Maywood, IL

James C. Folsom, M.D.,
Veterans Administration Medical Center, Topeka, KS

Howard H. Goldman, M.D., Ph.D.,
University of Maryland, Baltimore, MD

Philip Harber, M.D., M.P.H.,
University of California, Los Angeles, CA

William S. Haubrich, M.D.,
Scripps Clinic and Research Foundation, LaJolla, CA

William J. Kane, M.D.,
Northwestern University, Chicago, IL

Richard E. Kanner, M.D.,
University of Utah, Salt Lake City, UT

Paul E. Kaplan, M.D.,
University of Missouri, Columbia, MO

Arthur H. Keeney, M.D.,
University of Louisville, Louisville, KY

Philipp M. Lippe, M.D.,
Stanford University, San Jose, CA

Larry Livengood, M.D.,
private practice, Madison, WI

Herbert K.N. Luke, M.D.,
private practice, Honolulu, HA

Tom G. Mayer, M.D.,
University of Texas, Dallas, TX

Arthur T. Meyerson, M.D.,
Hahnemann University, Philadelphia, PA

Attilio D. Renzetti, M.D.,
University of Utah, Salt Lake City, UT

Joseph Sataloff, M.D.,
Jefferson University, Philadelphia, PA

George M. Smith, M.D., M.P.H.,
President, GM Smith Assoc., Inc., Bethesda, MD

Alfred B. Swanson, M.D.,
Michigan State University, Grand Rapids, MI

Genevieve de Groot Swanson, M.D.,
private practice, Grand Rapids, MI

James S. Taylor, M.D.,
Cleveland Clinic Foundation, Cleveland, OH

Ralph O. Wallerstein, M.D.,
University of California, San Francisco, CA

American Medical Association Staff

William R. Hendee, Ph.D.,
Vice President, Group on Science and Technology

Betty Jane Anderson, J.D.,
Associate General Counsel

Cathy Campbell,
Senior Secretary and Coordinator

Mark Oldach,
Design Manager

Alan L. Engelberg, M.D., M.P.H.
Editor and Director
Department of Preventive Medicine
American Medical Association

Foreword to the Second Edition

In 1956 the Board of Trustees of the American Medical Association (AMA) created an ad hoc Committee on Medical Rating of Physical Impairment to establish a series of practical guides for the rating of physical impairment of the various organ systems. As the scope of the Committee's work broadened, its name was changed to the Committee on Rating of Mental and Physical Impairment. From 1958 to 1970 the Committee published 13 separate "Guides to the Evaluation of Permanent Impairment" in *The Journal of the American Medical Association.*

In 1971 the AMA reviewed the Committee's *Guides* and published them as a single volume. By providing clinically sound and reproducible criteria for rating permanent impairment, the *Guides* have continued to be useful to physicians, attorneys and adjudicators in fulfilling their responsibilities to patients, clients, and applicants seeking benefits from agencies and programs serving the disabled.

In 1981 the AMA's Council on Scientific Affairs undertook a review of the *Guides* and established an advisory panel to determine the need for revision. At the suggestion of these consultants, 12 expert panels were established to update the clinical information that supports the impairment ratings. This second edition of the *Guides* is the result of their efforts combined with the efforts of many on the AMA's staff.

In this edition there are many changes. The chapter on the extremities, spine, and pelvis contains four new tables assigning impairment ratings to orthopedic conditions not mentioned in the first edition. Two chapters on the central and peripheral nervous systems in the first edition have become one, and the new chapter contains a section on impairment due to sleep and arousal disorders. This relatively recent field of clinical endeavor may be unfamiliar to users of the *Guides*; therefore, an appendix is included that briefly describes categories of sleep and arousal abnormalities, and gives examples of the impairments they may cause.

The chapter on the respiratory system has been modified extensively to include physiologic tests that reflect more accurately the degree of impairment. The chapter on the cardiovascular system is divided into sections on valvular heart disease, hypertensive cardiovascular disease, cardiomyopathies, arrhythmias, and peripheral vascular disease. Specific impairment criteria are given for each.

The chapter on the endocrine system features revised criteria for impairment due to diabetes mellitus. The chapters on the hematopoietic system, the visual system, the ear, nose and throat, the digestive system, the skin, and the reproductive and urinary systems have been modified to include more modern clinical examples and measurement techniques.

Finally the chapter on mental and behavioral disorders is written not only to stand by itself, but to be used in the assessment of mental impairment that may result from physical impairment. It emphasizes the need for rehabilitation before a rating of permanent impairment can be assigned.

The *Guides* continue to espouse the philosophy that all physical and mental impairments affect the whole person, and therefore, all impairment ratings should be combined to be expressed as impairment of the whole person. This is done with the aid of a "Combined Values Chart."

The AMA strongly urges that all readers become familiar with the proper use of the *Guides* and the proper terminology in the fields of impairment and disability. All users should read the Preface to the *Guides* and the two appendices on report preparation and terminology before using the *Guides*.

In addition to the members of the committees who devoted their time and gave of their knowledge to the revision of the *Guides*, many medical specialty societies, individual practitioners, and governmental agencies helped AMA's expert panels and staff add new and relevant information in this second edition.

The AMA acknowledges the contributions of the following members of the various panels whose efforts are largely responsible for the preparation of this new edition.

American Medical Association Council on Scientific Affairs

John R. Beljan, MD
George Bohigian, MD
Theodore Cooper, MD
William D. Dolan, MD
Ira R. Friedlander, MD
Ray W. Gifford, Jr, MD, Chairman
Michael B. Kastan
John H. Moxley, III, MD, Vice Chairman
Joseph H. Skom, MD
Rogers J. Smith, MD
James B. Snow, Jr, MD
C. John Tupper, MD

American Medical Association Staff

Leonard D. Fenninger, MD, Vice President,
Group on Medical Education and Scientific Policy

Betty Jane Anderson, JD, Associate General Counsel

Richard J. Jones, MD, Secretary
Council on Scientific Affairs

Environmental and Occupational Health Program
Theodore C. Doege, MD, MS, Program Director
Jermyn F. McCahan, MD, Senior Editor
Alan L. Engelberg, MD, MPH, Editor
Leatha A. Tiggelaar, Coordinator
Cathy A. Campbell
Barbara S. Jansson
Nancy T. O'Connor

Panel Members

Robert M. Adams, MD,
Stanford University, Palo Alto, CA

Robert G. Addison, MD,
Northwestern University, Chicago, IL.

William H. Anderson, MD,
University of Louisville, Louisville, KY

Budd Appleton, MD,
private practice, St. Paul, MN

Ronald A. Arky, MD,
Harvard University, Boston, MA

John L. Bell, MD,
Northwestern University, Chicago, IL

Harvey W. Bender, Jr, MD,
Vanderbilt University, Nashville, TN

Donald J. Birmingham, MD,
Wayne State University, Detroit, MI

Bernard R. Blais, MC,
Captain, United States Department of the Navy,
Washington, DC

Robert W. Cantrell, MD,
University of Virginia, Charlottesville, VA

Leon A. Carrow, MD,
Northwestern University, Chicago, IL

Francis I. Catlin, MD,
Baylor College of Medicine, Houston, TX

Oliver H. Dabezies, Jr, MD,
Tulane University, New Orleans, LA

Gilbert Daniels, MD,
Harvard University, Boston, MA

Jane Desforges, MD,
Tufts University, Boston, MA

Robert Dluhy, MD,
Harvard University, Boston, MA

Marvin I. Dunn, MD,
University of Kansas, Kansas City, KS

Jack R. Ewalt, MD,
Veterans Administration, Washington, DC

Thomas W. Farmer, MD,
University of North Carolina, Chapel Hill, NC

George M. Smith, MD,
private consultant, Bethesda, MD

James B. Snow, Jr, MD,
University of Pennsylvania, Philadelphia, PA

Arthur J. Spielman, PhD,
Albert Einstein College of Medicine, Bronx, NY

John A. Spittell, Jr, MD,
Mayo Clinic, Rochester, MN

James S. Taylor, MD,
Cleveland Clinic Foundation, Cleveland, OH

Gennaro M. Tisi, MD,
University of California, San Diego, CA

Theodore A. Tromovitch, MD,
University of California, San Francisco, CA

Ralph O. Wallerstein, MD,
University of California, San Francisco, CA

Hans Weill, MD,
Tulane University, New Orleans, LA

Elliott D. Weitzman, MD,
Cornell University, White Plains, NY (deceased)

Charles W. Whitmore, MD, LLB,
Health Sciences Education and Research
Corporation, Lynchburg, VA

Charles F. Wooley, MD,
Ohio State University, Columbus, OH

Dewey K. Ziegler, MD,
University of Kansas, Kansas City, KS

Chapter 1

Concepts of Impairment Evaluation

1.0 Introduction

The *AMA Guides to the Evaluation of Permanent Impairment* (the *Guides*) provides a reference framework within which physicians may evaluate and report medical impairment and within which nonmedical recipients of information about impairment may understand and make appropriate use of the medical information they receive.

The unique value of the *Guides* as *the* technical reference of choice for evaluation of medical impairment, which goes well beyond its broad scope of coverage (all body parts and systems), arises from the precise application of fundamental medical and scientific concepts; the systematic analysis that introduces each of the clinical chapters; the detail of the medical evaluation protocols; and the thorough state-of-the-art analyses that underlie the rating tables. In addition, a format for reports is described in Chapter 2 and summarized at the beginning of each clinical chapter to provide straightforward and well-structured guidelines so that reports about the same individual from different observers are likely to be of comparable content and completeness and may, therefore, be more easily analyzed and compared.

As is true of any other technical process, knowing the "rules," which in the case of the *Guides* are the specific procedures described in the clinical chapters, is not enough. The user of the *Guides*, both physicians and nonphysicians alike, must understand the concepts under which the "rules" have been developed and the intended approach for using them to achieve objective, accurate, fair, and reproducible evaluations of individuals with medical impairment. This chapter and Chapter 2 will enable the user to become familiar with the techniques and approach to evaluation of impairment embodied in the *Guides*.

1.1 Basic Considerations

Impairment—Disability—Handicap

Various terms used in the *Guides*, such as "impairment," "disability" and "handicap," appear in laws, regulations and policies of diverse origin without prior coordination of the ways in which they are used. It is no wonder, then, that there is uncertainty, if not controversy, about their meaning. The definitions used in the *Guides* seek to remedy this confusion through detailed description and delineation of the domain in which each term is applied, for it is the characteristics of the domain that are important, not the word used as the label. Accordingly, even when the terminology of the *Guides* may differ from or appear to be in conflict with that of a particular law, regulation or administrative system, analysis of the context in accordance with the following discussion should reveal how the principles embodied in the *Guides* may be interpreted and applied within the provisions of a particular disability system.

The accurate and proper use of medical information to assess impairment in connection with disability determinations depends on the recognition that, whereas impairment is a medical matter, disability arises out of the interaction between impairment and external demands. Consequently, as used in the *Guides*, "impairment" means an alteration of an individual's health status that is *assessed by medical means*; "disability," which is *assessed by nonmedical means*, means an alteration of an individual's capacity to meet personal, social, or occupational demands, or to meet statutory or regulatory requirements. Simply stated, "impairment" is what is wrong with the health of an individual; "disability" is the gap between what the individual can do and what the individual needs or wants to do.

An individual who is "impaired" is not necessarily "disabled." Impairment gives rise to disability only when the medical condition limits the individual's capacity to meet demands that pertain to nonmedical fields and activities.[1] On the other hand, if the individual is able to meet a particular set of demands, the individual is *not* "disabled" with respect to those demands, even though a medical evaluation may reveal impairment.

The concept of "handicap" is related to, yet independent of, both "impairment" and "disability," although it is sometimes used interchangeably with either of these terms. Under the provisions of Federal law,[2] an individual is identified as "handicapped" if that individual has an impairment that substantially limits one or more life activities, including work, has a record of such impairment, or is regarded as having such an impairment.[3] The terms of this definition are so indefinite and broad that, technically, almost any person who desires to do so might be included in the class of the handicapped under the law.

As a matter of practicality, however, a "handicap" may be operationally understood as being manifest in association with a "barrier" or obstacle to functional activity. An individual with limited functional capacity is handicapped if there are barriers to accomplishment of tasks or life activities that can be overcome only by compensating in some way for the effects of an impairment. Such compensation, or, more technically, "accommodation," normally entails the use of assistive devices (such as crutches, wheel chairs, hearing aids, optical magnifiers, prostheses, special tools or equipment), modification of the environment, and/or modification of tasks or activities (such as increased time for task completion, or special segmentation of tasks). Any

one these modalities, or all in combination, may be invoked to enable a handicapped person to overcome a barrier to an objective. If the individual is not able to accomplish a task or activity despite accommodation, or if there is no accommodation that will enable the accomplishment, then, in addition to being handicapped, the individual is also disabled. On the other hand, an impaired individual who is able to accomplish a task or activity without accommodation is, with respect to that task or activity, neither handicapped nor disabled.

For these reasons, it is difficult to overstate the importance of examining the context in which the terms "impairment," "disability," or "handicap" appear to avoid being misled by imprecise usage. For example, reference to a physician's evaluation of "disability" must be understood as a reference to a *medical* evaluation of an individual's health status, or, in the terms of the *Guides*, an evaluation of impairment. The physician does not determine industrial loss of use or economic loss for the purpose of paying a disability benefit.

Employability—Management/ Administrative Considerations

The concept of "employability" deserves special attention, for in an occupational setting, if an individual, within the boundaries of the medical condition, has the capacity with or without accommodation to meet the job demands and conditions of employment as defined by the employer, the individual is employable, and, consequently, not disabled. As an operational matter, employability is critically related to an individual's capacity to travel to and from work, to be at work, and to perform assigned tasks and duties for which the employer is willing to pay wages. If the individual has those capacities, even in the presence of impairment, then the individual is not disabled for that job. When these capacities are called into question, for whatever reason, the employer must carry out an "employability determination."

As in determination of disability, there are both administrative and medical components to the employability determination, the process by which an employer initially assesses an individual's qualifications and suitability for employment. On the administrative side, management will specifically assess performance capability to estimate the likelihood of a performance failure

---

1. The commonly used example of the impact of the loss of the fifth finger of the left hand illustrates the point. If the individual is a bank president, the occupational impact is likely to be negligible On the other hand, a concert pianist is likely to be totally disabled.

2. The Rehabilitation Act of 1973.

3. The law does not make clear by whom the individual must be "regarded" as being handicapped. There are cases on record in which an employer "accommodated" the individual even though there was no clear evidence or record of medical impairment. In these cases, it was determined that the individual was protected as handicapped under the law because the employer, by offering accommodation, had regarded the individual as handicapped.

as well as the likelihood of incurring a future liability in case of human failure. If neither likelihood of failure is too great, then the individual is considered to be employable in a particular job. This represents a fundamental "go" or "no go" determination that there is or is not a sufficient match between an individual and the job requirements to give further consideration to employment. It is different from a "desirability" determination, which would rank and compare the individuals who are employable.

During the course of employment, there is on-going reassessment of an individual's employability through monitoring of performance, conduct, and attendance. Employment continues until the employee leaves voluntarily or until a change gives rise to a deficiency in performance, conduct, or attendance so that retention in the job can no longer be justified. When an individual claims to be no longer employable, or disabled, because of a change in health, or alleges that a medical condition has caused a service deficiency, the employer has little choice but to conduct an employability determination and to assess the individual's capacity to travel to and from work, to be at work and to perform assigned tasks and duties. Disability, then, is the default result when it is determined that the individual lacks employability.

Employability—Medical Considerations

As noted above, an employable individual has the capacity to travel to and from work, to be at work, and to perform assigned tasks and duties. On the other hand, an individual who does not have the capacity, or who is unwilling, to travel to and from work, to be at work, and to perform assigned tasks and duties is not employable. The issue of disability arises from the critical questions of whether or not the service deficiency can be explained by a medical condition and whether or not the medical condition precludes, or warrants restriction from, traveling to and from work, being at work, or performing assigned tasks and duties. The answer is found in a "medical determination related to employability."

The first critical task in carrying out a medical determination related to employability is to learn about the job, specifically the expectations of the incumbent with respect to performance, physical activity, reliability, availability, productivity, expected duration of useful service life and any other criteria associated with qualification and suitability. Sufficiently detailed information from a job analysis will provide a basis upon which a physician determines exactly what kinds of medical information are needed; and to what degree of detail, to assess an individual's health with respect to demand criteria. Once the medical information needs are known, it is possible to develop a medical evaluation protocol, a set of instructions for performance of a medical evaluation designed to acquire that information.

However, a special medical evaluation may not be necessary, for, presumably, an individual who alleges disability would already be under the care of a personal physician, and if not, should be if the medical condition is interfering with life activities on or off the job. And, since a claimant bears the initial burden of proof, the place to start, then, is with review of medical information *already* available in the form of medical office and hospital records. Through this medium, the physician making the determination of employability may communicate with the personal physician to learn whatever is known about that individual's health so that, in accordance with established medical diagnostic criteria and generally accepted medical principles and practice, the two physicians may come to agreement about what is and is not known medically about the patient and determine what other information is necessary to resolve areas of medical uncertainty. This is nothing more or less than physicians do in the course of cooperative management of their patients. The practice of medicine is not an adversary process; and, consequently, by relying on communications and decisionmaking procedures ordinarily used by physicians, evaluations of impairment and medical determinations related to employability may be managed without confrontation between them. With respect to employability, then, the medical questions to be answered are whether or not medical documentation supports a conclusion that the individual's medical condition precludes travel to and from work, being at work, or performing assigned tasks and duties,[4] and, in the case of a service deficiency, whether or not the documentation provides reason to believe that the medical condition has either caused or contributed to the deficiency.

If review of the documentation does not show that the individual has met the required burden of proof, the employer or insurance company must decide whether or not acquisition of additional medical information is likely to enable the individual to do so. Or, there may be a need to verify clinical findings contained in the documentation provided. If so, the medical evaluation protocol will serve as a basis for a medical evaluation by *any* physician; for, in general, two

---

4. If the medical condition does not, for example, preclude daily travel to and from a physical therapy clinic, then it would be unlikely for the medical condition to preclude travel to and from place of work. Or, if an individual has not been restricted from shopping for and carrying groceries, from doing chores around the house, or from going to the movies, then there is little defense for a conclusion that the medical condition would warrant restriction from a similar level of activities in the workplace.

physicians examining the same patient under the same protocol will have approximately the same set of findings. Taken with the prior information, the results of this evaluation may be reviewed to reach conclusions that can then be compared with the demand criteria for the job. This can always be done with credibility and confidence, since the specifications for the medical evaluation are based on the demand criteria to begin with.

When approached in this way, the medical input into the employability determination will be quite independent of the individual's motivation to work, or lack of it. Moreover, because this process provides medical justification for the decision, a dispute over conflicting opinions of physicians about nonmedical matters need never occur.

1.2 Structure and Use of the *Guides*

Since any person has only one health status and only one life situation, given enough information about each, it is possible to understand the relationship and interaction between them. Moreover, because the evaluation of permanent impairment is not an isolated event but culminates the evolution of changes in health that result from injury or disease, the design of the *Guides* requires integration of already existing medical and nonmedical information with the results of a current clinical evaluation, carried out in accordance with the protocols of the *Guides*, to characterize fully and assess medical impairment. Accomplishment of this objective is based on utilization of three powerful tools that make up the fundamental components of the *Guides*.

First, Chapter 2 details with great precision the kinds of information needed to document the nature of an impairment and its consequences, specifies procedures for acquiring the information, and defines a structured format for analyzing, recording, and reporting the information. A summary of these requirements and procedures appears at the beginning of each clinical chapter.

Second, the clinical chapters contain definitive medical evaluation protocols, descriptions of specific procedures for evaluating a particular body part, function, or system, each developed by recognized medical specialty consultants. These protocols are defined in specific detail to ensure the acquisition of sufficient information to describe fully and characterize the current clinical status of a medical impairment.

Third, the clinical chapters contain reference tables specifically keyed to the evaluation protocols. If the protocols and tables have been followed, the clinical findings may be compared directly to the criteria and related to a percentage of impairment with confidence in the validity and acceptability of the determination.

Operationally, the key to effective and reliable evaluation of impairment is initially a review of clinical medical office and hospital records maintained by the physicians who have provided care and treatment since the onset of the medical condition. Such records comprise clinical notes of office visits, medical specialty consultation reports, hospital admission and discharge summaries, operative notes, pathology reports, laboratory test reports and the results of special tests and diagnostic procedures. Before formal evaluation is carried out under the *Guides*, analysis of the history and course of the medical condition, beginning with the circumstances of onset, and including findings on previous examinations, the course of treatment, responses to treatment, and the impact of the medical condition on life activities, must support a conclusion that an impairment is permanent and well stabilized.

This information gathering and analysis serves as the foundation upon which the evaluation of a permanent impairment is carried out. It is most important that the evaluator obtain all clinical information necessary to characterize fully the medical condition in accordance with requirements of the *Guides*; an incomplete or partial evaluation is not acceptable. Once this task is accomplished, the clinical findings may be compared to the clinical information already contained in the records about the individual. If the current findings are found to be consistent with the results of previous clinical evaluations performed by other observers, then, with complete confidence, they may be compared, as appropriate or required, with the reference tables to determine the percentage rating of the impairment. However, if the findings are not in substantial accordance with the information of record, then, until further clinical evaluation resolves the disparities, the rating step is meaningless and cannot be carried out.

This approach takes advantage of the fact that physicians normally communicate cooperatively with each other orally and in writing to determine what they do and do not know about a patient, and to determine further what additional information they need to resolve areas of medical uncertainty. It does not make sense, therefore, to manage cases in which there are differing "opinions" among physicians about the nature and degree of medical impairment by asking a nonmedical third party to adjudicate an issue of medical fact! Such differences are best handled through the ordinary process of everyday patient management. Then, with reference to the past medical documentation, the medical evaluation protocols contained in the clinical chapters and the reporting specifications of Chapter 2, the physician and nonphysician users of the *Guides* may verify that sufficient medical information has been assembled and reported to permit an assessment of an impairment, to justify any conclusions that are drawn, and to support a rating in accordance with the tables. At that point, it is a straightforward matter to verify whether or not a numerical rating of impairment is substantiated in accordance with the criteria contained in the *Guides*.

1.3 Medical Impairment and Workers' Compensation

In general, state and Federal workers' compensation laws are based on the concept that a worker who either sustains an injury or incurs an illness arising in the course of and out of employment is entitled to protection against financial loss without being required to sue the employer. In exchange for their having lost the right to sue, the workers' compensation system guarantees benefits to all workers who are covered under the law and who meet the criteria for award of benefits.

The types of payments that may be made when a claim is approved fall into three categories:

• payments to the claimant to compensate for lost wages due to temporary total disability;

• payment of medical bills; and

• payment to the claimant of an award for permanent disability, partial or total.

Up to this point, we have looked at disability as being related to functional capability or the lack of it. However, in the arena of disability benefits, disability, whether temporary or permanent, partial or total, is equivalent to economic loss for which the individual is to be compensated monetarily.

Payments are made for temporary total disability when the individual is unable to earn wages, return to work is expected, and the medical condition has not stabilized.[5] Temporary disability is partial when the individual returns to work but is not earning at the prior level.

A permanent disability award is normally independent of the individual's capacity to work and is formulated in terms of expected or presumed long-term or permanent economic loss associated with a permanent medical impairment, such as an amputation. Such an award may be paid according to a schedule that specifically associates impairment with certain body parts, functions, or systems; examples are amputations, loss of sight, and loss of hearing, and a schedule is defined in the workers' compensation law to equate the disability with a maximum number of weeks for which benefits are to be paid at a rate based on average weekly wages.

Rating of partial disability is necessary when a law, in recognition that the "loss of" or "loss of use of" the body part, function, or system may be less than total, requires determination of the proportion or percentage of loss. For example, in Maryland, the law says:

> In all cases where there has been an amputation of a part of any member of the body herein specified, or the *loss of use of* (emphasis added) any part thereof...the Commission shall allow compensation for such proportion of the total number of weeks allowed for the amputation or loss of use of the entire member as the affected or amputated portion bears to the whole.[6]

Moreover, because not all conditions that can arise out of an injury are accounted for in a schedule, back injuries, for example, there is likely to be a provision of the law similar to the following:

> In all other cases of disability other than those specifically enumerated disabilities[7]...which disability is partial in character, but permanent in quality, the Commission shall determine the portion or percentage by which the *industrial use* of the employee's body was *impaired* as a result of the injury and in determining such portion or percentage of impairment[8] resulting in industrial loss, the Commission shall take into consideration, among other things, the nature of the physical injury, the occupation, experience, training, and age of the injured employee, and shall award compensation in such proportion as the determined loss bears to 500 weeks...[9] (emphasis added)

---

5. In accordance with the earlier discussion, "temporary total disability" occurs when the medical condition precludes the individual from traveling to and from work, being at work, and performing assigned tasks and duties.

6. Workmen's Compensation Law of Maryland, Annotated, 1983, Art. 101, §36(3).

7. Note the context with which "disability" and "disabilies" are used. Clearly, the terms should be read as "impairment" and "impairments."

8. Should this read "disability"?

9. *Ibid.* Art. 101, *36(4)(a).*

While medical information is necessary for the decision process, a critical problem arises in the use of that information. Neither in this example nor in general is there a formula under which knowledge of the medical condition may be combined with knowledge of the other factors to calculate the percentage by which the industrial use of the employee's body is impaired. Accordingly, each commissioner or hearing official must come to a conclusion based on his or her own assessment of the available medical and nonmedical information.

It is evident that the *Guides* does not offer a solution for this problem, nor is it the intention that it do so. Each administrative or legal system that uses permanent impairment as a basis for disability rating needs to define its own process for translating knowledge of a medical condition into an estimate of the degree to which the individual's capacity to meet personal, social, or occupational demands, or to meet statutory or regulatory requirements, is limited by the impairment. We encourage each system not to make a "one-to-one" translation of impairment to disability, in essence creating a use of the *Guides* which is not intended.

Chapter 2 will emphasize that it is essential for the physician to provide the recipient of the medical information with more than a number that represents a percentage of impairment. To the extent that the physician provides a comprehensive medical picture in the form of a report formulated in accordance with (Figure 1), the user of the information will be able to determine how the medical information fits with all the other nonmedical information, thereby to reach a true understanding of the impact of the medical impairment on the claimant's future employability.

Chapter 2

Records and Reports

2.0 Introduction

A system for managing disability benefits is most effective when there is sufficient medical and nonmedical information to justify a decision and thereby to minimize or eliminate adversary confrontation. This chapter describes and analyzes how the tools contained in the *Guides*—its conceptual principles, medical evaluation protocols, rating reference tables and reporting procedures—taken together provide for consistent and reliable acquisition, analysis, communication and utilization of medical information.

One major objective of the *Guides* is to define the process of measuring and reporting medical impairment in sufficient detail so that physicians have the capability to collect, analyze, and report information about the medical impairment of claimants in accordance with a single set of standards. As noted in Chapter 1, two physicians following the same medical evaluation protocol to evaluate the same patient and using the same reference tables and reporting protocol should report very similar results and reach very similar conclusions. Moreover, if the clinical findings are completely described in the report, then any knowledgeable observer may compare the findings to the tables to determine the impairment rating. In this sense, "rating" is not a medical determination and, consequently, need not be done by a physician. However, because of its objective quality, no additional special weight or importance can be attached to the result, simply because a physician makes the comparison and reports the impairment rating.

Clearly, if the physicians have not obtained similar results and reached similar conclusions, there is a reference framework within which to resolve the discrepancies. Analysis of records and reports will disclose the areas of discrepancy. In such a case, the differences must occur in the clinical findings, which are *matters of fact, not opinion*, that can be verified by further observation of the claimant in accordance with the appropriate medical evaluation protocol. When the medical condition has become static or stabilized, the findings should be replicable in repeated examinations. If this is not the case, then the stability of the medical condition is in question, and there is no basis upon which to rate *permanent* impairment.

Compare this approach with the generally occurring practice in impairment or "disability" evaluation wherein each physician examines and reports without any protocol. In these cases, it is impossible to compare discrepant reports, for there can be no reasonable certainty that either physician has made *all* of the same observations as the other or has examined the same body parts or systems in a similar way. Quite commonly, the physicians have looked at different aspects of the same body part and have honestly reported their findings. For example, one physician may include measurement of rotation or lateral bend of the spine, whereas another may make no mention of having observed these movements. Or, one physician may report forward bend in terms of "reaches to 10 inches from the floor," and another may say of the same patient "forward bending limited to 80°." Or, in another case, one physician may report measurement of thigh circumferences showing a difference of more than 1 inch, and another may simply comment that there is no atrophy without having measured. Without standardization of both the evaluation and reporting procedures, the recipient of the information has a difficult choice to make in deciding which report to believe or which one deserves greater "weight." This outcome is neither reasonable nor fair and tends to give rise to inappropriate and avoidable adversary confrontations.

When physicians follow the *Guides* to measure and report their findings of impairment, then the recipients and users of this information may be held accountable to assess the results in accordance with the *Guides*. Because issues of medical fact should already have been settled by this stage in the process, the recipients should not find it necessary to (arbitrarily) give weight to or choose among conflicting "opinions" of physicians. By consulting the standardized medical evaluation protocols, the reference tables and the reporting protocol, the reviewer may verify with complete confidence whether or not all necessary information was collected. If so, the correctness of the rating may be verified by comparing the findings to the tables. In those cases where physicians disagree on the clinical findings, clearly further medical evaluation is necessary. It is *not* appropriate for the reviewer to overcome a deficiency in medical information by giving greater weight to the (unsupported) opinion of any of the physicians.

A simple number, the impairment rating, although it may have been derived from a well structured complex set of thorough observations, does not convey any information about the person or the impact of the impairment on the person's capacity to meet personal, social, or occupational demands. In fact, information is lost in arriving at the number. Consequently, the strength of the medical support for a disability determination is dependent on the completeness and reliability of the medical documentation submitted. Knowledge of the course of an individual's medical condition over time is essential in reaching an appropriate understanding of an individual's present health status. It is, therefore, essential that copies of existing medical office and hospital records be attached to the narrative report, even if the report itself discusses the past medical history and course of the condition. Because the impairment evaluation is not an isolated event but rather occurs in the

course of managing a medical condition, the disability reviewer will be able to determine whether or not the claim of disability makes sense over all and will be able to approach the question of disability as economic loss in a systematic and analytic fashion.

2.1 Medical Assessment of Impairment

Medical evaluation in accordance with the protocols of the *Guides*:
The first step in assessment of an impairment is a thorough medical evaluation with particular attention to the complete clinical and nonclinical history of the medical condition(s). Then, in accordance with the appropriate protocols of the *Guides*, clinical evaluation is carried out, supported by appropriate tests and diagnostic procedures. (Each clinical chapter of the *Guides* has been divided into numbered sections, so that in a report the evaluating physician can refer to the protocols described in appropriate sections. For example, a physician evaluating impairment of the cervical spine would refer to protocols in sections 3.3a through 3.3c Chapter 3.) When a medically sufficient evaluation is carried out in this way, the current clinical status of the individual will be documented. If the current findings are found to be consistent with the results of previous clinical evaluations performed by other observers, then, with complete confidence, they may be compared with the reference tables to determine the percentage rating of the impairment. However, if the findings are not in substantial accordance with the information of record, then, until further clinical evaluation resolves the disparities, the rating step is meaningless and cannot be carried out. The appropriate course at that point is further clinical evaluation to resolve the disparities by medical verification of the individual's current clinical condition.

Analysis of the findings:
The second step is analysis of the history and the clinical and laboratory findings to determine the nature and extent of the loss, loss of use of, or derangement of the affected body parts, systems, or functions.

Comparison of the results of analysis with the medical impairment criteria:
The third step is the comparison of the results of the analysis with the criteria that are specified in the *Guides* for the particular body part, system, or function. This process is distinct from the prior clinical evaluation and

need not be performed by the same physician doing that evaluation. Any knowledgeable physician or any other knowledgeable person may compare the clinical findings on a particular patient with the criteria in the *Guides*.

Rating of the whole person:

To support systems in which it is necessary because of legal or administrative requirements, the reference tables also take into account all relevant considerations in order to reach a "whole person" impairment rating. The final impairment value, whether the result of single or combined impairments, may be expressed in terms of the nearest 5 percent.

Impairment should not be considered "permanent" until clinical findings over the course of time support a conclusion that the medical condition is static or well stabilized. A physician who re-evaluates an individual's impairment must be aware that change may have occurred, even though the previous evaluator considered the impairment to be "permanent" at that time. For instance, the condition may have become worse as a result of aggravation (see Appendix A for the definition) or clinical progression, or it may have improved; regardless, the evaluator should assess the current state of the impairment in accordance with the criteria in the *Guides*.

The concept of "permanency" in disability programs may vary considerably; it usually relates to a provision in a contract, policy, or regulation in which the time limit for permanency of disability is defined.

Valid quantification of any change in impairment rating will depend on the reliability of the previous rating. If there were no valid rating previously, the adequacy of previous documentation about the condition could be used to estimate a rating according to the criteria in the *Guides*. If the evaluator does not have sufficient information to measure change accurately, the evaluator should not attempt to do so and should provide a narrative explanation of the reasons.

If *apportionment* is needed (see Appendix A for the definition), the analysis must consider the nature of the impairment and its possible relationship to each alleged factor and provide an explanation of the medical basis for all conclusions and opinions. To establish that a factor *could have* contributed to the impairment the analysis must include a discussion of the pathophysiology of the particular condition and of pertinent host characteristics. A conclusion that a factor *did* contribute to an impairment must rely on documentation of circumstances under which the factor was present, and verification that the type and magnitude of the factor were sufficient and had the necessary temporal relationship to the medical condition. The existence of medical impairment alone does not create a presumption of contribution by any factor with which the impairment is often associated. The establishment of nexus is a legal or administrative matter, not a medical matter.

Even when the impairment is well localized, its consequences cannot be understood without taking the person into account. As a consequence, attention to the full reporting format will provide the best opportunity for physicians to explain the health status of the claimant and the nature of the impairment for reviewers, claims examiners, hearing officials, and attorneys to understand the impairment and to relate to "industrial loss of use," or some similar concept and for the individual to pursue entitlement to any benefits that are deserved.

2.2 Reports

A clear, accurate, and complete report is essential to support a rating of permanent impairment. The kinds of information that should be expected by the reviewer of the report are the following:

Medical evaluation includes:

1. Narrative history of the medical condition(s) with specific reference to onset and course of the condition, findings on previous examination, treatments, and responses to treatment.

2. Results of the most recent clinical evaluation, including any of the following that were obtained:
- physical examination findings
- laboratory test results
- electrocardiogram
- radiographic studies
- rehabilitation evaluation
- mental status examination and psychological tests
- other special tests or diagnostic procedures

3. Assessment of current clinical status, and statement of plans for future treatment, rehabilitation and re-evaluation.

4. Diagnoses and clinical impressions.

5. Estimate of the expected date of full or partial recovery.

Analysis of the findings includes:

1. Explanation of the impact of the medical condition(s) on life activities.

2. Narrative explanation of the medical basis for any conclusion that the medical condition has, or has not, become static or well stabilized.

3. Explanation of the medical basis for a conclusion that the individual is, or is not, likely to suffer sudden or subtle incapacitation as a result of the medical condition.

4. Explanation of the medical basis for any conclusion that the individual is, or is not, likely to suffer injury or harm or further medical impairment by engaging in activities of daily living or any other activity necessary to meet personal, social, and occupational demands.

5. Explanation of any conclusion that restrictions or accommodations are, or are not, warranted with respect to daily activities or any other activities that are required to meet personal, social, and occupational demands. If restrictions or accommodations are necessary, there should be an explanation of their therapeutic or risk-avoiding value.

Comparison of the results of analysis with the impairment criteria includes:

1. Description of specific clinical findings related to each impairment, with reference to how the findings relate to the criteria described in the chapter. Reference to the absence of, or to the examiner's inability to obtain, pertinent data is essential.

2. Comparison of specific clinical findings to the specific criteria that pertain to the particular body system, as they are listed in the *Guides*.

3. Explanation of each percent of impairment rating, with reference to the applicable criteria.

4. Summary list of all impairment ratings.

On the following page is a standard form that may be used by the evaluator as a cover sheet for a report. This form may be reproduced without permission from the American Medical Association.

Report of Medical Evaluation (Permanent Medical Impairment)

To:

Re:

Case Number:

Date of Injury:

1. Past Medical History

			Yes	No
a. Medical Office Records	Reviewed			
	Enclosed			
b. Hospital Records	Reviewed			
	Enclosed			
c. From Patient				
d. From Other Source (describe)				

2. Clinical Evaluation

		Yes	No
a. Physical Examination			
	Report Enclosed		
b. Laboratory Tests			
	Reports Attached		
c. Special Tests and Diagnostic Procedures			
	Reports Attached		
d. Specialty Evaluations			
	Reports Attached		

3. Diagnoses

a.

b.

c.

4. Stability of the Medical Condition

_____ The clinical condition is not likely to improve with further active medical treatment or surgical intervention—medical maintenance care only is warranted

_____ Employability is not likely to improve with further active medical treatment or surgical intervention

_____ The degree of impairment is not likely to change by more than 3% within the next year

5. Impairment Evaluation—AMA Guides

(Attach a complete report of findings and narrative comments for each body part or system) Body Part/System	Protocol (Section) No.	Table No.

_____ This patient has been under my care from _____ to _____ .

_____ I have not provided care for this patient. I have seen this patient _____ time(s) for the purpose of evaluating medical impairment.

_____ , M.D.
(Signature)

Chapter 3

The Extremities, Spine, and Pelvis

3.0 Introduction

This chapter includes sections on the upper extremity, the lower extremity, the spine, and the pelvis. Each section considers techniques of measurement, includes tables for impairments due to restriction of active motion, ankylosis, amputations, and fractures. Also included are tables relating to specific disorders of body parts, and techniques for evaluating the peripheral nervous system and vasculature related to impairments of the upper and lower extremities.

The upper extremity, the lower extremity, the spine and the pelvis are each to be considered *a unit of the whole person.* The upper extremity may be divided into four sections: the hand, wrist, elbow, and shoulder. The normal hand has five digits: the thumb, index, middle, ring, and little fingers. The thumb has three joints: interphalangeal, metacarpophalangeal, and carpometacarpal. Each finger has three joints: the distal interphalangeal, proximal interphalangeal, and metacarpophalangeal joints.

The lower extremity may be divided into four sections: the foot; hind foot, which includes ankle and subtalar joints; knee; and hip. The foot has five digits: the great toe and the second, third, fourth, and fifth toes. The great toe has two joints: the interphalangeal and the metatarsophalangeal joints. The second, third, fourth, and fifth toes all have three joints: the distal interphalangeal, proximal interphalangeal, and metatarsophalangeal joints.

For the purpose of measuring restricted motion, the spine is divided into the cervical, thoracic, and lumbar regions. The cervical region has seven vertebrae, C1-C7. The thoracic region has 12 vertebrae, T1-T12. The lumbar region has five vertebrae, L1-L5. There may be congenital variations in the number of vertebrae.

The pelvis is composed of the pubis, ischium, and ilium that form the sides and the front and the sacrum and coccyx that form the rear.

Techniques of measurement should be simple, practical, and scientifically sound. For the examination of the upper and lower extremities, a large and a small portable goniometer are useful. For examination of the spine, either two mechanical inclinometers or a single, computerized inclinometer, which is capable of calculating compound joint motions, are needed. Procedures for testing restriction of active motion and ankylosis are described in the text and in the accompanying illustrations.

To determine restriction of motion, several measurements are necessary. If the subject cannot assume the prescribed neutral position for a joint, then the degree of deviation from the prescribed neutral position should be noted. If through attempted passive motion the examiner is unable to move the joint appreciably from that position, and the subject is unable actively to move the joint from that position as well, then the position of the joint is the degree of ankylosis of the joint. Finally, the full range of active motion should be carried out by the subject and measured by the examiner. For evaluating the extremities, the contralateral *uninvolved* joint should serve as a comparative standard against which the impaired joint is measured.

Additional testing procedures may be desirable in specific cases. However, in most instances the measurement techniques described in this chapter are adequate.

The measurements are converted to impairments by referring to the appropriate tables of the chapter.

Before using the information in this chapter, the reader is urged to review Chapters 1 and 2, which provide a general discussion of the purpose of the *Guides*, and of the situations in which they are useful; and which discuss techniques for the evaluation of the subject and for preparation of a report. The report should include the information found in the following outline, which is developed more fully in Chapter 2.

A. Medical Evaluation
1. Narrative history of medical conditions
2. Results of the most recent clinical evaluation
3. Assessment of current clinical status and statement of future plans
4. Diagnoses and clinical impressions
5. Expected date of full or partial recovery

B. Analysis of Findings
1. Impact of medical condition(s) on life activities
2. Explanation for concluding that the medical condition(s) has or has not become static or well-stabilized
3. Explanation for concluding that the individual is or is not likely to suffer from sudden or subtle incapacitation
4. Explanation for concluding that the individual is or is not likely to suffer injury or further impairment by engaging in life activities or by attempting to meet personal, social, and occupational demands
5. Explanation for concluding that accommodations and/or restrictions are or are not warranted

C. Comparison of Results of Analysis with Impairment Criteria
1. Description of clinical findings, and how these findings relate to specific criteria in the chapter
2. Explanation of each percent of impairment rating
3. Summary list of all impairment ratings
4. Overall rating of impairment of the whole person

3.1 The Hand and Upper Extremity

3.1a Introduction

For accurate impairment evaluation, a complete and detailed examination of the upper extremity is necessary and is facilitated by the use of a printed chart that lists the various tests and measurements in an orderly fashion (Figure 1). This chart may be reproduced without permission from the AMA. Methods for evaluating upper extremity impairment can be divided arbitrarily into anatomic, cosmetic, and functional categories. A combination of these methods is necessary to show an accurate profile of the patient's condition. Presently the most objective method of assessment is anatomic evaluation.

A system for evaluation of physical impairment in the hand and upper extremity due to amputation, sensory loss, abnormal motion, and ankylosis was developed and approved for international application by the International Federation of Societies for Surgery of the Hand. The hand and upper extremity section of this chapter is divided into regional evaluation of the thumb, finger, wrist, elbow, and shoulder. Each section considers techniques of measurement, and includes values for impairment from amputation, sensory loss, and abnormal motion. In addition, specific impairments of the upper extremity due to peripheral nerve and plexus lesions, and vascular problems will be discussed in this section. A method to combine and relate various impairments to the whole person is presented.

Nonpreferred Upper Extremity—Since the basic tasks of everyday living are more dependent upon the preferred upper extremity than upon the nonpreferred one, dysfunction of the nonpreferred extremity results in less impairment than dysfunction of the preferred. Therefore, when the impairment of an upper extremity has been determined to be between 5% and 50%, the value should be reduced by 5% if the impairment is of the nonpreferred extremity. If the determined value is 51% to 100%, the value should be reduced by 10% if the impairment is of the nonpreferred extremity. For example, a 60% impairment would become 60%−(60% x 10%) = 54%.

3.1b Principles and Methods of Impairment Evaluation

The most practical and useful approach to the evaluation of digit impairment is through comparison of the loss of function found to be present with that resulting from amputation. Total loss of motion or sensation of a digit, or ankylosis with severe malposition that renders the digit essentially useless, are considered about the same as amputation of the part. Ankylosis in the optimum functional position is given the least impairment. Sensory loss impairments are calculated as 50% of an amputation.

Principles of Evaluating Amputation
Amputation of the entire upper extremity, or 100% loss of the limb, is considered 60% impairment of the whole person (Figure 2). Amputations at levels below the elbow, distal to the biceps insertion and proximal to the metacarpophalangeal joint level, are considered to be a 95% loss of the upper extremity. Each digit is given a relative value to the whole hand: thumb, 40%; index and middle fingers, 20% each; ring and little fingers, 10% each.

Figure 1. Upper Extremity Impairment Evaluation Record

Name_____ Age_____ Sex □ M □ F   Dominant Hand □ R □ L   Date_____

Region	Abnormal Motion Measured Angles						Amputation Mark level of amputation	Sensory Loss Shade region of loss	Other Disorders	% Impairment	R	L
Thumb			Motion	Ank	% Imp		R L	R L		Abnormal Motion (add impairment values)		
	ADD.	R	cm	cm						Amputation		
		L	cm	cm						Sensory Loss		
	RAD. ABD.	R	°	°						Other Disorders		
		L	°	°						• Digit Impairment		
	OPP.	R	cm	cm						★ Hand Impairment		
		L	cm	cm								
			Flex	Ext	Ank	% Imp						
	MP	R										
		L										
	IP	R										
		L										
Index	MP	R								• Abnormal Motion		
		L								Amputation		
	PIP	R								Sensory Loss		
		L								Other Disorders		
	DIP	R								• Digit Impairment		
		L								★ Hand Impairment		
Middle	MP	R								• Abnormal Motion		
		L								Amputation		
	PIP	R								Sensory Loss		
		L								Other Disorders		
	DIP	R								• Digit Impairment		
		L								★ Hand Impairment		
Ring	MP	R								• Abnormal Motion		
		L								Amputation		
	PIP	R								Sensory Loss		
		L								Other Disorders		
	DIP	R								• Digit Impairment		
		L								★ Hand Impairment		
Little	MP	R								• Abnormal Motion		
		L								Amputation		
	PIP	R								Sensory Loss		
		L								Other Disorders		
	DIP	R								• Digit Impairment		
		L								★ Hand Impairment		

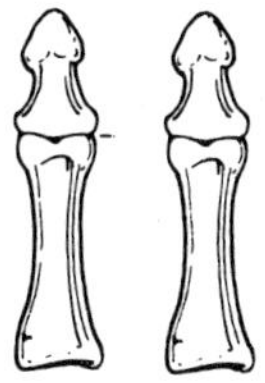

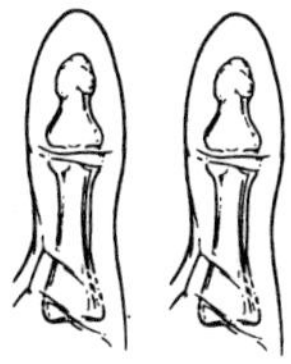

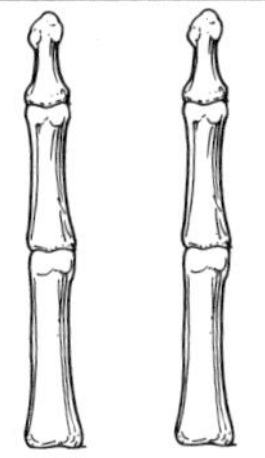

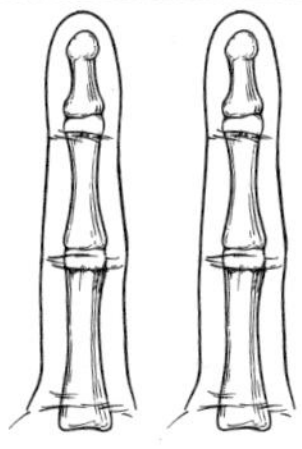

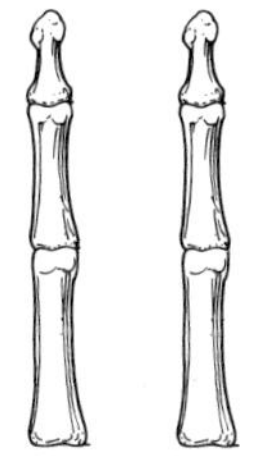

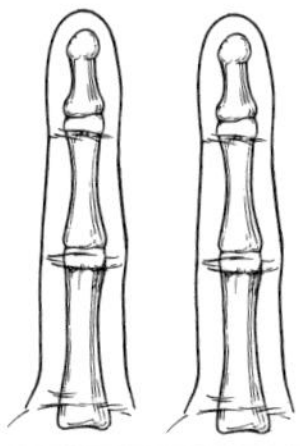

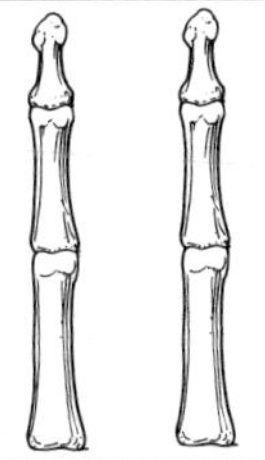

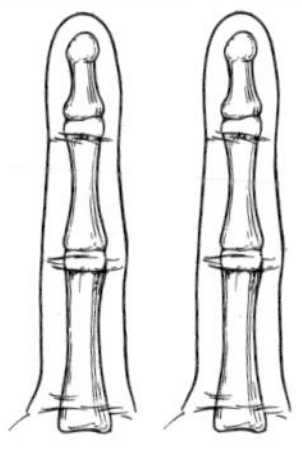

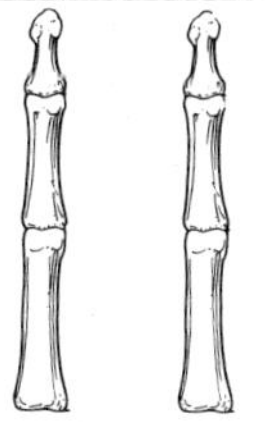

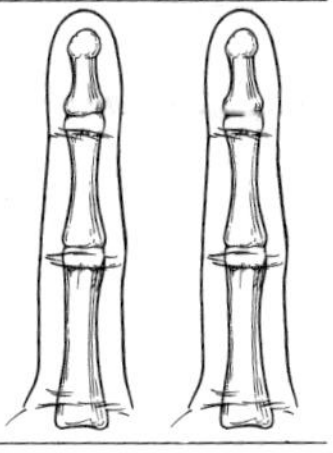

		R	L
Total Hand Impairment (add all values)	•		
Impairment of Upper Extremity (Table 2)			

• Use Combined Values Chart
★ Use Table 1 (Digit to Hand)

This form may be reproduced without permission from the American Medical Association.

Region	Abnormal Motion Measured Angles			Amputation Mark level of amputation	Other Disorders	Upper Extremity Impairment	
Wrist		Flex	Ext	Ank			R	L
	R							
	L							
		RD	UD	Ank				
	R							
	L							
Elbow		Flex	Ext	Ank			R	L
	R							
	L							
		PRO	SUP	Ank				
	R							
	L							
Shoulder		Flex	Ext	Ank			R	L
	R							
	L							
		ADD	ABD	Ank	100% Impairment of Extremity			
	R							
	L							
		IN ROT	EX ROT	Ank				
	R							
	L							

	Upper Extremity Impairment	
Peripheral Nerve and/or Peripheral Vascular Disorders (Describe; see §§ 3.1i & 3.1j).	R	L
• Total of Upper Extremity Impairments from Hand, Wrist, Elbow and Shoulder (Combined Values Chart)	R	L
Impairment of the Whole Person (Table 3)	R	L

Amputation through each portion of a digit is given a relative value loss to the entire digit: digit metacarpophalangeal, 100%; thumb interphalangeal, 50%; finger proximal interphalangeal, 80%; finger distal interphalangeal, 45% (Figure 3). Amputation of all digits at the metacarpophalangeal joint level is considered to be 100% impairment of the hand, or 90% of the upper extremity. Since loss of the entire upper extremity equals 60% impairment of the whole person, 90% impairment of the upper extremity equals 54% impairment of the whole person. By principle of progressive multiplication of percentage values, impairment of each digit or portion thereof can be related to the hand, to the upper extremity, and eventually to the whole person (Tables 1, 2, and 3).

Principles of Evaluating Sensory Loss of the Digits
Any loss resulting from sensory deficit contributing to permanent impairment must be unequivocal and permanent. Sensibility is determined by the two-point discrimination test (Figure 4). This test is performed with a paper clip opened and bent into a caliper. With the subject's eyes closed, the examiner lightly touches the caliper points to the digit in the longitudinal axis on the radial or ulnar side. The subject indicates whether one or two points are felt. A varied series of one or two points is applied. If the subject cannot distinguish between one point and two points at a distance of at least 10mm in two out of three applications, sensation is impaired.

Sensory loss on the dorsal surface of the digits is not considered impairing. Complete loss of palmar sensation of a digit is considered to be a 50% impairment of the digit. Partial palmar *transverse* sensory loss is calculated as the percentage value of that portion of the digit (see Figure 8 for the thumb and Figure 19 for the fingers). Partial *longitudinal* sensory loss values are based on the relative importance of the side of the digit for sensory function in hand activities (see Figure 5 and Tables 4 and 5).

See the section on Impairment of the Upper Extremity Due to Peripheral Nervous System Disorders for evaluation of sensory loss above the digits and motor loss in the entire upper extremity.

Principles of Evaluating Abnormal Motion
The range of motion should be recorded on the principle that the neutral position equals 0°. In this method, all joint motions are measured from zero as the starting position, and the degree of motion is added in the direction the joint moves from this point. Active motion is obtained with full flexion or extension muscle force. Passive motion is measured after normal soft tissue resistance to movement is overcome. The term "extension" is used for motions opposite to flexion to the zero starting position. If extension exceeds the zero

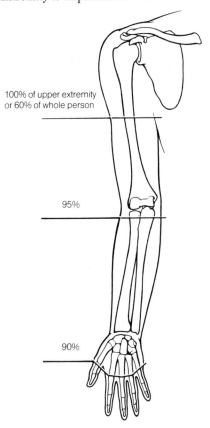

Figure 2. Relationship of Impairments of the Upper Extremity to Impairments of the Whole Person

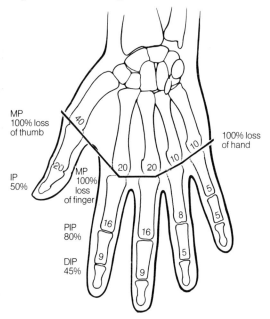

Figure 3. Relationships of Various Amputations to Impairments of the Digits and Hand

Relative Values to Hand:
Thumb = 40%
Index and Middle Fingers = 20% each
Ring and Little Fingers = 10% each

Table 1. Relationship of Impairment of the Digits to Impairment of the Hand

% Impairment of Thumb	Hand	% Impairment of Index or Middle Finger	Hand	% Impairment of Ring or Little Finger	Hand
0- 1	0	0- 2	0	0- 4	0
2- 3	1	3- 7	1	5- 14	1
4- 6	2	8- 12	2	15- 24	2
7- 8	3	13- 17	3	25- 34	3
9- 11	4	18- 22	4	35- 44	4
12- 13	5	23- 27	5	45- 54	5
14- 16	6	28- 32	6	55- 64	6
17- 18	7	33- 37	7	65- 74	7
19- 21	8	38- 42	8	75- 84	8
22- 23	9	43- 47	9	85- 94	9
24- 26	10	48- 52	10	95-100	10
27- 28	11	53- 57	11		
29- 31	12	58- 62	12		
32- 33	13	63- 67	13		
34- 36	14	68- 72	14		
37- 38	15	73- 77	15		
39- 41	16	78- 82	16		
42- 43	17	83- 87	17		
44- 46	18	88- 92	18		
47- 48	19	93- 97	19		
49- 51	20	98-100	20		
52- 53	21				
54- 56	22				
57- 59	23				
59- 61	24				
62- 63	25				
64- 66	26				
67- 68	27				
69- 71	28				
72- 73	29				
74- 76	30				
77- 78	31				
79- 81	32				
82- 83	33				
84- 86	34				
87- 88	35				
89- 91	36				
92- 93	37				
94- 96	38				
97- 98	39				
99-100	40				

Note: Impairment of the hand contributed by a digit may be rounded to the nearest 5 percent only when it is the *sole* impairment involved. See Table 2 for converting hand impairment to upper extremity impairment.

Figure 4. Two-Point Discrimination Test for Sensory Loss

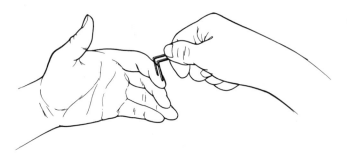

starting position, it is referred to as "hyperextension" and is expressed with the (+) symbol. Incomplete motion of extension from a flexed position to zero starting position, or extension lag, is expressed with the (−) symbol. For example, finger joint flexion contracture of 15° with flexion to 45° would be recorded as −15° to 45°. A finger joint that has 15° of hyperextension to 45° of flexion would be recorded as +15° to 45° (Figure 6). The plus and minus signs have no mathematical significance. They are used to highlight the concepts of "hyperextension" (that is, a larger range of motion than is normal, therefore "+") and extension lag (that is, a loss of extension from the flexed position, therefore "−").

"A = E + F" Method for Impairment Evaluation Definitions and Principles

• Measured flexion angle V_{flex} = largest possible angle to achieve by flexion.

• Measured extension angle V_{ext} = smallest possible angle to achieve by extension.

Example: If the metacarpophalangeal joint moves from 0° extension to 90° flexion, then V_{flex} = 90° and V_{ext} = 0°. In this case, 90° is also the largest theoretical V_{flex} and 0° the smallest theoretical V_{ext}.

• When joint flexion is decreased, F (loss of flexion) = (largest theoretical V_{flex})−(measured V_{flex}).

Example: If the metacarpophalangeal joint has 60° flexion, F = 90° − 60° = 30°.

• Similarly, the E (loss of extension) = (measured V_{ext})−(smallest theoretical V_{ext}).

Example: If the metacarpophalangeal joint has -20° extension, E = 20° − 0° = 20°.

With decreasing flexion and extension, V_{flex} and V_{ext} will finally meet at the same point on the arc of motion, or $V_{flex} = V_{ext}$. When this occurs, there is ankylosis, or total loss of potential arc of motion. Therefore

• A (Ankylosis, or total loss of motion) = E (loss of extension) + F (loss of flexion), or A = E + F.

Example: If the metacarpophalangeal joint has 40° anky-losis in flexion: $V_{ext} = V_{flex}$ = 40°; E = 40°; F = 90° −40° = 50°; A = 40° + 50° = 90°. Note that A always equals the normal, full range of motion of the joint.

Furthermore, impairment of finger motion can be caused by a loss of extension (E), with or without loss

Table 2. Relationship of Impairment of the Hand to Impairment of the Upper Extremity

% Impairment of Hand	Upper Extremity	% Impairment of Hand	Upper Extremity	% Impairment of Hand	Upper Extremity	% Impairment of Hand	Upper Extremity	% Impairment of Hand	Upper Extremity	% Impairment of Hand	Upper Extremity
0 =	0	18 =	16	35 =	32	53 =	48	70 =	63	88 =	79
1 =	1	19 =	17	36 =	32	54 =	49	71 =	64	89 =	80
2 =	2			37 =	33			72 =	65		
3 =	3	20 =	18	38 =	34	55 =	50	73 =	66	90 =	81
4 =	4	21 =	19	39 =	35	56 =	50	74 =	67	91 =	82
		22 =	20			57 =	51			92 =	83
5 =	5	23 =	21	40 =	36	58 =	52	75 =	68	93 =	84
6 =	5	24 =	22	41 =	37	59 =	53	76 =	68	94 =	85
7 =	6			42 =	38			77 =	69		
8 =	7	25 =	23	43 =	39	60 =	54	78 =	70	95 =	86
9 =	8	26 =	23	44 =	40	61 =	55	79 =	71	96 =	86
10 =	9	27 =	24	45 =	41	62 =	56	80 =	72	97 =	87
11 =	10	28 =	25	46 =	41	63 =	57	81 =	73	98 =	88
12 =	11	29 =	26	47 =	42	64 =	58	82 =	74	99 =	89
13 =	12			48 =	43			83 =	75		
14 =	13	30 =	27	49 =	44	65 =	59	84 =	76	100 =	90
		31 =	28			66 =	59				
15 =	14	32 =	29	50 =	45	67 =	60	85 =	77		
16 =	14	33 =	30	51 =	46	68 =	61	86 =	77		
17 =	15	34 =	31	52 =	47	69 =	62	87 =	78		

Note: Impairment of the upper extremity contributed by the hand may be rounded to the nearest 5 percent only when it is the *sole* impairment involved. Consult Table 3 for converting upper extremity impairment to whole person impairment.

of flexion (F), or ankylosis (A). The restricted motion impairment percentages are called $I_E\%$, $I_F\%$, and $I_A\%$, respectively, and are functions of the angle (V) measured at examination.

- I_E is a function of V_{ext} and is 0% when V_{ext} reaches its smallest theoretical value.

- I_F is a function of V_{flex} and is 0% when V_{flex} reaches its largest theoretical value.

- I_A is a function of V when $V_{ext} = V_{flex}$; similarly, $I_A\% = I_E\% + I_F\%$. Note that the impairment value for ankylosis ($I_A\%$) varies according to the angle at which $V_{ext} = V_{flex}$, even as A always equals the full range of motion of the joint.

Impairment values for loss of motion of the fingers, thumb, wrist, elbow, and shoulder are derived from the basic formulas described above.

When there is more than one impairment (e.g., abnormal motion, sensation, or amputation) to a given unit, such as the finger, these impairments must be combined before the conversion to the larger unit, such as the hand, is made. These can then be related to the hand, upper extremity, and the whole person. Multiple regional impairments, as in the hand, wrist, elbow, and shoulder, are expressed in terms of impairment of the upper extremity and are combined using the Combined Values Chart.

Figure 5. Impairment of Hand Due to Partial Longitudinal Sensory Loss*

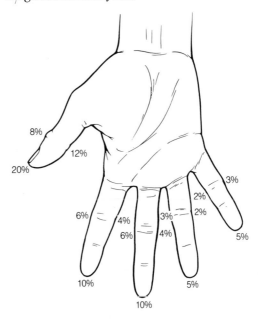

*Based on complete loss of palmar sensation of a digit equal to 50% impairment of the digit.

Table 3. Relationship of Impairment of the Upper Extremity to Impairment of the Whole Person

% Impairment of Upper Extremity		Whole Person	% Impairment of Upper Extremity		Whole Person	% Impairment of Upper Extremity		Whole Person
0	=	0	35	=	21	70	=	42
1	=	1	36	=	22	71	=	43
2	=	1	37	=	22	72	=	43
3	=	2	38	=	23	73	=	44
4	=	2	39	=	23	74	=	44
5	=	3	40	=	24	75	=	45
6	=	4	41	=	25	76	=	46
7	=	4	42	=	25	77	=	46
8	=	5	43	=	26	78	=	47
9	=	5	44	=	26	79	=	47
10	=	6	45	=	27	80	=	48
11	=	7	46	=	28	81	=	49
12	=	7	47	=	28	82	=	49
13	=	8	48	=	29	83	=	50
14	=	8	49	=	29	84	=	50
15	=	9	50	=	30	85	=	51
16	=	10	51	=	31	86	=	52
17	=	10	52	=	31	87	=	52
18	=	11	53	=	32	88	=	53
19	=	11	54	=	32	89	=	53
20	=	12	55	=	33	90	=	54
21	=	13	56	=	34	91	=	55
22	=	13	57	=	34	92	=	55
23	=	14	58	=	35	93	=	56
24	=	14	59	=	35	94	=	56
25	=	15	60	=	36	95	=	57
26	=	16	61	=	37	96	=	58
27	=	16	62	=	37	97	=	58
28	=	17	63	=	38	98	=	59
29	=	17	64	=	38	99	=	59
30	=	18	65	=	39	100	=	60
31	=	19	66	=	40			
32	=	19	67	=	40			
33	=	20	68	=	41			
34	=	20	69	=	41			

Note: Impairment of the whole person contributed by the upper extremity may be rounded to the nearest 5 percent only when it is the *sole* impairment involved.

Figure 6. Definitions and Relative Values of Flexion, Extension, and Hyperextension, in Degrees

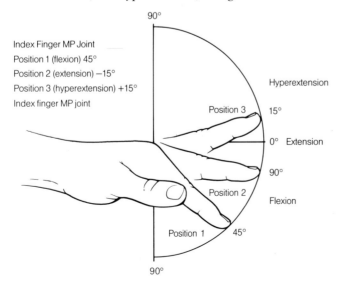

Index Finger MP Joint
Position 1 (flexion) 45°
Position 2 (extension) −15°
Position 3 (hyperextension) +15°
Index finger MP joint

3.1c Thumb

Amputation

- Determine the length of thumb remaining after amputation and consult Figure 7 to find the impairment of that digit.

- Amputations through the metacarpal bone are considered 100% impairment of the thumb and are not given extra values.

Example: A thumb amputation through the proximal metaphysis of the proximal phalanx is equivalent to 90% impairment of the thumb.

Sensory Loss
Transverse Sensory Loss (both digital nerves involved)

- Determine the level of palmar sensory loss and consult Figure 8 to find the sensory impairment of the thumb.

- Sensory loss proximal to the metacarpophalangeal joint is given the same impairment as a loss at the metacarpophalangeal joint and is not given extra value.

Example: A transverse sensory loss at the level of the thumb interphalangeal joint is equivalent to a 25% impairment of the thumb.

Longitudinal Sensory Loss (one digital nerve involved)

- Determine the level of sensory loss and consult Figure 8 as if it were a transverse sensory loss impairment.

- Convert this transverse sensory loss to a longitudinal sensory impairment by using Table 4.

Example: A longitudinal ulnar sensory loss at the level of the thumb interphalangeal joint is a 15% impairment of the thumb.

Abnormal Motion

The thumb has four functional units of motion, each contributing a relative value to the total thumb function:

1. Flexion/extension of the metacarpophalangeal and interphalangeal joints (20% of the total value of thumb motion). On a 100% scale, a relative value of 55% is given to the metacarpophalangeal joint and of 45% to the interphalangeal joint. This is equivalent to 55% x 20% =11% for the metacarpophalangeal joint, and 45% x 20% = 9% for the interphalangeal joint.

2. Adduction (20% of total motion value).

3. Radial abduction (10% of total motion value).

4. Opposition (50% of total motion value).

Table 4. Conversion of Transverse Sensory Loss (Impairment) to Longitudinal Sensory Loss (Impairment) for the Thumb and Little Finger (Values in % of Digit Impairment)

Transverse Sensory Loss %	Longitudinal Sensory Loss %	
	Ulnar Digital Nerve	**Radial Digital Nerve**
50	30	20
45	27	18
40	24	16
35	21	14
30	18	12
25	15	10
20	12	8
15	9	6
10	6	4
5	3	2

Interphalangeal Joint—Flexion and Extension

1. Measure the maximum flexion and extension and record the goniometer readings (Figures 9 & 10). Round the figure to the nearest 10°.

2. From Figure 11, match the measured flexion and extension degrees (V) to their corresponding impairments of flexion (I_F%) and extension (I_E%).

3. *Add* values of flexion and extension impairment to obtain thumb interphalangeal joint motion impairment.

4. If the interphalangeal joint is ankylosed, measure the position and match it to the corresponding ankylosis (I_A%) impairment in Figure 11. Ankylosis in the functional position (20° flexion) is given the lowest impairment value (4%).

Example: Thumb interphalangeal joint has +10° extension and 50° flexion:
I_E% = 0% I_F% = 2%
0% + 2% = 2% impairment of the thumb interphalangeal joint motion

Example: Thumb interphalangeal joint ankylosis in 80° flexion: I_A% = 9%, or complete impairment of the thumb interphalangeal joint motion.

Metacarpophalangeal Joint—Flexion and Extension

• Measure the maximum flexion and extension and record the goniometer readings (Figures 12 & 13). Round the figures to the nearest 10°.

• From Figure 14, match the measured flexion and extension degrees (V) to their corresponding impairments of flexion (I_F%) and extension (I_E%).

Figure 7. Impairment Due to Amputation of Thumb at Various Lengths

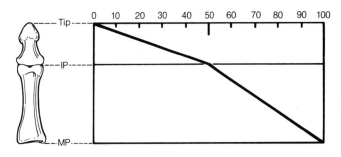

Amputation of Thumb (% Impairment)

Figure 8. Impairment Due to Transverse Sensory Loss of Thumb at Various Lengths

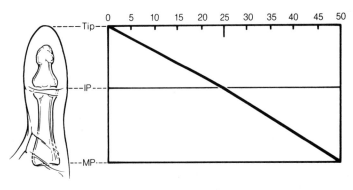

Transverse Sensory Loss of Thumb (% Impairment)

Figure 9. Neutral Position of Thumb IP Joint

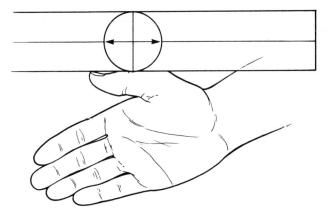

Figure 10. Flexion of Thumb IP Joint

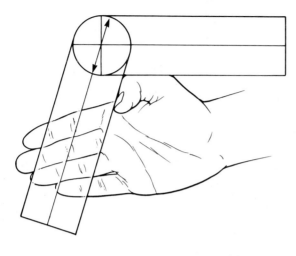

Figure 11. Chart of Thumb IP Joint Impairments

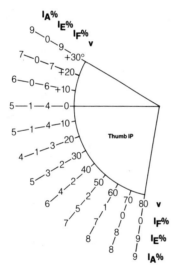

$I_A\%$ = impairment due to ankylosis
$I_E\%$ = impairment due to loss of extension
$I_F\%$ = impairment due to loss of flexion
V   = degrees of motion or ankylosis

• *Add* values of flexion and extension impairment to obtain thumb metacarpophalangeal joint motion impairment.

• If the metacarpophalangeal joint is ankylosed, measure the position and match it to the corresponding ankylosis ($I_A\%$) impairment in Figure 14.

Ankylosis in the functional position (20° flexion) is given the lowest impairment value (5%).

Example: Thumb metacarpophalangeal joint has +10° extension and 40° flexion:
$I_E\% = 0\%$ $I_F\% = 2\%$
0% + 2% = 2% impairment of the thumb metacarpophalangeal joint motion.

Example: Thumb metacarpophalangeal joint ankylosis in 60° flexion: $I_A\% = 11\%$, or complete impairment of the thumb metacarpophalangeal joint motion.

When both joints are involved:
• *Add* the percentage impairment of the interphalangeal joint with that of the metacarpophalangeal joint to obtain the thumb flexion/extension impairment.

• For joint ankylosis, impairments are added in a similar fashion.

Example: Interphalangeal joint impairment 2% and metacarpophalangeal joint impairment 2%:
2% + 2% = 4% flexion/extension impairment of the thumb.

Example: Ankylosis impairment of the interphalangeal joint 9% and metacarpophalangeal joint 11%: 9% + 11% = 20% ankylosis impairment of the thumb, or total loss of motion at both joints.

Adduction
• Measure and record the smallest possible distance in centimeters (cm) from the flexor crease of the thumb interphalangeal joint to the distal palmar crease over the metacarpophalangeal joint of the little finger (Figure 15).

• Consult Table 6 to determine percent of thumb impairment contributed by adduction.

Example: Adduction measured at 4 cm is equivalent to 4% impairment to the thumb.

Radial Abduction
• Measure and record the largest possible angle in degrees formed by the first and second metacarpals during maximum active radial abduction (Figure 16).

Table 5. Conversion of Transverse Sensory Loss (Impairment) to Longitudinal Sensory Loss (Impairment) for the Index, Middle, and Ring Fingers (Values in % of Finger Impairment)

Transverse Sensory Loss %	Longitudinal Sensory Loss %	
	Ulnar Digital Nerve	Radial Digital Nerve
50	20	30
45	18	27
40	16	24
35	14	21
30	12	18
25	10	15
20	8	12
15	6	9
10	4	6
5	2	3

- Consult Table 7 to determine percent of thumb impairment contributed by radial abduction.

Example: Radial abduction measured at 20° is equivalent to 7% impairment to the thumb.

Opposition
- Measure and record the largest possible distance in centimeters (cm) from the flexor crease of the thumb interphalangeal joint to the distal palmar crease directly over the third metacarpophalangeal joint (Figure 17).

- Consult Table 8 (p. 26) to determine percent of thumb impairment contributed by opposition.

Example: Opposition measured at 4 cm is equivalent to 10% impairment to the thumb.

When more than one abnormal motion is involved:
- Measure and record thumb motion impairments of flexion/extension, adduction, radial abduction, and opposition as described above.

- *Add* these values directly to determine abnormal thumb motion impairment.

Note: Because the relative value of each thumb functional unit has been taken into consideration in the impairment values to the total thumb, impairment values of each thumb motion are *added* directly together, whereas those for the fingers are calculated by using the Combined Values Chart. If the maximum impairment for each motion unit is reached, the sum would be 100% impairment, or total loss of thumb motion.

Example: Thumb flexion/extension impairment of 4%, adduction impairment of 4%, abduction of 0%, and opposition impairment of 10%, or 4% + 4% + 0% + 10% = 20% motion impairment to the thumb.

Figure 12. Neutral Position of Thumb MP Joint

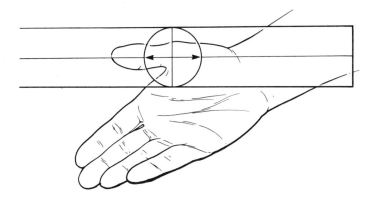

Figure 13. Flexion of Thumb MP Joint

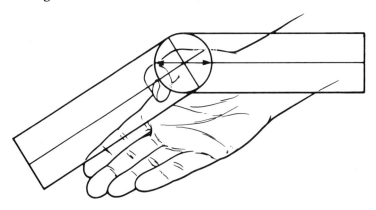

Figure 14. Chart of Thumb MP Joint Impairments

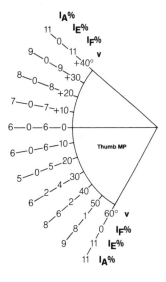

$I_A\%$ = impairment due to ankylosis
$I_E\%$ = impairment due to loss of extension
$I_F\%$ = impairment due to loss of flexion
V = degrees of motion or ankylosis

Table 6. Impairment Due to Abnormal Motion and Ankylosis of Thumb Adduction

Abnormal Motion
Average range of motion is 8 centimeters (cm).
Value to total range of motion is 20%.

Adduction from neutral position (0 cm) to:	Length of Motion Lost	Retained	% Impairment of Thumb
0 cm	8 cm	0 cm	20
1 cm	7 cm	1 cm	13
2 cm	6 cm	2 cm	8
3 cm	5 cm	3 cm	6
4 cm	4 cm	4 cm	4
5 cm	3 cm	5 cm	3
6 cm	2 cm	6 cm	1
7 cm	1 cm	7 cm	0
8 cm	0 cm	8 cm	0

Ankylosis

Adduction ankylosed at:	% Impairment of Thumb
0 cm (neutral position)	20
1 cm	19
2 cm	17
3 cm	15
4 cm	10
5 cm	15
6 cm	17
7 cm	19
8 cm	20

Table 7. Impairment Due to Abnormal Motion and Ankylosis of Thumb Radial Abduction

Abnormal Motion
Average range of motion is 50°.
Value to total range of motion is 10%.

Radial adduction from neutral (0°) position to:	Degree of Motion Lost	Retained	% Impairment of Thumb
0°	50°	0°	10
10°	40°	10°	9
20°	30°	20°	7
30°	20°	30°	3
40°	10°	40°	1
50°	0°	50°	0

Ankylosis

Radial abduction ankylosed at:	% Impairment of Thumb
0°	10
10°	10
20°	10
30°	10
40°	10
50°	10

Thumb flexion/extension ankylosis impairment of 20%, adduction impairment of 20%, abduction impairment of 10%, and opposition impairment of 50%, or 20% + 20% + 10% + 50% = 100% motion impairment to the thumb.

Combining Thumb Amputation, Sensory, and Abnormal Motion Impairments
• Measure separately and record the impairment of the thumb contributed by amputation, sensory loss, and abnormal motion as described above.

Note: If an amputation affects the measurement of abnormal motion, then only the amputation impairment is given. For example, amputation proximal to the interphalangeal joint will affect measurements of adduction and opposition. Impairment is given only for the amputation.

• Combine the impairment values using the Combined Values Chart to ascertain impairment of the thumb.

• Use Tables 1, 2, and 3 to relate thumb impairment to impairments of the hand, upper extremity, and the whole person.

Example: Thumb amputation impairment of 30%, sensory impairment of 10%, abnormal motion impairment of 10%:
30% combined with 10% = 37%;
37% combined with 10% = 43% thumb impairment.
  This is equivalent to 17% impairment of the hand, 15% impairment of the upper extremity, and 9% impairment of the whole person.

Figure 15. Measuring Thumb Adduction

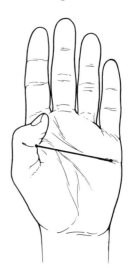

3.1d Fingers

Amputation
• Determine the length of the finger remaining after amputation and consult Figure 18 to determine the impairment of that digit.

• Amputations through the metacarpal bone are considered 100% impairment of the finger and are not given extra values.

Example: The index finger amputated through the proximal interphalangeal joint is equivalent to 80% finger impairment.

Sensory Loss
Transverse Sensory Loss (both digital nerves involved)
• Determine the level of palmar sensory loss and consult Figure 19 to find the sensory impairment of the finger.

• Sensory loss proximal to the metacarpophalangeal joint is given the same impairment as a loss at the metacarpophalangeal joint and is not given extra values.

Example: A transverse sensory loss at the level of the index finger proximal interphalangeal joint is a 40% finger impairment.

Longitudinal Sensory Loss (one digital nerve involved)
• Determine the level of sensory loss and consult Figure 19 as if it were a transverse sensory loss impairment.

• Convert this transverse sensory loss to a longitudinal sensory impairment by using Table 5 for the index, middle and ring fingers, and Table 4 for the little finger.

Example: A longitudinal radial sensory loss at the level of the index finger proximal interphalangeal joint is a 24% impairment of the index finger.

Abnormal Motion
Distal Interphalangeal Joint—Flexion and Extension
• Measure the maximum flexion and extension and record the goniometer readings (Figures 20 & 21). Round the figures to the nearest 10°.

• From Figure 22 (p. 28), match the measured flexion and extension degrees (V) to their corresponding impairments of flexion (I_F%) and extension (I_E%).

• *Add* the values of flexion and extension impairment to obtain finger distal interphalangeal joint motion impairment.

• If the distal interphalangeal joint is ankylosed, measure the position and match it to the corresponding ankylosis (I_A%) impairment in Figure 22 (p. 28). Ankylosis in the functional position (20° flexion) is given the lowest impairment value (30%).

Figure 16. Radial Abduction of Thumb

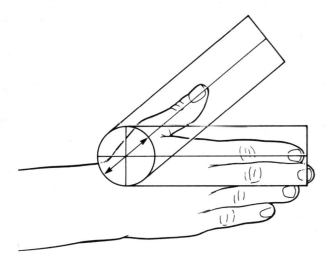

Figure 17. Measuring Thumb Opposition

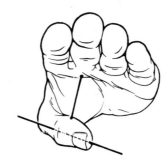

Table 8. Impairment Due to Abnormal Motion and Ankylosis of Thumb Opposition

Abnormal Motion
Average range of motion is 8 centimeters (cm).
Value to total range of motion is 50%.

Opposition from neutral position (0 cm) to:	Length of Motion Lost	Retained	% Impairment of Thumb
0 cm	8 cm	0 cm	50
1 cm	7 cm	1 cm	35
2 cm	6 cm	2 cm	25
3 cm	5 cm	3 cm	15
4 cm	4 cm	4 cm	10
5 cm	3 cm	5 cm	6
6 cm	2 cm	6 cm	3
7 cm	1 cm	7 cm	1
8 cm	0 cm	8 cm	0

Ankylosis

Opposition ankylosed at:	% Impairment of Thumb
0 cm	50
1 cm	45
2 cm	40
3 cm	35
4 cm	30
5 cm	25
6 cm	27
7 cm	30
8 cm	32

Example: Middle finger distal interphalangeal joint has -10° extension and 50° flexion:
$I_E\% = 2\%$ $I_F\% = 10\%$
2% + 10% = 12% impairment of the middle finger distal interphalangeal joint motion.

Example: Distal interphalangeal joint ankylosis in 30° flexion: $I_A\% = 33\%$ impairment of the distal interphalangeal joint motion.

Proximal Interphalangeal Joint—Flexion and Extension

• Measure the maximum flexion and extension and record the goniometer readings (Figures 23 and 24, p.29). Round the figures to the nearest 10°.

• From Figure 25 (p. 29), match the measured flexion and extension degrees (V) to their corresponding impairments of flexion ($I_F\%$) and extension ($I_E\%$).

• *Add* the values of flexion and extension impairment to obtain finger proximal interphalangeal joint motion impairment.

• If the proximal interphalangeal joint is ankylosed, measure the position and match it to the corresponding ankylosis ($I_A\%$) impairment in Figure 25 (p. 29). Ankylosis in the functional position (40° flexion) is given the lowest impairment value (50%).

Example: Middle finger proximal interphalangeal joint measures -20° extension and 60° flexion:

$I_E\% = 7\%$ $I_F\% = 24\%$
7% + 24% = 31% impairment of the middle finger proximal interphalangeal joint motion.

Example: Proximal interphalangeal joint ankylosis in 40° flexion: $I_A\%$ − 50% impairment of the proximal interphalangeal joint motion.

Metacarpophalangeal Joint—Flexion and Extension

• Measure the maximum flexion and extension and record the goniometer readings (Figures 26 & 27, p.30). Round the figures to the nearest 10°.

• From Figure 28 (p. 30), match the measured flexion and extension degrees (V) to their corresponding impairments of flexion ($I_F\%$) and extension ($I_E\%$).

• *Add* the values of flexion and extension impairment to obtain finger metacarpophalangeal joint motion impairment.

• If the metacarpophalangeal joint is ankylosed, measure the position and match it to the corresponding ankylosis ($I_A\%$) impairment (Figure 28, p.30). Ankylosis in the functional position (30° flexion) is given the lowest impairment value (45%).

Example: Middle finger metacarpophalangeal joint has 0° extension and 50° flexion:
$I_E\% = 5\%$ $I_F\% = 22\%$
5% + 22% = 27% impairment of the middle finger metacarpophalangeal joint motion.

Figure 18. Impairments Due to Amputation of Finger at Various Lengths

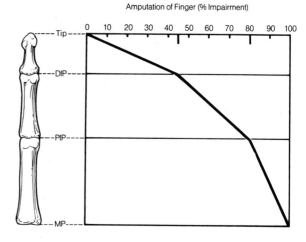

Amputation of Finger (% Impairment)

Example: Metacarpophalangeal joint ankylosis in 30° flexion: $I_A\% = 45\%$ impairment of the metacarpophalangeal joint motion.

When more than one finger abnormal motion is involved:

• Determine the flexion/extension impairments of the three joints of the finger as described above.

• Use the Combined Values Chart to obtain the impairment of the entire finger.

Example: Middle finger distal interphalangeal joint impairment of 12%, proximal interphalangeal joint impairment of 31%, and metacarpophalangeal joint impairment of 27%: 12% combined with 31% = 39%; 39% combined with 27% = 55% motion impairment of the finger.

Combining Finger Amputation, Sensory, and Abnormal Motion Impairments

• Determine the impairment of the finger contributed by amputation, sensory loss, and abnormal motion as described above.

• Combine the impairment values using the Combined Values Chart to ascertain the finger impairment.

• Use Tables 1, 2, and 3 to relate finger impairment to the hand, upper extremity, and the whole person.

Example: Middle finger amputation impairment of 20%, sensory impairment of 10%, and abnormal motion impairment of 10%:

20% combined with 10% = 28%; 28% combined with 10% = 35% finger impairment.

This equates to 7% impairment of the hand, 6% of the upper extremity, and 4% of the whole person.

Combining Multiple Digit Involvement

• If two or more digits of the hand are involved, measure separately and record the combined impairment for each digit as described above.

• Using Table 1, find the hand impairment contributed by each digit.

• *Add* the hand impairment value of each digit to obtain the total hand impairment.

• Using Tables 2 and 3, the hand impairment can be related to the upper extremity and the whole person.

Example:

% Impairment of the Digit	% Impairment of the Hand
10 of thumb	4
20 of index finger	4
30 of middle finger	6
40 of ring finger	4
50 of little finger	5
(4% +4% +6% +4% +5% = 23%)	23

23% of hand impairment is equivalent to 21% impairment of the upper extremity, and 12% of the whole person.

Figure 19. Impairments Due to Transverse Sensory Loss of Finger at Various Levels

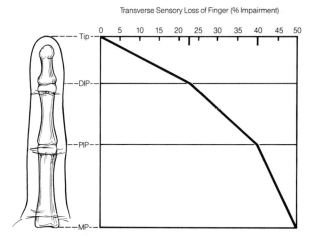

Figure 20. Neutral Position of Finger DIP Joint

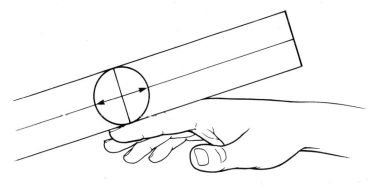

Figure 21. Flexion of Finger DIP Joint

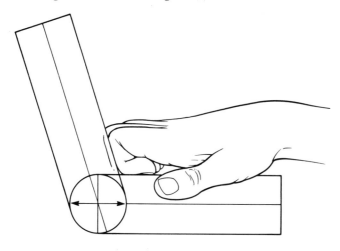

3.1e Wrist

Amputation
• Determine the level of amputation about the wrist (Figure 2).

• Amputations at levels below the biceps insertion and proximal to the metacarpophalangeal joint are considered to be 90% to 95% impairment of the upper extremity, depending on the location.

• Use Table 3 to relate impairment of the upper extremity to impairment of the whole person.

Example: An amputation at the wrist joint level is a 92% impairment of the upper extremity, and 55% impairment of the whole person.

Abnormal Motion
The wrist has two units of motion, each contributing a relative value to its function. Complete loss of wrist function is considered a 60% impairment of the upper extremity. Flexion/extension is considered to be 70% of wrist motion, or 42% of the upper extremity. Radial/ulnar deviation is considered to be 30% of wrist motion, or 18% of the upper extremity.

Joint—Flexion and Extension
• Measure the maximum flexion and extension and record the goniometer readings (Figures 29 & 30, p. 31). Round the figures to the nearest 10°.

• From Figure 31 (p. 32), match the measured flexion and extension degrees (V) to their corresponding impairments of flexion ($I_F\%$) and extension ($I_E\%$).

• *Add* flexion and extension impairment values to obtain the impairment of the upper extremity.

• If the wrist is ankylosed, measure the position and match it to the corresponding ankylosis ($I_A\%$) impairment in Figure 31 (p. 32). Ankylosis in the functional position (10° extension to 10° flexion) is given the lowest value, or 21% impairment of motion. Wrist ankylosis in 60° flexion or 60° extension is a 100% loss of wrist flexion/extension function. This is equivalent to a 70% impairment of wrist motion and 42% impairment of the upper extremity.

Example: Wrist extension of 10° and flexion of 10°:
$I_E\%$ = 8% impairment of the upper extremity.
$I_F\%$ = 8% impairment of the upper extremity.
8% + 8% = 16% impairment of the upper extremity.

Example: Wrist ankylosis in 40° flexion: $I_A\%$ = 33% upper extremity impairment.

Joint—Radial and Ulnar Deviation
• Measure the maximum radial and ulnar deviation and record the goniometer readings (Figures 32 & 33, p. 32). Round the figures to the nearest 10°.

• From Figure 34 (p. 33), match the measured ulnar and radial deviation degrees (V) to their corresponding impairment of radial deviation ($I_{RD}\%$) and ulnar deviation ($I_{UD}\%$).

• *Add* the impairment values of radial and ulnar deviation to obtain the impairment of the upper extremity.

Figure 22. Chart of Finger DIP Joint Impairments

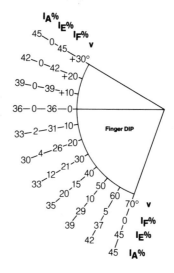

$I_A\%$ = impairment due to amputation
$I_E\%$ = impairment due to loss of extension
$I_F\%$ = impairment due to loss of flexion
V   = degrees of motion or ankylosis

• If the wrist is ankylosed, measure the position and match it to the corresponding ankylosis impairment value (I_A%) in Figure 34 (p. 33). Ankylosis in the functional position (0° to 10° ulnar deviation) is given the lowest value, or 9% impairment of motion. Wrist ankylosis in either 30° ulnar deviation or 20° radial deviation is a 100% loss of wrist lateral deviation function. This is equivalent to a 30% impairment of wrist motion and 18% impairment of the upper extremity.

Example: Ulnar deviation 0° and radial deviation 10°:
I_{UD}% = 5% impairment of the upper extremity.
I_{RD}% = 2% impairment of the upper extremity.
5% + 2% = 7% impairment of the upper extremity.

Example: Wrist ankylosis in 15° radial deviation: I_A% = 16% impairment of the upper extremity.

Combining Wrist Abnormal Motion Impairments
• Determine the impairments of the upper extremity contributed by abnormal wrist motions (flexion/ extension and radial/ulnar deviation) as described above.

Note: Impairments of pronation and supination are ascribed to the elbow.

• Because the relative value of each wrist functional unit has been taken into consideration in the impairment charts, impairments of flexion/extension and radial/ ulnar deviation are *added* to determine the impairment of the upper extremity.

• Use Table 3 to relate impairment of the upper extremity to impairment of the whole person.

Example: Wrist flexion/extension impairment of 16% and wrist radial/ulnar deviation impairment of 7%:
16% + 7% = 23% impairment of the upper extremity and 14% impairment of the whole person.

Example: Wrist ankylosis in 0° flexion and 0° lateral deviation:
Flexion I_A% = 21%   Lateral deviation I_A% = 9%
21% + 9% = 30% impairment of the upper extremity and 18% impairment of the whole person.

3.1f Elbow

Amputation
• Determine the level of amputation about the elbow (Figure 2).

• Amputations at levels below the axilla and proximal to the biceps insertion are considered to be 95% to 100% impairment of the upper extremity, depending on the location.

Figure 23. Neutral Position of Finger PIP Joint

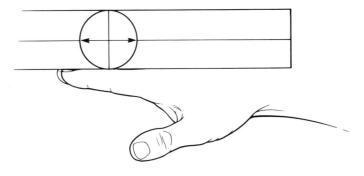

Figure 24. Flexion of Finger PIP Joint

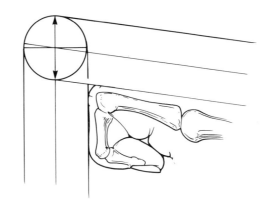

Figure 25. Chart of Finger PIP Joint Impairments

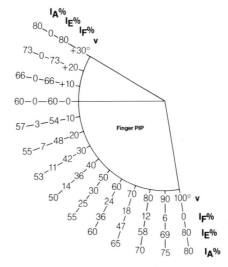

I_A% = impairment due to ankylosis
I_E% = impairment due to loss of extension
I_F% = impairment due to loss of flexion
V   = degrees of motion or ankylosis

Figure 26. Neutral Position of Finger MP Joint

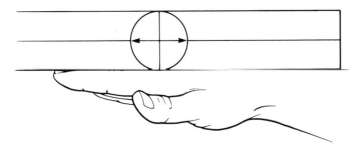

Figure 27. Flexion of Finger MP Joint

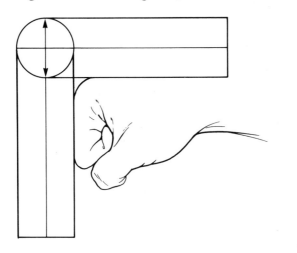

Figure 28. Chart of Finger MP Joint Impairments

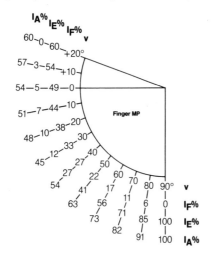

$I_A\%$ = impairment due to ankylosis
$I_E\%$ = impairment due to loss of extension
$I_F\%$ = impairment due to loss of flexion
V   = degrees of motion or ankylosis

• Use Table 3 to relate impairment of the upper extremity to impairment of the whole person.

Example: An amputation at the elbow joint level is a 96% impairment of the upper extremity, or 58% impairment of the whole person.

Abnormal Motion

The elbow joint has two units of motion, each contributing a relative value to its function. Complete loss of elbow function is considered a 70% impairment of the upper extremity. Flexion/extension is considered to be 60% of elbow motion, and 42% of the upper extremity. Pronation/supination is considered to be 40% of elbow motion and 28% of the upper extremity.

Flexion and Extension

• Measure the maximum flexion and extension and record the goniometer readings (Figure 35, p. 33). Round the figures to the nearest 10°.

• From Figure 36 (p. 34), match the measured flexion and extension degrees (V) to their corresponding impairments of flexion ($I_F\%$) and extension ($I_E\%$).

• *Add* the impairment values of flexion and extension.

• If the elbow is ankylosed, measure the position and match it to the corresponding ankylosis impairment ($I_A\%$) in Figure 36 (p. 34). Anklyosis in the functional position (80° flexion) is given the lowest value, or 21% impairment. Ankylosis in either 0° extension or 140° flexion is a 100% loss of elbow flexion/extension function. This is equivalent to a 60% impairment of the elbow, and a 42% impairment of the upper extremity.

Example: Elbow extension −40° and flexion 75°:
$I_E\%$ = 4% impairment of the upper extremity.
$I_F\%$ = 15% impairment of the upper extremity.
4% + 15% = 19% impairment of the upper extremity.

Example: Elbow ankylosis in 140° flexion: $I_A\%$ = 42% impairment of the upper extremity.

Pronation and Supination

• Measure the maximum pronation and supination and record the goniometer readings (Figure 37, p. 34). Round the figures to the nearest 10°.

• From Figure 38 (p. 34), match the measured flexion and extension degrees (V) to their corresponding impairments of pronation ($I_P\%$) and supination ($I_S\%$).

• *Add* the impairment values of pronation and supination to obtain the impairment of the upper extremity.

• If the elbow is ankylosed, measure the position and match it to the corresponding ankylosis impairment (I_A%) in Figure 38 (p. 34). Ankylosis in the functional position (20° pronation) is given the lowest value, or 8% impairment. Ankylosis in 80° pronation or supination is considered to be 100% impairment of the elbow rotation function. This is equivalent to a 40% impairment of elbow motion, and 28% impairment of the upper extremity.

Example: Pronation 30° and supination 10°:
I_P% = 3% impairment of the upper extremity.
I_S% = 3% impairment of the upper extremity.
3% + 3% = 6% impairment of the upper extremity.

Example: Elbow ankylosis in 80° supination: I_A% = 28% impairment of the upper extremity.

Combining Impairments Due to Abnormal Motion of the Elbow Joint
• Determine the impairment of the upper extremity contributed by abnormal elbow motions (flexion/extension and pronation/supination) as described above.

• Because the relative value of each elbow function unit has been taken into consideration in the charts, impairment values of each elbow motion are *added* to determine the impairment of the upper extremity.

• Use Table 3 to relate impairment of the upper extremity to impairment of the whole person.

Example: Elbow flexion/extension impairment of 19% and pronation/supination impairment of 6%.
19% + 6% = 25% impairment of the upper extremity, and 15% impairment of the whole person.

Example: Elbow ankylosis in 140° flexion and 80° supination:
Flexion I_A% = 42% Supination I_A% = 28%
42% + 28% = 70% impairment of the upper extremity, and 42% impairment of the whole person.

3.1g Shoulder

Amputation
• Amputations at the shoulder level are considered 100% impairment of the upper extremity.

• Use Table 3 to relate impairment of the upper extremity to impairment of the whole person.

Example: Amputation at the shoulder joint is 100% impairment of the upper extremity, and 60% impairment of the whole person.

Abnormal Motion
The shoulder has three motion planes, each contributing a relative value to its function. Complete loss of shoulder function is considered to be a 60% impairment of the upper extremity. Flexion is considered to be

---

Figure 29. Flexion of Wrist

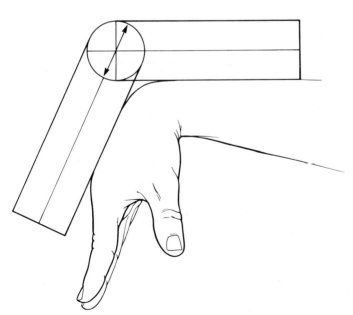

Figure 30. Extension of Wrist

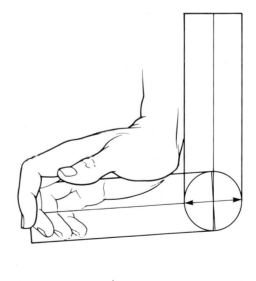
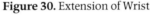

Figure 31. Chart of Wrist Flexion/Extension Impairments

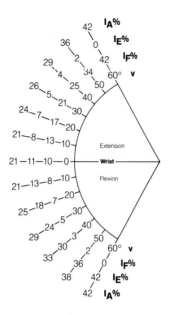

$I_A\%$ = impairment due to ankylosis
$I_E\%$ = impairment due to extension
$I_F\%$ = impairment due to flexion
V = degree of motion or ankylosis

40% of shoulder motion and extension 10% of shoulder motion. Therefore, flexion/extension is considered to be 50% of shoulder motion, or 30% of the upper extremity. Abduction is considered to be 20% of shoulder motion and adduction 10% of shoulder motion. Therefore, abduction/adduction is considered to be 30% of shoulder motion, or 18% of the upper extremity. Internal rotation is considered to be 10% of shoulder motion and external rotation 10% of shoulder motion. Therefore, internal/external rotation is considered to be 20% of shoulder motion, or 12% of the upper extremity.

Flexion and Extension

• Measure the maximum flexion and extension and record the goniometer readings (Figures 39 & 40, p. 35). Round the figures to the nearest 10°.

• From Figure 41 (p. 36), match the measured flexion and extension degrees (V) to their corresponding impairments to determine the upper extremity impairment due to loss of shoulder flexion ($I_F\%$) and extension ($I_E\%$).

• *Add* the impairment values for flexion and extension to obtain the impairment of the upper extremity.

Figure 32. Radial Deviation of Wrist

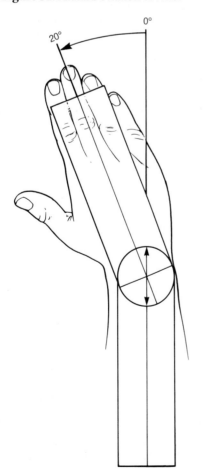

Figure 33. Ulnar Deviation of Wrist

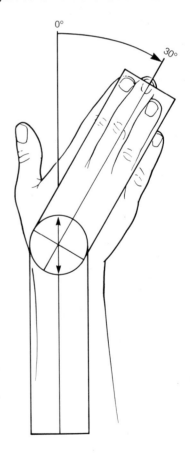

• If the shoulder is ankylosed, measure the position and match it to the corresponding ankylosis (I_A%) impairment in Figure 41 (p. 36). Ankylosis in the functional position (25° flexion) is given the lowest value, or 15% impairment. Ankylosis in 50° extension or 180° flexion are both a 100% loss of flexion/extension function. This is equivalent to a 50% loss of shoulder function, or 30% impairment of the upper extremity.

Example: Shoulder flexion 90° and extension 0°:
I_F% = 6% impairment of the upper extremity.
I_E% = 3% impairment of the upper extremity.
6% + 3% = 9% impairment of the upper extremity.

Example: Shoulder ankylosis of 50° extension: I_A% = 30% impairment of the upper extremity.

Abduction and Adduction
• Measure the maximum abduction and adduction and record the goniometer readings (Figure 42, p. 36). Round the figures to the nearest 10°.

• From Figure 43 (p. 37), match the measured abduction and adduction degrees (V) to their corresponding impairments to determine the impairment of the upper extremity due to loss of shoulder abduction (I_{ABD}%) and adduction (I_{ADD}%).

• *Add* abduction and adduction impairment values to obtain the impairment of the upper extremity.

• If the shoulder is ankylosed, measure the position and match it to the corresponding ankylosis (I_A%) impairment value in Figure 43 (p. 37). Ankylosis in the functional position (50° abduction) is given the lowest value, or 9% impairment. Ankylosis in either 50° adduction or 180° abduction is a 100% loss of abduction/adduction function. This is equivalent to a 30% loss of shoulder function, or 18% impairment of the upper extremity.

Example: Shoulder abduction 100° and adduction 0°:
I_{ABD}% = 4% impairment of the upper extremity.
I_{ADD}% = 1% impairment of the upper extremity.
4% + 1% = 5% impairment of the upper extremity.

Example: Shoulder ankylosis of 180° abduction: I_A% = 18% impairment of the upper extremity.

Internal and External Rotation
• Measure the maximum internal and external rotation and record the goniometer readings (Figures 44 and 45, pp. 37-38). Round the figures to the nearest 10°.

• From Figure 46 (p. 38), match the measured internal and external rotation degrees (V) to their corresponding impairment values to determine the impairment of the upper extremity to loss of shoulder internal rotation (I_{IR}%) and external rotation (I_{ER}%).

Figure 34. Chart of Wrist Lateral Deviation Impairments

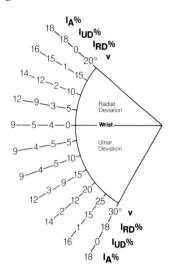

I_A% = impairment due to ankylosis
I_E% = impairment due to extension
I_F% = impairment due to flexion
V   = degree of motion or ankylosis

Figure 35. Flexion/Extension of Elbow

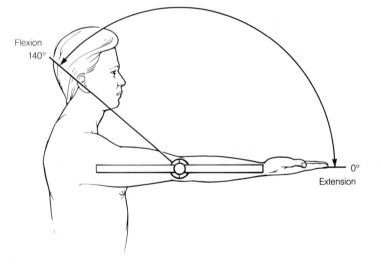

Figure 36. Chart of Elbow Flexion/Extension Impairments

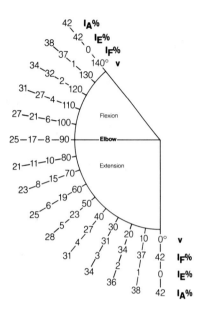

$I_A\%$ = impairment due to ankylosis
$I_E\%$ = impairment due to extension
$I_F\%$ = impairment due to flexion
V   = degree of motion or ankylosis

- *Add* internal and external rotation impairment values to obtain the impairment of the upper extremity.

- If the shoulder is ankylosed, measure the position and match it to the corresponding ankylosis impairment value ($I_A\%$) in Figure 46 (p. 38). Ankylosis in the functional position (20° external rotation) is given the lowest value, or 6% impairment. Ankylosis in either 90° internal or external rotation is a 100% loss of shoulder rotation function. This is equivalent to a 20% loss of shoulder function, or 12% impairment of the upper extremity.

Example: Shoulder internal rotation 40° and external rotation 50°:
$I_{IR}\%$ = 1% impairment of the upper extremity.
$I_{ER}\%$ = 1% impairment of the upper extremity.
1% + 1% = 2% impairment of the upper extremity.

Example: Shoulder ankylosis in 90° external rotation:
$I_A\%$ = 12% impairment of the upper extremity.

Combining Impairments Due to Abnormal Motions of the Shoulder Joint
- Determine the impairments of the upper extremity

Figure 37. Elbow Pronation and Supination

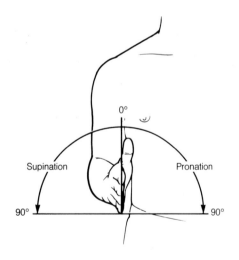

Figure 38. Chart of Elbow Pronation/Supination Impairments

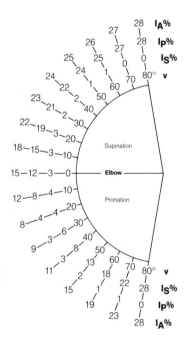

$I_A\%$ = impairment due to ankylosis
$I_P\%$ = impairment due to loss of pronation
$I_S\%$ = impairment due to loss of supination
V   = degree of motion or ankylosis

contributed by abnormal shoulder motions (flexion/extension, abduction/ adduction, and internal/external rotation) as described above.

- Because the relative value of each shoulder functional unit has been taken into consideration in the charts, impairment values of each shoulder motion are *added* to determine the impairment of the upper extremity.

- Use Table 3 to relate impairment of the upper extremity to impairment of the whole person.

Example: Shoulder flexion/extension impairment 9%, abduction/adduction impairment 5%, and internal/external rotation impairment 2%: 9% + 5% + 2% = 16% impairment of the upper extremity, and 10% impairment of the whole person.

Example: Shoulder ankylosis in 0° extension, 0° adduction and 0° rotation:
Extension $I_A\% = 24\%$; adduction $I_A\% = 14\%$; rotation $I_A\% = 7\%$.
24% + 14% + 7% = 45% impairment of the upper extremity, and 27% impairment of the whole person.

3.1h Combining Regional Impairments to Obtain Impairment of the Whole Person

- Determine the impairments of each region (hand, wrist, elbow, and shoulder joints) as described above.

- Use the Combined Values Chart to combine impairments of the upper extremity contributed by each region. *Note:* Digit and hand impairments must be converted to impairments of the upper extremity before regional impairments can be combined.

- Use Table 3 to convert impairment of the upper extremity to impairment of the whole person.

Example: An upper extremity that has sustained multiple injuries has regional impairments of: 50% of thumb, 10% of index finger, 5% of the upper extremity due to the wrist, and 2% of the upper extremity due to the elbow. Using Table 1, a 50% thumb impairment and a 10% index finger impairment convert to 20% and 2% impairment of the hand, respectively. These are *added* to obtain a 22% impairment of the hand. Using Table 2,

Figure 39. Flexion of Shoulder

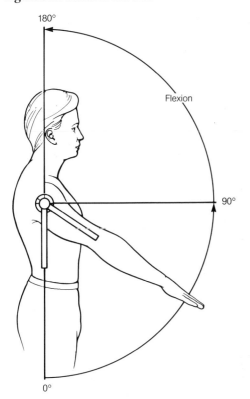

Figure 40. Extension of Shoulder

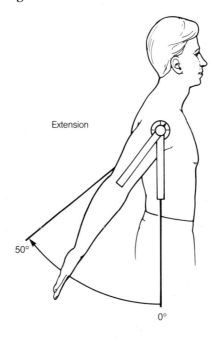

a 22% impairment of the hand is equivalent to a 20% impairment of the upper extremity. Using the Combined Values Chart 20% combined with 5% = 24%; 24% combined with 2% = 26% impairment of the upper extremity, and a 16% impairment of the whole person (Table 3).

3.1i Impairment of the Upper Extremity Due to Peripheral Nervous System Disorders

The peripheral spinal nerves constitute an intricate system that serves as the conductor of neural impulses traveling in both directions between the spinal cord and other tissues of the body and through which many important bodily functions are regulated. For descriptive purposes, the peripheral spinal nerves may be classified according to their site of origin from the spinal cord and their function (Table 9). The sensory nerves and their roots of origin are shown in Figure 47.

Method of Evaluation: Permanent impairment related to a peripheral spinal nerve may be described as an alteration of sensory or motor function that has become static or well-stabilized after an appropriate course of medical management and rehabilitation therapy for a period of time sufficient to permit regeneration and other physiologic recovery. In order to evaluate impairment resulting from the effects of peripheral spinal nerve lesions, it is necessary to determine the extent of loss of function due to (a) sensory deficit, pain or discomfort; and (b) loss of muscle strength and altered fine motor control of muscles of the part. Although atrophy, vasomotor and trophic changes, reflex changes, and certain characteristic deformities are also effects of peripheral nerve lesions, it is not necessary to evaluate all of these separately, because they would be reflected in the sensory disturbance, loss of muscle strength, or altered fine motor control.

Note: Restrictions of motion and ankyloses may result from peripheral spinal nerve impairments. Consideration was given to such impairments when the percentage values set forth in this section were derived. Therefore, if an impairment results strictly from a peripheral nerve lesion, the evaluator *should not* apply the impairment values from both Sections 3.1a through 3.1g and this section, because this would result in a duplication and a multiplying of the impairment rating. However, when restricted motion or ankylosis exists but cannot be attributed to sensory involvement or

Figure 41. Chart of Shoulder Flexion/Extension Impairments

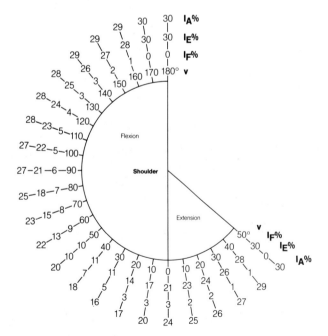

I$_A$% = impairment due to ankylosis
I$_E$% = impairment due to loss of extension
I$_F$% = impairment due to loss of flexion
V   = degrees of motion or ankylosis

Figure 42. Shoulder Abduction and Adduction

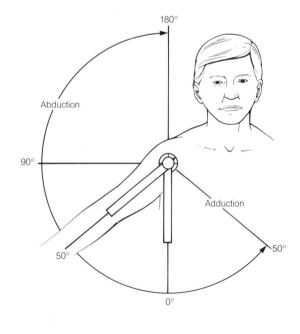

muscle weakness, then values from Sections 3.1a through 3.1g may be combined with values of this section using the Combined Values Chart.

It is necessary for the physician to establish as accurately as possible the anatomic distribution of sensory and/or motor loss and verify that the distribution relates to a specific peripheral spinal nerve or nerves before determining the percentage of permanent impairment. The diagnosis is based firmly on the patient's signs and symptoms. With a carefully obtained history, a thorough medical and neurological examination, and appropriate laboratory aids, the physician should characterize the pain, discomfort, and loss of sensation occurring in the areas innervated by the affected nerve, and also the degree of muscle strength and fine motor control that has been lost.

Pain: The pain associated with peripheral spinal nerve impairment, and particularly with that of the median nerve, sometimes has a constant burning quality. This pain is described as a major or a minor causalgia in accordance with its severity, and it is evaluated on the same percentage basis as are other types of pain. Major causalgia that persists despite appropriate treatment can result in loss of function of the affected extremity and impairment that is as great as 100%.

In evaluating pain that is associated with peripheral spinal nerve disorders, the physician should consider: (a) how the pain interferes with the individual's performance of the activities of daily living; (b) to what extent the pain follows the defined anatomical pathways of the root, plexus, or peripheral nerve; and (c) to what extent the description of the pain indicates that it is caused by a peripheral spinal nerve abnormality. That is, the pain should correspond to other kinds of disturbances of the involved nerve or nerve root.

Complaints of pain that cannot be characterized as above are not considered within the scope of this section (for a discussion of categories of pain and their characterization, see Appendix B). The examiner must determine whether the sensory or motor deficit is due to involvement of one or more nerve roots or of one or more peripheral nerves in order to use the appropriate table. Table 12 relates to nerve roots, Table 13 relates to the brachial plexus, and Table 14 relates to the peripheral nerves affecting the upper extremity.

A grading scheme and procedure for determining impairment of a body part that is affected by pain, discomfort, or loss of sensation are found in Tables 10a and 10b, respectively.

Example: Following an injury to his elbow, a worker was left with pain and a loss of sensation that prevented activity and caused minor causalgia in the medial aspect of his right forearm (preferred side).

Figure 43. Chart of Shoulder Abduction/Adduction Impairments

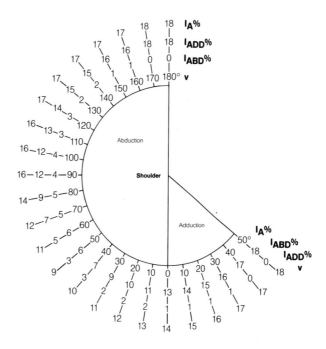

I_A%   = impairment due to ankylosis
I_{ADD}% = impairment due to loss of adduction
I_{ABD}% = impairment due to loss abduction
V   = degrees of motion or ankylosis

Figure 44. Shoulder Internal Rotation

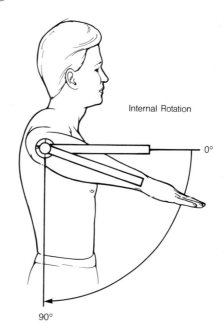

Figure 45. Shoulder External Rotation

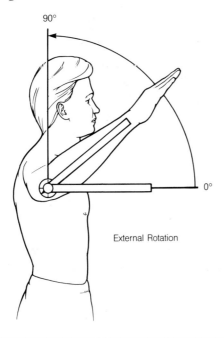

Figure 46. Chart of Shoulder Internal/External Rotation Impairments

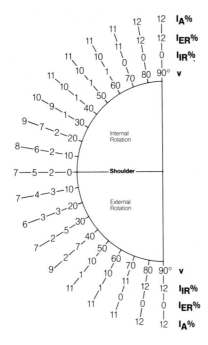

$I_A\%$ = impairment due to ankylosis
$I_{ER}\%$ = impairment due to loss of external rotation
$I_{IR}\%$ = impairment due to loss of internal rotation
V   = degrees of motion or ankylosis

1. Area of involvement is medial aspect of right forearm; see Figure 47.

2. Nerve involved is medial antebrachial cutaneous nerve; see Table 9.

3. Maximum loss of function due to loss of sensation or pain is 5%; see Table 14.

4. Gradation of decreased sensation or pain is 65% to 80%; see Table 10.

5. Therefore, impairment of the upper extremity is 80% x 5%, or 4%.

Strength: Involvement of peripheral spinal nerves or nerve roots may lead to paralysis or to weakness of the muscles supplied by them as well as to characteristic sensory changes. In the case of weakness, the patient often will attempt to substitute stronger muscles to accomplish the desired motion. Thus, the physician should have an understanding of the muscles that are involved in the performance of the various movements of the body and its parts.

Muscle testing, including tests for strength, duration, repetition of contraction, and function, aids evaluation of the functions of specific nerves. Muscle testing is based on the principle of gravity and resistance, that is, the ability to raise a segment of the body through its range of motion against gravity and to hold the segment at the end of its range of motion against resistance. In interpreting muscle testing, comparable muscle functions on both sides of the body should be considered.

A grading scheme and procedure for determining impairment of a body part that is affected by loss of strength are found in Tables 11a and 11b, respectively.

Example: In an injury, a patient sustained a subluxation of the right shoulder, which was reduced to its anatomical position as seen on radiographs. The patient could abduct the shoulder fully against gravity and some resistance, starting with the arm alongside the body while in a standing position.

1. Motion involved is abduction of the shoulder.

2. Muscle performing the motion is the deltoid; see Table 9.

3. Maximum loss of function due to loss of strength of the axillary nerve is 35%; see Table 4.

4. Gradation of loss of strength is 5% to 20%; see Table 11.

5. Therefore, impairment of the upper extremity is 20% x 35%, or 7%.

Table 9. Origins and Functions of the Peripheral Nerves of the Upper Extremity Emanating from the Brachial Plexus (Cervical 5 to 8 and Thoracic 1)

Nerves of Plexus	Primary Branches	Secondary Branches	Function
Muscular branches	Unnamed		Motor to Longus colli, scaleni, and Subclavius
Dorsal scapular			Motor to Rhomboideus major and minor, Levator scapulae
Long thoracic			Motor to Serratus anterior
Suprascapular			Motor to Supraspinatus and Infraspinatus
Lateral anterior thoracic			Motor to Pectoralis major
Medial anterior thoracic			Motor to Pectoralis major and minor
Upper subscapular			Motor to Subscapularis
Lower subscapular			Motor to Teres major and Subscapularis
Thoracodorsal			Motor to Latissimus dorsi
	Teres minor br		Motor to Teres minor
	Posterior		Motor to Teres minor and posterior part of Deltoid
Axillary		Upper lateral brachial-cutaneous	Sensory to skin over lower two-thirds of Deltoid
	Anterior		Motor to central and anterior parts of Deltoid
Medial brachial cutaneous			Sensory to anteromedial surface of arm (with intercostobrachial)
Medial antebrachial cutaneous			Sensory to anteromedial surface of arm and ulnar surface of forearm
Musculocutaneous	Unnamed		Motor to Coracobrachialis, Biceps brachili, Brachialis .
	Lateral antebrachial cutaneous		Sensory to radial surface of forearm
	Unnamed	Cubital fossa and forearm branches	Motor to Pronator terres, Flexor carpi radialis, Palmaris longus, Flexor digitorum sublimus
	Anterior interosseus		Motor to radial half of Flexor digitorum profundus of the index and middle fingers, Flexor pollicis longus, Pronator quadratus
	Palmar cutaneous		Sensory to radial surface of palm
Median	Common palmar radial digital	Thenar muscular branch	Motor to Abductor pollicis brevis, Flexor pollicis brevis and Oppens pollicis
		Proper palmar digitals (1st, 2nd, 3rd)	Motor to first Lumbrical; sensory to first web space, to palmar and distal dorsal surfaces of thumb, and to index palmar surface and distal dorsal surface on on radial side
	Common palmar central digital	Proper palmar digital (4th)	Motor to second Lumbrical; sensory to 2nd web space and to palmar surfaces and distal dorsal surfaces of contiguous sides of index and middle fingers
	Common palmar ulnar digital	Proper palmar digital (5th)	Sensory to 3rd web space and to palmar surfaces and distal dorsal surfaces of contiguous sides of middle and ring fingers
	Unnamed		Motor to Flexor carpi ulnaris, ulnar half of Flexor digitorum profundus of ring and little fingers
	Palmar and dorsal cutaneous		Sensory to ulnar half of hand, little finger and ulnar half of ring finger
Ulnar	Superficial palmar		Motor to Palmaris brevis
	Deep palmar		Motor to Abductor pollicis, deep head of Flexor pollicis brevis, Abductor digiti quinti, Flexor digiti quinti brevis, Opponens digiti quinti, third and fourth Lumbricals, all Interossei
	Unnamed		Motor to Triceps, Anconeus, Brachioradialis, Extensor carpi radialis longus, Brachialis
	Ulnar collateral		Motor to medial head of Triceps brachii
	Posterior brachial cutaneous		Sensory to posteromedial surface of arm (with intercostobrachial) as far as olecranon
Radial	Posterior lower lateral brachial cutaneous		Sensory to distal anterolateral surface of arm
	Antebrachial cutaneous		Sensory to dorsal surface of arm and forearm and distal posterolateral one-third of arm
	Superficial and dorsal digitals		Sensory to dorsum of radial one-half of wrist and hand; thumb, index, middle and radial one-half of ring finger to middle phalanx
	Posterior interosseous		Motor to Extensor carpi radialis brevis, Supinator, Extensor digitorum communis, Extensor digiti quinti proprius, Extensor carpi ulnaris, Extensor pollicis longus, Extensor pollicis brevis, Abductor pollic longus, Extensor indicis proprius

After the individual values for loss of function due to sensory deficit, pain, or discomfort, and loss of function due to loss of strength have been determined, the impairment to the part of the body or to the whole person is calculated by combining the values using the Combined Values Chart.

Determination of Impairment: The order in which permanent impairment of the peripheral spinal nerves will be discussed is (1) the spinal nerve roots; (2) the brachial plexus; and (3) the named spinal nerves.

The Spinal Nerve Roots

The roots of the spinal nerves can be impaired by various diseases or by injuries that produce partial or complete, and unilateral or bilateral, effects. The degree of permanent impairment resulting from a spinal nerve root dysfunction would be reflected in the loss of function of the named spinal nerves having fibers from the specific nerve root. Since the named spinal nerves have fibers from more than one root, a dysfunction affecting two or more roots that supply fibers to the same nerves usually will be more impairing than a combination of the individual root impairment values (see section on brachial plexus).

Table 12 provides values for the spinal nerve roots that are most frequently involved in permanent impairment of the upper extremity. The values given are for unilateral involvement only. Where there is bilateral involvement, the values should be combined, using the Combined Values Chart at the end of the book.

Values for impairment of a specific spinal nerve root that is not mentioned should be determined by taking into consideration the values that are suggested for a nerve having fibers from the specific nerve root. The reader should refer to the "The Named Spinal Nerves."

Example: A 42-year-old right handed man fell 30 feet and landed on his upper back. He complained of neck pain radiating down his right arm. Examination revealed 20% sensory loss of the C5 area and 50% loss of strength of the muscles innervated by C5.

1. 20% of 5% (see Table 12) equals 1% loss of function due to sensory deficit, pain, or discomfort.

2. 50% of 30% equals 15% loss of function due to loss of strength.

3. 1% combined with 15% equals 16% impairment of the right upper extremity.

Table 10. Grading Scheme and Procedure for Determining Impairment of Affected Body Part Due to Pain, Discomfort, or Loss of Sensation

a. Grading Scheme

Description	Grade
1. No loss of sensation or no spontaneous abnormal sensations	0%
2. Decreased sensation with or without pain, which is forgotten during activity	5-25%
3. Decreased sensation with or without pain, which interferes with activity	30-60%
4. Decreased sensation with or without pain, which may prevent activity (minor causalgia)	65-80%
5. Decreased sensation with severe pain, which may cause outcries as well as prevent activity (major causalgia)	85-95%
6. Decreased sensation with pain, which may prevent all activity	100%

b. Procedure

1. Identify the area of involvement, using the dermatome chart.
2. Identify the nerve(s) that innervate the area(s).
3. Find the value for maximum loss of function of the nerve(s) due to pain or loss of sensation or pain, using the appropriate table.*
4. Grade the degree of decreased sensation or pain according to the grading scheme above.
5. Multiply the value of the nerve (from the appropriate table) by the degree of decreased sensation or pain.

*Table 12 for nerve roots; Table 13 for brachial and lumbosacral plexuses; Table 14 for peripheral nerves.

Table 11. Grading Scheme and Procedure for Determining Impairment of Affected Body Part Due to Loss of Strength

a. Grading Scheme

Description	Grade
1. Complete range of motion against gravity and full resistance	0%
2. Complete range of motion against gravity and some resistance, or reduced fine movements and motor control	5-20%
3. Complete range of motion against gravity, and only without resistance	25-50%
4. Complete range of motion with gravity eliminated	55-75%
5. Slight contractibility, but no joint motion	80-90%
6. No contractibility	100%

b. Procedure

1. Identify the motion involved, such as flexion, extension, etc.
2. Identify the muscle(s) performing the motion.
3. Determine the nerve(s) that innervate the muscle(s), and find the value for maximum percent loss, due to loss of strength, according to the appropriate table.*
4. Grade degree of loss of strength according to the grading scheme above.
5. Multiply the value of the nerve (from the appropriate table) by the degree of loss of strength.

*Table 12 for nerve roots; Table 13 for brachial plexus; Table 14 for peripheral nerves.

Figure 47. Sensory Nerves of the Upper Extremity and Their Roots of Origin

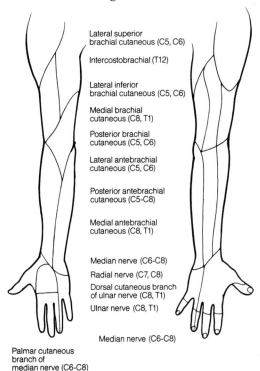

Lateral superior brachial cutaneous (C5, C6)

Intercostobrachial (T12)

Lateral inferior brachial cutaneous (C5, C6)

Medial brachial cutaneous (C8, T1)

Posterior brachial cutaneous (C5, C6)

Lateral antebrachial cutaneous (C5, C6)

Posterior antebrachial cutaneous (C5-C8)

Medial antebrachial cutaneous (C8, T1)

Median nerve (C6-C8)
Radial nerve (C7, C8)
Dorsal cutaneous branch of ulnar nerve (C8, T1)
Ulnar nerve (C8, T1)

Median nerve (C6-C8)

Palmar cutaneous branch of median nerve (C6-C8)

4. 16% impairment of the preferred upper extremity equals 10% impairment of the whole person (see Table 3).

The Brachial Plexus

Impairment due to brachial plexus injury or disease can be determined by evaluating the various functions that are lost. The brachial plexus innervates the shoulder girdle and upper extremity. It is formed by the anterior primary divisions of the fifth, sixth, seventh, and eighth cervical and first thoracic roots. Through anastamoses, these roots unite to form three primary trunks (Figure 48). The clinical importance of the trunks lies in the fact that lesions of them give rise to easily recognized syndromes of the upper trunk, middle trunk, and lower trunk.

The Named Spinal Nerves

The named spinal nerves most frequently associated with impairment of the upper extremity are found in Table 14. The absence of some of the named spinal nerves and their impairment values indicates that impairment associated with those particular nerves seldom occurs or is considered to be of little significance.

The percentages are expressed in terms of unilateral involvement. When there is bilateral involvement,

Table 12. Unilateral Spinal Nerve Root Impairment Affecting the Upper Extremity

Nerve Root Impaired	Maximum % Loss of Function Due to Sensory Deficit, Pain or Discomfort	Maximum % Loss of Function Due to Loss of Strength	% Impairment of Upper Extremity*
C-5	5	30	0-34
C-6	8	35	0-40
C-7	5	35	0-38
C-8	5	45	0-48
T-1	5	20	0-24

*See Tables 10 and 11 for grading schemes for deriving the percent impairment of the upper extremity due to sensory deficit or loss of strength. See Table 3 for converting upper extremity impairments to whole person impairment. Conversion to whole person impairment should be made only when all impairments involving the upper extremity have been combined.

Table 13. Unilateral Brachial Plexus Impairment

	Maximum % Loss of Function Due to Sensory Deficit, Pain or Discomfort	Maximum % Loss of Function Due to Loss of Strength	% of Impairment Upper Extremity*	Whole Person
Brachial Plexus	100	100	0-100	0-60
Upper Trunk (C-5, C-6) (Duchenne-Erb)	25	70	0-78	0-47
Middle Trunk (C-7)	5	35	0-38	0-23
Lower Trunk (C-8, T-1) (Klumpke-Dejerine)	20	70	0-76	0-46

*See Tables 10 and 11 for grading schemes for deriving the percent impairment of the upper extremity due to sensory deficit or loss of strength. See Table 3 for converting impairment of the upper extremity to impairment of the whole person. Conversion to whole person impairment should be made *Only* when all impairments involving the one upper extremity have been combined.

the unilateral impairments should be determined separately and each converted to whole person impairment. Finally, the unilateral values are combined by using the Combined Values Chart.

Figure 49 is a schematic diagram of the major peripheral motor nerves of the upper extremities.

3.1j Impairment Due to Vascular Disorders of the Upper Extremity

Table 15 provides a classification of impairments due to peripheral vascular disease. When amputation due to peripheral vascular disease is involved, the impairment due to amputation should be evaluated according to Section 3.1c, 3.1d, 3.1e, 3.1f or 3.1g, and combined with the appropriate value in Table 15, using the Combined Values Chart. Note that the values in Table 15 relate to impairment of the upper extremity.

3.1k Impairment Due to Other Disorders of the Upper Extremity

Other derangements can contribute to impairment of the hand and upper extremity and should be considered in the final impairment determination, including bone and joint deformities (including postreconstructive

Table 14. Specific Unilateral Spinal Nerve Impairment Affecting the Upper Extremity

Nerve	Maximum % Loss of Function Due to Sensory Deficit, Pain, or Discomfort	Maximum % Loss of Function Due to Loss of Strength	% Impairment of Upper Extremity*		% Impairment of the Digit
Anterior thoracics (pectoral)	0	5	0- 5		
Axillary (circumflex)	5	35	0-38		
Dorsal scapular	0	5	0- 5		
Long thoracic (posterior thoracic n., external respiratory n. of Bell, n. to serratus anterior)	0	15	0-15		
Medial antebrachial cutaneous	5	0	0- 5		
Medial brachial cutaneous	5	0	0- 5		
Median (above midforearm)	40	55	0-73		
Median (below midforearm)	40	35	0-61		
Branch to radial side of thumb	7	0	0- 7	=	0-20
Branch to ulnar side of thumb	11	0	0-11	=	0-30
Branch to radial side of index finger	5	0	0- 5	=	0-30
Branch to ulnar side of index finger	4	0	0- 4	=	0-20
Branch to radial side of middle finger	5	0	0- 5	=	0-30
Branch to ulnar side of middle finger	4	0	0- 4	=	0-20
Branch to radial side of ring finger	3	0	0- 3	=	0-30
Musculocutaneous	5	25	0-29		
Radial (musculospiral) (Upper arm with loss of triceps) wrist placed in position of function	5	55	0-57		
Radial (musculospiral) (with sparing of triceps) wrist placed in position of function	5	40	0-43		
Subscapular (upper and lower)	0	5	0- 5		
Suprascapular	5	15	0-19		
Thoracordorsal (long subscapular; nerve to latissimus dorsi)	0	10	0-10		
Ulnar (above midforearm)	10	35	0-42		
Ulnar (below midforearm)	10	25	0-33		
Branch to ulnar side of ring finger	2	0	0- 2	=	0-20
Branch to radial side of little finger	2	0	0- 2	=	0-20
Branch to ulnar side of little finger	3	0	0- 3	=	0-30

*See Tables 10 & 11 for grading schemes for determining impairment of upper extremity due to sensory deficit or loss of strength.

See Table 3 for converting impairment of upper extremity to impairment of whole person.

Note: Conversion to whole person impairment should by made *only* when all impairments involving the one upper extremity have been combined.

Figure 49. Motor Innervation of the Upper Extremity

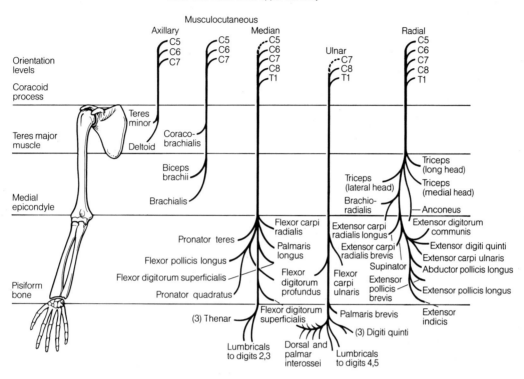

Motor Innervation of the Upper Extremity

surgery) and musculotendinous disorders. Impairments due to skin disorders of the upper extremity, including scars, are evaluated according to the criteria in Chapter 13.

Table 16 shows relative impairment values of the upper extremity for the *loss of function* of the hand, wrist, elbow and shoulder due to the conditions described below. This table is distinct from Figure 2, which shows *values for amputation* at these levels. Table 17 more finely converts upper extremity joint abnormalities to impairment of the digit, hand, upper extremity and whole person, using the relative impairments of Table 16.

Bone and Joint Deformities
Joint Crepitation with Motion

Joint crepitation with motion can reflect synovitis or cartilage degeneration. The impairment degree is multiplied by the relative value of the joint.

The evaluator must use appropriate judgment to avoid duplication of impairments when other findings, such as synovial hypertrophy or carpal collapse with

Figure 48. Brachial Plexus

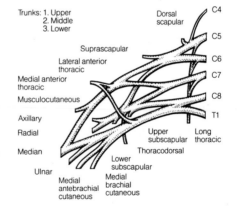

Table 15. Impairment of the Upper Extremity Due to Peripheral Vascular Disease

Class 1 (0-5% Impairment)	Class 2 (10-35% Impairment)	Class 3 (40-60% Impairment)	Class 4 (70-85% Impairment)	Class 5 (90-100% Impairment)
The patient experiences neither intermittent claudication nor pain at rest; **and** The patient experiences only transient edema; **and**	The patient experiences intermittent claudication on severe usage of the upper extremity; **or** There is persistent edema of a moderate degree, incompletely controlled by elastic supports; **or**	The patient experiences intermittent claudication on moderate upper extremity usage; **or** There is marked edema that is only partially controlled by elastic supports; **or**	The patient experiences intermittent claudication on mild upper extremity usage; **or** The patient has marked edema that cannot be controlled by elastic supports; **or**	The patient experiences severe and constant pain at rest; **or** There is vascular damage as evidenced by signs such as amputation at or above the wrists of two extremities, or amputation of all digits of two or more extremities with evidence of persistent vascular disease or of persistent, wide-spread, or deep ulceration involving two or more extremities;
On physical examination, not more than the following findings are present: loss of pulses; minimal loss of subcutaneous tissue of fingertips; calcification of arteries as detected by radiographic examination; asymptomatic dilation of arteries or of veins, not requiring surgery and not resulting in curtailment of activity; **or**	There is vascular damage as evidenced by a sign, such as that of a healed, painless stump of an amputated digit showing evidence of persistent vascular disease, or of a healed ulcer; **or**	There is vascular damage as evidenced by a sign, such as healed amputation of two or more digits of one extremity, with evidence of persisting vascular disease or superficial ulceration; **or**	There is vascular damage as evidenced by signs such as an amputation at or above a wrist, or amputation of two or more digits of two extremities with evidence of persistent vascular disease, or persistent widespread or deep ulceration involving one extremity; **or**	**or**
Raynaud's phenomenon that occurs with exposure to temperatures lower than 0°C (32°F) but is readily controlled by medication.	Raynaud's phenomenon occurs on exposure to temperatures lower than 4°C (39°F), but is controlled by medication.	Raynaud's phenomenon occurs on exposure to temperatures lower than 10°C (50°F), and it is only partially controlled by medication.	Raynaud's phenomenon occurs on exposure to temperatures lower than 15°C (59°F), and it is only partially controlled by medication.	Raynaud's phenomenon occurs on exposure to temperatures lower than 20°C (68°F) and is poorly controlled by medication.

arthritic changes, are present. The latter findings could indicate a greater severity of the same underlying pathological process and take precedence over joint crepitation, which should not be rated in these instances.

Joint Crepitation Severity	% Joint Impairment
Mild: Inconstant during active ROM*	10
Moderate: Constant during active ROM	20
Severe: Constant during passive ROM	30

*ROM = Range of Motion

Example: Mild joint crepitation of the carpometacarpal joint of the thumb would result in 10% x 80% = 8% impairment of the thumb, 3% impairment of the hand, 3% impairment of the upper extremity, and 2% impairment of the whole person (numbers are rounded to the nearest whole percent).

Joint Swelling Due to Synovial Hypertrophy	% Joint Impairment
Mild	10
Moderate	20
Severe	30

Digit Lateral Deviation

The longitudinal alignment of the DIP, PIP, or MP joint is measured in degrees during maximum active extension. Since lateral deviation at any level affects the longitudinal arch of the digit, the entire digit is considered impaired. If this is the sole impairment, the lateral deviation impairment is multiplied by the relative value of the digit to the hand to calculate hand impairment. If the digit has other impairments, the lateral deviation impairment value is combined using the Combined Values Chart.

Ulnar or Radial Deviation	% Digit Impairment
Mild: Less than 10°	10
Moderate: 10° to 30°	20
Severe: Greater than 30°	30

Example: 35° ulnar deviation at the proximal interphalangeal joint of the little finger following a ligamentous injury. Range of motion at that joint is −20° extension to 30° flexion.

1. Ulnar deviation impairment of the little finger = 30%.

2. Motion impairment of the little finger PIP joint:
$I_E\% = 7\%$ $I_F\% = 42\%$
$7\% + 42\% = 49\%$ motion impairment (see Figure 25).

3. 30% combined with 49% = 64% impairment of the little finger, which is 6% impairment of the hand, and 5% impairment of the upper extremity (see Tables 1 and 2).

Digit Rotational Deformity
Rotational deformity of the distal, middle, or proximal phalanx is measured during maximum active flexion of the finger. It expresses a malrotation of the normal axial alignment of the phalanx. Rotational deformity at any level affects the entire digit function, and the impairment percentage is applied to the entire digit. If other impairments of the same digits are present, rotational deformity impairment is combined using the Combined Values Chart.

Rotational Deformity	% Digit Impairment
Mild: Less than 15°	20
Moderate: 15° to 30°	40
Severe: Greater than 30°	60

Example: A 20° pronation deformity of the index finger is present following a healed fracture of the second metacarpal.

1. Rotational impairment of the index finger = 40%.

2. Relative value of the index finger to the hand = 20% (Table 1).

3. Hand impairment is 40% x 20% = 8%; this is equivalent to a 7% impairment of the upper extremity (Table 2).

Table 16. Relative Impairment Values for Loss of Function at Various Levels of the Upper Extremity

Level	% Impairment of the Upper Extremity	% Impairment of the Whole Person
Hand	90	54
Wrist	60	36
Elbow	70	42
Shoulder	60	36

Persistent Joint Subluxation and Dislocation
When persistent joint subluxation or dislocation results in restricted motion, impairment percentages for lack of motion *only* are given to avoid duplication in the rating. If there is no restricted motion, the following table is used:

Persistent Joint Subluxation or Dislocation	% Joint Impairment
Mild: Can be completely reduced manually	20
Moderate: Cannot be completely reduced manually	40
Severe: Cannot be reduced	60

Joint Instability
Excessive passive mediolateral motion is evaluated by comparing normal joint stability and graded according to its degree of severity. The percentage of impairment is then multiplied by the relative value of the joint. If other impairment percentages of the same joint are present, the values are combined using the Combined Values Chart.

Table 17. Impairment Values for Digits, Hand, Upper Extremities, and Whole Person for Disorders of Specific Joints

Joints	% Impairment of Unit	% Impairment of Hand	% Impairment of Upper Extremity	% Impairment of Whole Person
Shoulder Glenohumeral	–	–	60	36
Elbow Ulnohumeral	–	–	50	30
Proximal Radioulnar	–	–	20	12
Wrist Radiocarpal	–	–	40	24
Distal Radioulnar	–	–	20	12
Thumb Carpometacarpal	80	32	29	17
Metacarpophalangeal	11	4	4	2
Interphalangeal	9	4	3	2
Index and Middle Metacarpophalangeal	100	20	18	11
Proximal interphalangeal	80	16	14	8
Distal interphalangeal	45	9	8	5
Ring and Little Metacarpophalangeal	100	10	9	5
Proximal interphalangeal	80	8	7	4
Distal interphalangeal	45	4	4	2

Table 18. Impairments of Upper Extremity Due to Carpal Instability Patterns

Radiographic Findings	% Impairment of Upper Extremity		
	Mild (6%)	Moderate (12%)	Severe (18%)
Radioscaphoid angle (Scaphoid)	40°-60°	60°-70°	>70°
Radiolunate angle (Lunate)	<10°	10°-30°	>30°
Carpal height collapse	0%-5%	5%-10%	>10%
Carpal translation	Mild	Moderate	Severe
Arthritic changes	Mild	Moderate	Severe

Joint Instability	% Joint Impairment
Mild: Less than 10°	20
Moderate: 10° to 20°	40
Severe: Greater than 20°	60

Example: 15° passive radial deviation of thumb IP joint due to collateral ligament injury in a poor candidate for surgery.

1. 15° radial instability = 40% joint impairment.

2. IP joint relative value to thumb motion = 9%.

3. Thumb impairment is 40% x 9% = 4% (rounded); since the thumb relative value to the hand is 40%, this represents a 4% x 40% = 2% hand impairment (Table 1), or 2% x 90% = 2% upper extremity impairment (Table 2).

Wrist and Elbow Joint Lateral Deviation

These angles are measured with the wrist or elbow in maximal active extension. The degree of severity is multiplied by the relative value of the joint to the upper extremity to obtain upper extremity impairment due to lateral deviation. If other impairments of the same joint are present they are combined using the Combined Values Chart. After all impairments for either the wrist or elbow joint have been tabulated, they are combined with any other upper extremity impairment using the Combined Values Chart.

Lateral Deviation Severity	% Joint Impairment
Mild: Less than 20°	10
Moderate: 20° to 30°	20
Severe: Greater than 30°	30

Example: Elbow injury with medial collateral ligament and radial head fracture, treated with simple radial head resection. One year later the patient has 25° lateral deviation of the elbow.

1. 25° lateral deviation of the elbow = 20% impairment of the elbow. Elbow joint relative value = 70% of upper extremity, which equates to 20% x 70% = 14% impairment of the upper extremity.

2. Radial head resection = 8% impairment of upper extremity (see Arthroplasty Impairment, Table 19).

3. Total elbow impairment is 14% combined with 8% = 21% impairment of the upper extremity.

Carpal Instability

Carpal instability patterns resulting from lunate or scaphoid pathology can be classified as mild, moderate, or severe, based on the severity of radiographic findings. The proximal carpal row represents half of the value of the wrist, or 30% of the upper extremity. Therefore, a gradation of mild (20%), moderate (40%), or severe (60%) would represent upper extremity impairments of 6%, 12%, and 18%, respectively. The values can be combined with other upper extremity impairments due to wrist abnormalities using the Combined Values Chart.

In using Table 18, apply only the greatest impairment value determined by the radiographic findings. *Do not* combine or add impairment values.

Example: Radioscaphoid angle of 60°, radiolunate angle of 5°, and arthritic changes are moderate. The greatest impairment is 12% (moderate) for either the radioscaphoid angle or the arthritic changes. Therefore, the impairment of the upper extremity for carpal instability is 12%.

Arthroplasty

Simple resection arthroplasty is given 40% of the impairment of the upper extremity due to loss of function of a joint; implant arthroplasty is given 50% of the impairment of the upper extremity due to loss of function of a joint. Table 19 provides impairment ratings for the upper extremity for arthroplasty of specific joints, based on these values. Arthroplasty impairment may be combined with impairments due to restricted range of motion, using the Combined Values Chart (*Note:* Range of motion impairments must be brought to the level of the upper extremity before combining can occur). Following arthrodesis procedures, impairment is rated only according to the Ankylosis section of the appropriate table(s) in Sections 3.1c through 3.1g.

Example: Total wrist replacement with flexion 30° and extension 20°.

1. Wrist implant arthroplasty = 30% impairment of upper extremity (Table 19).

2. $I_F\% = 5\%$ impairment of upper extremity.
$I_E\% = 7\%$ impairment of upper extremity.
$5\% + 7\% = 12\%$ motion impairment (see Figure 31).

3. 30% combined with 12% = 38% impairment of the upper extremity.

Example: Implant resection arthroplasty of metacarpophalangeal joints of index, middle, and ring fingers with a range of motion of -10° extension to 70° flexion for each. Fusion of index proximal interphalangeal joint at 40° flexion and simple resection arthroplasty of thumb carpometacarpal joint with fusion of thumb metacarpophalangeal joint at 20° flexion.

1. Index finger:
• PIP joint fusion at 40° flexion: $I_A\% = 50\%$ impairment of the finger (Figure 25).

• MP joint implant arthroplasty = 50% impairment of the index finger MP joint.

• MP joint -10° extension: $I_E\% = 7\%$ impairment of the index finger; 70° flexion: $I_F\% = 11\%$ impairment of the index finger (Figure 28); 7% + 11% = 18% impairment of the index finger due to MP joint motion.

• Index finger impairment is found using the Combined Values Chart: 50% combined with 50% = 75%; 75% combined with 18% = 80% impairment of the index finger.

• The index finger represents 20% of the hand; therefore 80% x 20% = 16% impairment of the hand (Table 1).

2. Middle finger:
• MP joint implant arthroplasty = 50% impairment of the middle finger MP joint.

• MP joint -10° extension: $I_E\% = 7\%$ impairment of the middle finger; 70° flexion: $I_F\% = 11\%$ impairment of the middle finger (Figure 28); 7% + 11% = 18% impairment of the middle finger due to MP joint motion.

• Middle finger impairment is found using the Combined Values Chart: 50% combined with 18% = 59% impairment of the middle finger.

• The middle finger represents 20% of the hand; therefore, 59% x 20% = 12% impairment of the hand (Table 1).

3. Ring finger:
• Calculations for the ring finger are the same as above and combine to 59% impairment of the ring finger.

• The ring finger represents 10% of the hand; therefore, 59% x 10% = 6% impairment of the hand (Table 1).

4. Thumb:
• CMC joint resection arthroplasty: 40% of CMC joint, or 40% x 80% = 32% impairment of the thumb.

• Fusion of MP joint at 20° flexion: $I_A\% = 5\%$ impairment of the thumb (Figure 14).

• Thumb joint impairments are *added* directly: 32% + 5% = 37% impairment of the thumb.

• The thumb represents 40% of the hand; therefore, 37% x 40% = 15% impairment of the hand (Table 1).

5. Total hand impairment is calculated by ADDING hand impairments derived for each digit:
Index (16%) + middle finger (12%) + ring finger (6%) + thumb (15%) = 49% impairment of the hand.

• The hand represents 90% of the upper extremity; therefore, 49% x 90% = 44% impairment of the upper extremity.

Musculotendinous Impairments
Intrinsic Tightness
Intrinsic tightness in the hand may be demonstrated by a test described by Bunnell. Hyperextension of the metacarpophalangeal (MP) joint in a normal hand still allows passive flexion of the proximal interphalangeal (PIP) joint. If the intrinsic muscles are tight or contracted,

---

Table 19. Impairment of the Upper Extremity Following Arthroplasty of Specific Bones or Joints

Level of Arthroplasty*	Resection Arthroplasty % Impairment of Upper Extremity	Implant Arthroplasty % Impairment of Upper Extremity
Shoulder	24	30
Total elbow	28	35
Radial head (isolated)	8	10
Total wrist	24	30
Ulnar head (isolated)	8	10
Proximal carpal row	12	15
Carpal bones	12	15
Thumb**		
Carpometarcarpal	11	14
Metacarpophalangeal	1	2
Interphalangeal	1	2
*Index or middle fingers****		
Metacarpophalangeal	7	9
Proximal interphalangeal	6	7
Distal interphalangeal	3	4
*Ring or little fingers****		
Metacarpophalangeal	3	4
Proximal interphalangeal	3	3
Distal interphalangeal	2	2

*If more than one level is involved, combine from distal to proximal using the Combined Values Chart.

**If more than one thumb joint is involved, *add* impairments.

***If more than one joint is involved in the same finger, combine impairments using the Combined Values Chart. If multiple digits are involved, *add* the impairment value for each digit.

Figure 50. Patient's Position for Evaluation of Toes

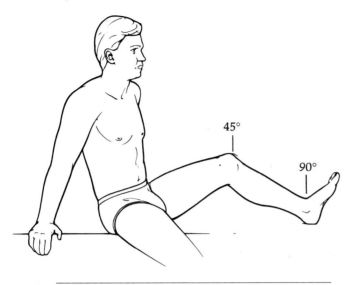

Figure 51. Neutral Position of IP Joint of Great Toe

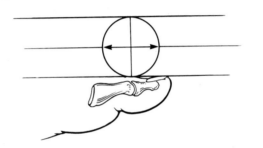

Figure 52. Flexion of Great Toe

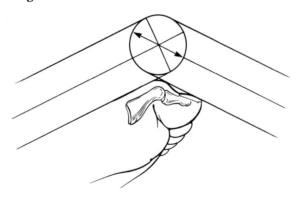

the available stretch of these muscles is taken up by the hyperextended position of the MP joint, and passive flexion of the PIP joint will be difficult.

Intrinsic tightness impairment is combined with other impairments of the same digit using the Combined Values Chart. Finger impairment is converted to hand impairment using Table 1.

Intrinsic Tightness Severity

(Passive flexion of PIP joint with MP joint hyperextended)	% Digit Impairment
Mild: PIP flexion 80° to 60°	20
Moderate: PIP flexion 59° to 20°	40
Severe: PIP flexion less than 20°	60

Constrictive Tenosynovitis

Impairment due to constrictive tenosynovitis is combined with other impairments at the level of the digit using the Combined Values Chart. The digit impairment is converted to hand impairment with Table 1.

Constrictive Tenosynovitis Severity	% Digit Impairment
Mild: Inconstant triggering during active ROM*	20
Moderate: Constant triggering during active ROM	40
Severe: Constant triggering during passive ROM	60

*ROM: Range of Motion

Tendons

The severity of extensor tendon subluxation at the metacarpophalangeal joint is combined with other impairments of the same digit using the Combined Values Chart. The finger impairment is converted to hand impairment with Table 1.

Extensor Tendon Subluxation Severity	% Joint Impairment
Mild: Ulnar subluxation on MP flexion only	10
Moderate: Reducible tendon subluxation in the intermetacarpal groove	20
Severe: Nonreducible tendon subluxation in the intermetacarpal groove	30

3.2 The Lower Extremity

Note: For the purposes of impairment evaluation, ankylosis is defined as either: (a) complete absence of motion, or (b) planar restriction of motion preventing the subject from reaching the neutral position of motion in that plane. Using an impairment rating of ankylosis excludes the simultaneous use of the abnormal motion measurements from the same table. For example, an individual whose hip joint forward flexion ranges from 50° to 90° is considered to have an ankylosis at 50°, which is 67% impairment of the lower extremity. An exception to this rule is the knee, for which extension lag is taken into account (see Table 35).

3.2a Toes

Interphalangeal Joint of the Great Toe—
Flexion and Extension
Abnormal Motion

• Place the patient's foot in the neutral position (Figure 50). Note the 45° angle of the knee and the 90° angle of the ankle.

• Center the goniometer next to the interphalangeal joint (Figure 51). Record the goniometer reading.

• With the patient plantar-flexing the great toe as far as possible (Figure 52), follow the range of motion with the goniometer arm. Record the angle that subtends the arc of motion.

• Consult the Abnormal Motion Section of Table 20 to determine the impairment of the great toe.

Example: 10° active flexion from neutral position or from maximum extension is equivalent to 30% impairment of the great toe.

Ankylosis

• Place the goniometer base as if measuring the neutral position (Figure 51). Measure the deviation from the neutral position with the goniometer arm and record the reading.

• Consult the Ankylosis Section of Table 20 to determine the impairment of the great toe.

Example: The interphalangeal joint with ankylosis at 10° flexion is equivalent to 55% impairment of the great toe.

Amputation

• Amputations distal to the interphalangeal joint are expressed as a percentage of the amputation values of that joint.

Example: If 50% of the distal phalanx of the large toe is amputated, the impairment is 50% x 75% = 38% impairment of the toe.

Metatarsophalangeal Joint of the Great Toe—
Dorsi-flexion
Abnormal Motion

• Place the patient in the neutral position (Figure 50). Note the 45° angle of the knee and the 90° angle of the ankle.

• Center the goniometer under the metatarsophalangeal joint (Figure 53). Record the goniometer reading.

• With the patient dorsi-flexing the great toe, follow the range of motion with the goniometer arm (Figure 54). Record the angle that subtends the arc of motion.

• Consult the Abnormal Motion Section of Table 21 to determine the impairment of the great toe.

Example: 20° active dorsi-flexion from neutral position (0°) is equivalent to 21% impairment of the great toe.

• *Add* the impairment values of the great toe contributed by dorsi-flexion and plantar-flexion. Their sum is the impairment of the great toe contributed by abnormal motions of the metatarsophalangeal joint.

Table 20. Impairment Due to Amputation, Abnormal Motion and Ankylosis of the Interphalangeal Joint of the Great Toe

Amputation			% Impairment of Great Toe
At Joint			75

Abnormal Motion
Average range of *Flexion-Extension* is 30°
Value to total range of joint motion is 100%

Flexion from neutral position (0°) to:	Degrees of Joint Motion Lost	Retained	% Impairment of Great Toe
0°	30°	0°	45
10°	20°	10°	30
20°	10°	20°	15
30°	0°	30°	0

Ankylosis	% Impairment of Great Toe
Joint ankylosed at:	
0° (neutral position)	45
*10°	55
20°	65
30° (full flexion)	75

*position of function

Figure 53. Neutral Position of MP Joint of Great Toe

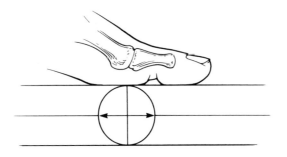

Figure 54. Dorsi-flexion of Great Toe

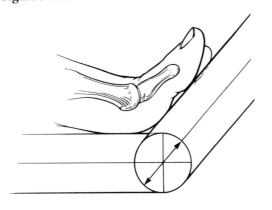

Figure 55. Neutral Position of MP Joint of Great Toe

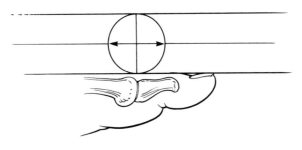

Figure 56. Plantar-flexion of Great Toe

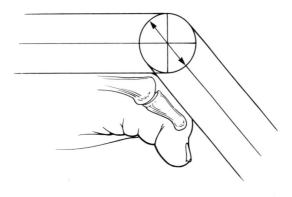

Ankylosis

• Place the goniometer base as if measuring the neutral position (Figure 53). Measure the deviation from neutral position with the goniometer arm and record the reading.

• Consult the Ankylosis Section of Table 21 to determine the impairment of the great toe.

Example: The metatarsophalangeal joint with ankylosis at 20° dorsi-flexion is equivalent to 62% impairment of the great toe.

Amputation

• Amputations distal to the metatarsophalangeal joint and proximal to the interphalangeal joint are expressed as a percentage between 100% and 75%.

Example: If 50% of the proximal phalanx of the large toe is amputated, the impairment is 75% + (50% x 25%) = 88%.

Metatarsophalangeal Joint of the Great Toe–
Plantar-flexion
Abnormal Motion

• Place the patient in the neutral position (Figure 50).

• Center the goniometer over the metatarsophalangeal joint (Figure 55). Record the goniometer reading. Note that the goniometer is rotated 180° from its position for testing dorsi- flexion.

• With the patient plantar-flexing the great toe (Figure 56), follow the range of motion with the goniometer arm. Record the angle that subtends the arc of motion.

• Consult the Abnormal Motion Section of Table 22 to determine the impairment of the great toe.

Example: 20° active plantar-flexion from neutral position (0°) is equivalent to 7% impairment of the great toe.

• *Add* the impairment values contributed by abnormalities of dorsi-flexion and plantar-flexion. Their sum represents impairment of the great toe contributed by the metatarsophalangeal joint.

Ankylosis

• Place the goniometer base as if measuring the neutral position (Figure 55). Measure the deviation from the neutral position with the goniometer arm and record the reading.

• Consult the Ankylosis Section of Table 22 to determine the impairment of the great toe.

Example: The metatarsophalangeal joint with ankylosis at 20° plantar-flexion is equivalent to 85% impairment of the great toe.

Great Toe—Both Joints Involved

Measure separately and record the impairment of the great toe contributed by each joint. Then, combine the impairment values using the Combined Values Chart to determine the impairment of the great toe contributed by both joints.

Example: Description	% **Impairment** of Great Toe
Interphalangeal joint with ankylosis at 10° flexion	55
Metatarsophalangeal joint with ankylosis at 20° dorsi-flexion	<u>62</u>
(62% combined with 55% = 83%)	83

Example: Description	% **Impairment** of Great Toe
Amputation at interphalangeal joint	75
Metatarsophalangeal joint with 20° active dorsi-flexion from neutral position (0°)	21
Metatarsophalangeal joint with 20° active plantar-flexion from neutral position (0°)	<u>7</u>
(21% + 7% = 28% combined with 75% = 82%)	82

Finally, consult Table 23 to determine impairment of the foot that is contributed by the great toe; in these examples, the impairment of the foot would be 15%.

Distal Interphalangeal Joint of the Second Through Fifth Toes—Dorsi- and Plantar-flexion
Abnormal Motion
• Abnormal motion is not measurable

Ankylosis
• Place the goniometer base as if measuring the neutral position (Figure 57). Measure the deviation from the

Table 21. Impairment Due to Amputation, Abnormal Motion and Ankylosis of the Metatarsophalangeal Joint of the Great Toe—Dorsi-flexion

Amputation	% **Impairment of** **Great Toe**
At Joint	100

Abnormal Motion
Average range of *Dorsi-Plantar-Flexion* is 80°
Value to total range of joint motion is 100%

Dorsi-flexion **from neutral** **position (0°) to:**	**Degrees of** **Joint Motion** Lost	Retained	% **Impairment of** **Great Toe**
0°	50°	0°	34
10°	40°	10°	28
20°	30°	20°	21
30°	20°	30°	14
40°	10°	40°	7
50°	0°	50°	0

Ankylosis	
Joint ankylosed at:	% **Impairment of** **Great Toe**
0° (neutral position)	55
*10°	49
20°	62
30°	74
40°	87
50° (full dorsi-flexion)	100

Arthroplasty at joint: 25%, combined with impairment value for either ankylosis, or loss of range of motion, if present

*position of function

Table 22. Impairment Due to Amputation, Abnormal Motion and Ankylosis of the Metatarsophalangeal Joint of the Great Toe—Plantar-flexion

Amputation	% **Impairment of** **Great Toe**
At Joint	100

Abnormal Motion
Average range of *Dorsi-Plantar-Flexion* is 80°
Value to total range of joint motion is 100%

Plantar-flexion **from neutral** **position (0°) to:**	**Degrees of** **Joint Motion** Lost	Retained	% **Impairment of** **Great Toe**
0°	30°	0°	21
10°	20°	10°	14
20°	10°	20°	7
30°	0°	30°	0

Ankylosis	
Joint ankylosed at:	% **Impairment of** **Great Toe**
0° (neutral position)	55
10°	70
20°	85
30° (full plantar flexion)	100

Figure 57. Neutral Position of DIP Joint of Small Toe

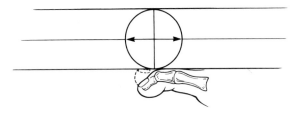

Figure 58. Hammer Toe Ankylosis of Little Toe

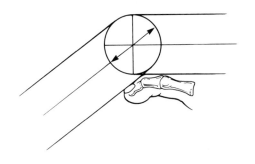

Figure 59. Neutral Position of PIP Joint of Small Toes

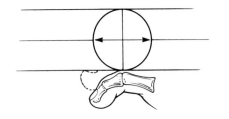

Figure 60. Plantar-flexion Ankylosis of Small Toes

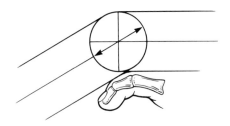

neutral position with the goniometer arm (Figure 58), and record the reading.

• Consult the Ankylosis Section of Table 24 to determine the impairment of the toe.

Amputation
• Amputations distal to the distal interphalangeal joint are expressed as a percentage of 45%.

Example: If 50% of the distal phalanx is amputated, the impairment is 50% x 45% = 22% of the toe.

Proximal Interphalangeal Joint of the Second through Fifth Toes—Dorsi-and Plantar-flexion Abnormal Motion
• Abnormal motion is not measurable.

Ankylosis
• Place the goniometer base as if measuring the neutral position (Figure 59). Measure the deviation from the neutral position with the goniometer arm (Figure 60), and record the reading.

• Consult the Ankylosis Section of Table 25 to determine the impairment of the toe.

Amputation
• Amputations distal to the proximal interphalangeal joint and proximal to the distal interphalangeal joint are expressed as a percentage between 45% and 80%.

Example: If 50% of the middle phalanx is amputated, the impairment is 45% + (50% x 35%) = 63%.

Metatarsophalangeal Joint of the Second through Fifth Toes—Dorsi- and Plantar-flexion Abnormal Motion
• Place patient in the neutral position (Figure 50).

Table 23. Relationship of Impairment of the Great Toe to Impairment of the Foot

% Impairment of			% Impairment of		
Great Toe		Foot	Great Toe		Foot
0– 2	=	0	53– 57	=	10
3– 8	=	1	58– 62	=	11
9–13	=	2			
14–19	=	3	63– 68	=	12
			69– 73	=	13
20–24	=	4	74– 79	=	14
25–30	=	5	80– 84	=	15
31–35	=	6			
36–41	=	7	85– 90	=	16
			91– 95	=	17
42–46	=	8	96–100	=	18
47–52	=	9			

Note: Impairment of the foot contributed by the great toe may be rounded to the nearest 5% only when it is the *sole* impairment involved.

Consult Table 32 for converting foot impairment to lower extremity impairment.

• Dorsi-flexion: Center the goniometer beneath the metatarsophalangeal joint of the toe being tested (Figure 61a). Record the goniometer reading. With the patient dorsi-flexing the toe as far as possible (Figure 61b), follow the range of motion with the goniometer arm. Record the angle that subtends the arc of motion.

• Plantar-flexion: Center the goniometer over the metatarsophalangeal joint of the toe being tested (Figure 61c). Record the goniometer reading. Starting from the neutral position with patient plantar-flexing the toe as far as possible (Figure 61d), follow the range of motion with the goniometer arm. Record the angle that subtends the arc of motion.

• Consult the Abnormal Motion Section of Tables 26-29 to determine the impairment of the toe.

Example: 20° active dorsi-flexion from neutral position (0°) is equivalent to 14% impairment of the second toe (Table 26).

• *Add* the toe impairment values contributed by dorsi-flexion and plantar-flexion. The sum of these values is the impairment of the toe.

Ankylosis
• Place the goniometer base as if measuring the neutral position (Figure 61a or 61c). Measure the deviation from the neutral position with goniometer arm and record the reading.

• Consult the Ankylosis Section of Tables 26-29 to determine the impairment of the toe.

Example: A metatarsophalangeal joint with ankylosis at 20° dorsi-flexion is equivalent to 75% impairment of the second toe (Table 26).

Amputation
• Amputations distal to the metatarsophalangeal joint and proximal to the proximal interphalangeal joint are expressed as a percentage between 100% and 80%.

Example: If 50% of the proximal phalanx is amputated, the impairment is 80% + (50% x 20%) = 90%.

Second Through Fifth Toes—Two or More Joints
Measure separately and record the impairment of the toe contributed by each joint. Then, combine the impairment values using the Combined Values Chart to determine the impairment of the toe contributed by two or more joints.

Example: **Description** Second Toe	**% Impairment of Toe**
Amputation at distal interphalangeal joint	45
Proximal interphalangeal joint with ankylosis in neutral position	45
Metatarsophalangeal joint with 20° active dorsi-flexion from neutral position	14
Metatarsophalangeal joint with 20° active plantar-flexion from neutral position	7
(14% + 7% = 21%; 21% combined with 45% = 57%; 57% combined with 45% = 76%)	76

Finally, consult Table 30 to determine the impairment of the foot contributed by the toe. In the example, foot impairment would be 2%.

Table 24. Impairment Due to Amputation, Abnormal Motion and Ankylosis of the Distal Interphalangeal Joint of the 2nd Through 5th Toe—Dorsi-Plantar-flexion

Amputation	% Impairment of Toe
At Joint	45

Abnormal Motion	
No functional value	

Ankylosis	
Joint ankylosed in:	% Impairment of Toe
Dorsi-flexion	45
*Neutral position	30
Plantar-flexion (hammer toe)	45

*position of function

Table 25. Impairment Due to Amputation, Abnormal Motion and Ankylosis of the Proximal Interphalangeal Joint of the 2nd Through 5th Toe—Dorsi-Plantar-flexion

Amputation	% Impairment of Toe
At Joint	80

Abnormal Motion	
No functional value	

Ankylosis	
Joint ankylosed in:	% Impairment of Toe
Dorsi-flexion	80
*Neutral position	45
Plantar-flexion	80

*position of function

Figure 61. Neutral Positions & Dorsi- & Plantar-flexion of Small Toes

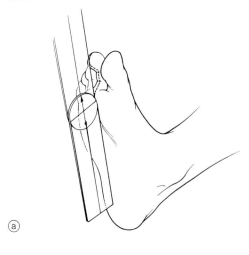

(a)

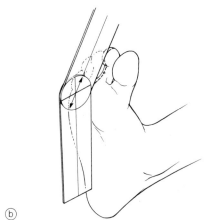

(b)

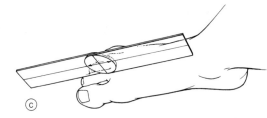

(c)

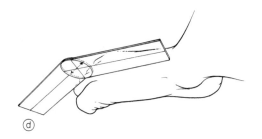

(d)

Foot—Involvement of Two or More Toes

Measure separately and record the impairment of each toe involved. Then, measure separately and record the impairment of the foot as contributed by each toe.

   Add all the impairment values. Their sum equals the impairment of the foot.

Example:

Description	% Impairment of Foot
10% impairment of great toe	2
20% impairment of second toe	1
30% impairment of third toe	1
40% impairment of fourth toe	1
50% impairment of fifth toe	2
(2%+1%+1%+1%+2%=7%)	7

Table 26. Impairment Due to Amputation, Abnormal Motion and Ankylosis of the Metatarsophalangeal Joint of the Second Toe—Dorsi-Plantar flexion

Amputation		% Impairment of Second Toe
At Joint		100

Abnormal Motion
Average range of *Dorsi-Plantar Flexion* is 70°
Value to total range of joint motion is 100%

Dorsi-flexion from neutral position (0°) to:	Degrees of Joint Motion Lost	Retained	% Impairment of Second Toe
0°	40°	0°	29
10°	30°	10°	21
20°	20°	20°	14
30°	10°	30°	7
40°	0°	40°	0

Plantar-flexion from neutral position (0°) to:			
0°	30°	0°	21
10°	20°	10°	14
20°	10°	20°	7
30°	0°	30°	0

Ankylosis

Joint ankylosed at:	% Impairment of Second Toe
* 0° (neutral position)	50
10°	63
20°	75
30°	88
40° (full dorsi-flexion)	100

Joint ankylosed at:	% Impairment of Second Toe
* 0° (neutral position)	50
10°	67
20°	83
30° (full plantar-flexion)	100

*position of function

Finally, consult Table 31 to determine the impairment of the foot that is contributed by combinations of impairment of the toes, and consult Table 32 (p. 58) to determine the impairment of the lower extremity.

For example, mid-tarsal joint ankylosis results in 10% impairment of the foot and 7% impairment of the lower extremity.

3.2b Hind Foot

Dorsi- and Plantar-flexion (Ankle Joint Primarily) Abnormal Motion

• Place the patient in the neutral position (Figure 62).

• Center the goniometer over the lateral malleolus (Figure 63). Note that the goniometer base lies along the axis

of the tibia. Record the goniometer reading with the goniometer arm parallel to the sole of the foot.

• Dorsi-flexion: With the patient dorsi-flexing the foot as far as possible, follow the range of motion with the goniometer arm. Record the angle that subtends the arc of motion.

• Plantar-flexion: Starting from the neutral position with the patient plantar-flexing the foot as far as possible, follow the range of motion with the goniometer arm. Record the angle that subtends the arc of motion.

• Retest the range of dorsi- and plantar-flexion of the foot with the knee flexed to 45°. If the arcs of motion are different from those obtained previously, then the averages of the results represent the angles to be used in determining the impairment of the lower extremity.

Table 27. Impairment Due to Amputation, Abnormal Motion and Ankylosis of the Metatarsophalangeal Joint of the Third Toe—Dorsi-Plantar flexion

Amputation			% Impairment of Third Toe
At Joint			100

Abnormal Motion
Average range of *Dorsi-Plantar Flexion* is 50°
Value to total range of joint motion is 100%

Dorsi-flexion from neutral position (0°) to:	Degrees of Joint Motion Lost	Retained	% Impairment of Third Toe
0°	30°	0°	30
10°	20°	10°	20
20°	10°	20°	10
30°	0°	30°	0

Plantar-flexion from neutral position (0°) to:			
0°	20°	0°	20
10°	10°	10°	10
20°	0°	20°	0

Ankylosis

Joint ankylosed at:	% Impairment of Third Toe
* 0° (neutral position)	50
10°	67
20°	83
30° (full dorsi-flexion)	100

Joint ankylosed at:	
* 0° (neutral position)	50
10°	75
20° (full plantar-flexion)	100

*position of function

Table 28. Impairment Due to Amputation, Abnormal Motion and Ankylosis of the Metatarsophalangeal Joint of the Fourth Toe—Dorsi-Plantar flexion

Amputation			% Impairment of Fourth Toe
At Joint			100

Abnormal Motion
Average range of *Dorsi-Plantar Flexion* is 30°
Value to total range of joint motion is 100%

Dorsi-flexion from neutral position (0°) to:	Degrees of Joint Motion Lost	Retained	% Impairment of Fourth Toe
0°	20°	0°	33
10°	10°	10°	17
20°	0°	20°	0

Plantar-flexion from neutral position (0°) to:			
0°	10°	0°	17
10°	0°	10°	0

Ankylosis

Joint ankylosed at:	
* 0° (neutral position)	50
10°	75
20° (full dorsi-flexion)	100

Joint ankylosed at:	
* 0° (neutral position)	50
10° (full plantar-flexion)	100

*position of function

Table 29. Impairment Due to Amputation, Abnormal Motion and Ankylosis of the Metatarsophalangeal Joint of the Fifth Toe—Dorsi-Plantar flexion

Amputation	% Impairment of Fifth Toe
At Joint	100

Abnormal Motion
Average range of *Dorsi-Plantar Flexion* is 20°
Value to total range of joint motion is 100%

Dorsi-flexion from neutral position (0°) to:	Degrees of Joint Motion Lost	Retained	% Impairment of Fifth Toe
0°	10°	0°	50
10°	0°	10°	0

Plantar-flexion from neutral position (0°) to:			
0°	10°	0°	50
10°	0°	10°	0

Ankylosis

Joint ankylosed at:	% Impairment of Fifth Toe
* 0° (neutral position)	50
10° (full dorsi-flexion)	100

Joint ankylosed at:	
* 0° (neutral position)	50
10° (full plantar-flexion)	100

*position of function

Consult the Abnormal Motion Section of Table 33 to determine the impairment of the lower extremity.

Example: 10° active dorsi-flexion from neutral position (0°) is equivalent to 4% impairment of the lower extremity.

• *Add* impairment values contributed by dorsi-flexion and plantar-flexion. Their sum is the impairment of the lower extremity contributed by abnormalities of dorsi-flexion and plantar-flexion of the hind foot.

Note: There may also be impairment of inversion or eversion, the value for which should be *added* (see below).

Ankylosis
• Place the goniometer base as if measuring the neutral position (Figure 62). Measure the deviation from the neutral position with the goniometer arm and record the reading.

• Consult the Ankylosis Section of Table 33 to determine the impairment of the lower extremity.

Example: A hind foot with ankylosis at 10° dorsi-flexion is equivalent to 50% impairment of the lower extremity.

Figure 62. Neutral Position of Hind Foot for Dorsi-and Plantar-flexion

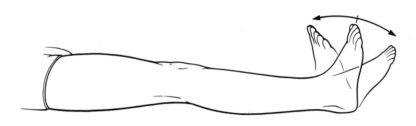

Figure 63. Dorsi- and Plantar-flexion of Hind Foot

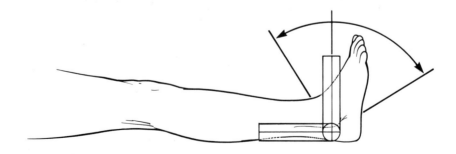

Table 30. Relationship of Impairments of Second Through Fifth Toes to Impairment of the Foot

% Impairment of Each Toe	% Impairment of Foot
0- 16	0
17- 49	1
50- 83	2
84-100	3

Note: Impairment of the foot contributed by the toe may be rounded to the nearest 5 percent only when it is the *sole* impairment involved. Consult Table 32 for converting foot impairment to lower extremity impairment.

Table 31. Impairment of the Foot Due to Amputation and Ankylosis of Multiple Digits

Digit(s) Involved	% Impairment of Foot			
	Amputated	Ankylosed in		
		Full Extension	Position of Function	Full Flexion
Great	18	14	13	18
Great, Second	21	17	15	21
Great, Second, Third	24	20	17	24
Great, Second, Fourth	24	20	17	24
Great, Second, Fifth	24	20	17	24
Great, Second, Third, Fourth	27	23	19	27
Great, Second, Third, Fifth	27	23	19	27
Great, Second, Fourth, Fifth	27	23	19	27
Great, Second, Third, Fourth, Fifth	30	26	21	30
Great, Third	21	17	15	21
Great, Third, Fourth	24	20	17	24
Great, Third, Fifth	24	20	17	24
Great, Third, Fourth, Fifth	27	23	19	27
Great, Fourth	21	17	15	21
Great, Fourth, Fifth	24	20	17	24
Great, Fifth	21	17	15	21
Second	3	3	2	3
Second, Third	6	6	4	6
Second, Third, Fourth	9	9	4	9
Second, Third, Fifth	9	9	6	9
Second, Third, Fourth, Fifth	12	12	8	12
Second, Fourth	6	6	4	6
Second, Fourth, Fifth	9	9	6	9
Second, Fifth	6	6	4	6
Third	3	3	2	3
Third, Fourth	6	6	4	6
Third, Fourth, Fifth	9	9	6	9
Third, Fifth	6	6	4	6
Fourth	3	3	2	3
Fourth, Fifth	6	6	4	6
Fifth	3	3	2	3

Figure 64. Neutral Position of Hind Foot for Inversion and Eversion

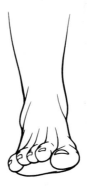

Figure 65. Inversion of Hind Foot

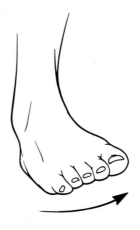

Figure 66. Eversion of Hind Foot

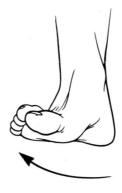

Table 32. Relationship of Impairment of the Foot to Impairment of the Lower Extremity

% Impairment of		% Impairment of		% Impairment of	
Foot	Lower Extremity	Foot	Lower Extremity	Foot	Lower Extremity
0 = 0		34 = 24		68 = 48	
1 = 1		35 = 25		69 = 48	
2 = 1		36 = 25		70 = 49	
3 = 2		37 = 26		71 = 50	
4 = 3		38 = 27		72 = 50	
5 = 4		39 = 27		73 = 51	
6 = 4		40 = 28		74 = 52	
7 = 5		41 = 29		75 = 53	
8 = 6		42 = 29		76 = 53	
9 = 6		43 = 30		77 = 54	
10 = 7		44 = 31		78 = 55	
11 = 8		45 = 32		79 = 55	
12 = 8		46 = 32		80 = 56	
13 = 9		47 = 33		81 = 57	
14 = 10		48 = 34		82 = 57	
15 = 11		49 = 34		83 = 58	
16 = 11		50 = 35		84 = 59	
17 = 12		51 = 36		85 = 60	
18 = 13		52 = 36		86 = 60	
19 = 13		53 = 37		87 = 61	
20 = 14		54 = 38		88 = 62	
21 = 15		55 = 39		89 = 62	
22 = 15		56 = 39		90 = 63	
23 = 16		57 = 40		91 = 64	
24 = 17		58 = 41		92 = 64	
25 = 18		59 = 41		93 = 65	
26 = 18		60 = 42		94 = 66	
27 = 19		61 = 43		95 = 67	
28 = 20		62 = 43		96 = 67	
29 = 20		63 = 44		97 = 68	
30 = 21		64 = 45		98 = 69	
31 = 22		65 = 46		99 = 69	
32 = 22		66 = 46		100 = 70	
33 = 23		67 = 47			

Note: Impairment of the lower extremity as contributed by the foot may be rounded to the nearest 5% only when it is the *sole* impairment involved.

Consult Table 42 for converting lower extremity impairment to whole person impairment.

Figure 67. Neutral Position of Knee

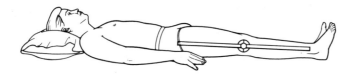

Figure 68. Flexion of Knee

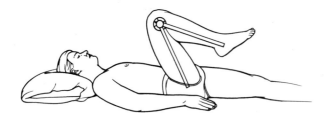

Note: There may also be impairment of dorsi- and plantar-flexion, which should be *added* to impairment of inversion and eversion.

Inversion and Eversion (Subtalar Joint Primarily)
Abnormal Motion
- Place the patient in the neutral position (Figure 64). The plane of the foot is at a right angle to the lower leg. The goniometer is not used.
- Inversion: Starting from the neutral position with the patient inverting the foot (Figure 65), record the range of motion by estimating the arc described by the plantar surface of the foot as it turns.
- Eversion: With the patient everting the foot (Figure 66), record the range of motion by estimating the arc described by the plantar surface of the foot as it turns.
- Consult the Abnormal Motion Section of Table 34 to determine the impairment of the lower extremity.

Example: A foot with 20° inversion from neutral position (0°) is equivalent to 2% impairment of the lower extremity.

- *Add* impairment values contributed by inversion and eversion. Their sum represents the impairment of the lower extremity contributed by abnormal inversion and eversion of the hind foot.

Ankylosis
- Estimate the angle of ankylosis by observing the angle of the plane formed by the plantar surface of the foot.
- Consult the Ankylosis Section of Table 34 to determine the impairment of the lower extremity.

Example: A hind foot with ankylosis of 20° inversion is equivalent to 57% impairment of the lower extremity.

Hind Foot—Two Ranges of Motion
Abnormal Motion
Measure separately and record the impairment of the lower extremity that is contributed by each range of motion. *Add* the impairment values of the lower extremity contributed by all ranges of motion. Their sum is the impairment of the lower extremity contributed by the ankle and subtalar joints.

Example: Description	% **Impairment of Lower Extremity**
10° active dorsi-flexion	4
10° active plantar-flexion	11
10° active inversion	4
10° active eversion	2
(4% +11% +4% +2% = 21%)	21

Ankylosis

Measure separately and record the impairment of the lower extremity that is contributed by ankylosis in each position. The larger impairment value represents the impairment of the lower extremity that is contributed by ankylosis of the ankle and subtalar joints.

Example: Description	% **Impairment of** Lower Extremity
Ankylosis at 10° dorsi-flexion	50
Ankylosis at 10° inversion	43

The larger value is 50%; therefore, the lower extremity has 50% impairment due to the ankylosis.

3.2c Knee Joint

Flexion and Extension
Abnormal Motion

• Place the patient in the neutral position (Figure 67).

• Center the goniometer next to the knee joint (Figure 67). Record the goniometer reading with one arm of the goniometer along the axis of the femur and the other arm along the axis of the lower leg. Maintain this relationship of the arms as motion is carried out. Record any deviation from the neutral position, which would indicate limitation of knee joint extension.

• With the patient flexing the knee as far as possible, follow the range of motion with the goniometer arm. Record the angle that subtends the arc of motion (Figure 68).

• Retest the flexion of the knee with the patient in a sitting position. If the arc of motion is different from that obtained previously, then the average of the results represents the value to be used in determining impairment of the lower extremity.

• Consult the Abnormal Motion Section of Table 35. *Add* the percentages for flexion loss and limitation of extension to determine impairment of the lower extremity.

Note: If there is inability to extend the knee beyond 50° flexion, for weight-bearing purposes the degree of impairment is equivalent to that for amputation and no additional impairment value should be given for loss of range of motion.

Example: 70° flexion from neutral position (0°) is equivalent to 28% impairment of the lower extremity.

Example: Flexion to 100° with extension limited to 30° is equivalent to 35% impairment of the lower extremity (18% plus 17%, Table 35).

Ankylosis

• Place the goniometer base as if measuring the neutral position (Figure 67). Measure the deviation from neutral position with the goniometer arm extending along the lower leg and record the reading.

• Consult the Ankylosis Section of Table 35 to determine the impairment of the lower extremity.

Example: A knee joint with ankylosis at 20° flexion is equivalent to 60% impairment of the lower extremity.

Table 36 lists impairment ratings for other disorders of the knee.

Table 33. Impairment Due to Amputation, Abnormal Motion and Ankylosis of the Hind Foot (Ankle Joint Primarily)—Dorsi-Plantar Flexion

Amputation	% Impairment of Lower Extremity
At Joint	70

Abnormal Motion
Average range of *Dorsi-Plantar Flexion* is 60°
Value to total range of joint motion is 70%

Dorsi-flexion from neutral position (0°) to:	Degrees of Joint Motion Lost	Retained	% Impairment of Lower Extremity
0°	20°	0°	7
10°	10°	10°	4
20°	0°	20°	0

Plantar-flexion from neutral position (0°) to:			
0°	40°	0°	14
10°	30°	10°	11
20°	20°	20°	7
30°	10°	30°	4
40°	0°	40°	0

Ankle instability due to lateral collateral ligament loss	25
Ankle instability due to medial collateral ligament loss	15

Ankylosis

Joint ankylosed at:	% Impairment of Lower Extremity
* 0° (neutral position)	30
10°	50
20° (full dorsi-flexion)	70

Joint ankylosed at:	
* 0° (neutral position)	30
10°	40
20°	50
30°	60
40° (full plantar-flexion)	70

Arthroplasty of joint: 25%, combined with impairment value for either ankylosis or loss of range of motion, if present.

*position of function

Table 34. Impairment Due to Amputation, Abnormal Motion and Ankylosis of the Hind Foot (Subtalar Joint Primarily)—Inversion-Eversion

Amputation	% Impairment of Lower Extremity
At Joint	70

Abnormal Motion
Average range of *Inversion-Eversion* is 50°
Value to total range of joint motion is 30%

Inversion from neutral position (0°) to:	Degrees of Joint Motion Lost	Retained	% Impairment of Lower Extremity
0°	30°	0°	5
10°	20°	10°	4
20°	10°	20°	2
30°	0°	30°	0

Eversion from neutral position (0°) to:			
0°	20°	0°	4
10°	10°	10°	2
20°	0°	20°	0

Ankylosis

Joint ankylosed at:	% Impairment of Lower Extremity
* 0° (neutral position)	10
10°	43
20°	57
30° (full inversion)	70

Joint ankylosed at:	
* 0° (neutral position)	10
10°	50
20° (full eversion)	60

*position of function

Figure 69. Neutral Position for Right Hip

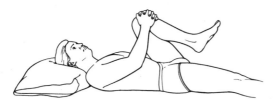

Figure 70. Placement of Goniometer at Right Hip

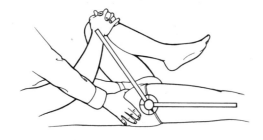

3.2d Hip Joint

Forward Flexion
Abnormal Motion
• Place the patient in the neutral position (Figure 69) with the opposite hip flexed and held to lock the pelvis. The leg to be tested is extended in a relaxed position.

• Place the goniometer next to the hip joint (Figure 70). Record the goniometer reading. With the patient flexing the hip to be tested as far as possible (Figure 71), follow the range of motion with the goniometer arm until the superior iliac spine begins to move. Record the angle that subtends the arc of motion.

• Consult the Abnormal Motion Section of Table 37 to determine the impairment of the lower extremity.

Example: 20° forward flexion from neutral position (0°) is equivalent to 14% impairment of the lower extremity.

Ankylosis
• Place the goniometer base as if measuring the neutral position (Figure 69). Measure the deviation from neutral position with the goniometer arm and record the reading.

• Consult the Ankylosis Section of Table 37 to determine the impairment of the lower extremity.

Example: A hip joint with ankylosis at 25° forward flexion is equivalent to 50% impairment of the lower extremity.

Hip Joint—Backward Extension
Abnormal Motion
• Place the patient in the neutral position (Figure 72).

• Center the goniometer next to the hip (Figure 72) and record the reading.

• With the patient raising the leg as far as possible (Figure 73), follow the range of motion with the goniometer arm. Record the angle that subtends the arc of motion.

• Consult the Abnormal Motion Section of Table 38 to determine the impairment of the lower extremity.

Example: 20° active backward extension from neutral position (0°) is equivalent to 2% impairment of the lower extremity.

• *Add* the impairment values contributed by forward flexion and backward extension. Their sum represents the impairment of the lower extremity contributed by abnormal forward flexion and backward extension of the hip.

Ankylosis

• Place the goniometer base as if measuring the neutral position (Figure 72). Measure the deviation from neutral position with the goniometer arm and record the reading.

Table 35. Impairment Due to Amputation, Abnormal Motion and Ankylosis of the Knee Joint

Amputation	% Impairment of Lower Extremity
At Joint	90

Abnormal Motion*
Average range of *Flexion-Extension* is 150°
Value to total range of joint motion is 100%

Retained active flexion of:	% Impairment of Lower Extremity
0°	53
10°	49
20°	46
30°	42
40°	39
50°	35
60°	32
70°	28
80°	25
90°	21
100°	18
110°	14
120°	11
130°	7
140°	4
150°	0

Extension back to (extension lag):	% Impairment of Lower Extremity
0° (neutral position)	0
10°	1
20°	7
30°	17
40°	27
50° to 150° (full flexion)	90

Ankylosis

Joint ankylosed at:	% Impairment of Lower Extremity
0° (neutral position)	53
**10°	50
20°	60
30°	70
40°	80
50° to 150° (full flexion)	90

*If a permanent groin-to-ankle orthosis is required for extension stability, there is a 50% impairment of the lower extremity, although there may be full range of motion of the knee joint. This rating does not apply to any other types of local knee bracing.

**position of function

Table 36. Impairment Ratings of the Lower Extremity For Other Disorders of the Knee

Disorder	Impairment of Lower Extremity*
1. Patellectomy (with loss of power)	5-15%, combined with impairment for loss of motion**
2. Torn meniscus and/or meniscectomy	0-10%, for one meniscus; 0-25% for both menisci; combined with impairment for loss of motion
3. Knee replacement arthroplasty	20%, if in optimum position
4. Patella replacement only	Same as for patellectomy
5. Arthritis due to any etiology, including trauma; chondromalacia	0-20%, according to deformity
6. Anterior cruciate ligament loss	0-15%, combined with impairment, for loss of motion
7. Posterior cruciate ligament loss	0-15%, combined with impairment for loss of motion
8. Collateral ligament loss	10% for moderate instability 20% for marked instability
9. Post-traumatic varus deformity (if over 15°)	10%, combined with impairment for loss of motion
10. Post-traumatic valgus deformity (if over 20°)	10%, combined with impairment for loss of motion

*See Table 35 for impairment ratings for loss of motion.
**The combining of any impairment value in this table with impairment for loss of motion is to be done using the Combined Values Chart

Figure 71. Forward Flexion of Right Hip

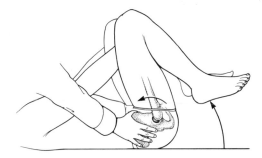

Table 37. Impairment Due to Amputation, Abnormal Motion and Ankylosis of the Hip Joint—Forward Flexion

Amputation	% Impairment of Lower Extremity
At Joint	100

Abnormal Motion
Average range of *Forward Flexion-Backward Extension* is 130°
Value to total range of joint motion is 33%

Forward flexion from neutral position (0°) to:	Degrees of Joint Motion Lost	Retained	% Impairment of Lower Extremity
0°	100°	0°	18
10°	90°	10°	16
20°	80°	20°	14
30°	70°	30°	12
40°	60°	40°	11
50°	50°	50°	9
60°	40°	60°	7
70°	30°	70°	5
80°	20°	80°	4
90°	10°	80°	2
100°	0°	100°	0

Ankylosis

Joint ankylosed at:	% Impairment of Lower Extremity
0° (neutral position)	70
10°	62
20°	54
* 25°	50
30°	53
40°	60
50°	67
60°	73
70°	80
80°	87
90°	93
100° (full forward flexion)	100

*position of function

Figure 72. Neutral Position for Extension of Hip

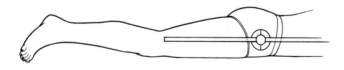

Figure 73. Extension of Hip

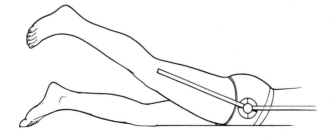

• Consult the Ankylosis Section of Table 38 to determine the impairment of the lower extremity.

Example: A hip joint with ankylosis at 20° backward extension is equivalent to 90% impairment of the lower extremity.

Hip Joint—Abduction and Adduction
Abnormal Motion
• Place the patient on a table in the neutral position (Figure 74) with the opposite hip flexed and held to lock the pelvis. The leg to be tested is extended in a relaxed position.

• Center the goniometer over the hip joint (Figure 74). Record the goniometer reading. Consider 90° as the neutral point.

• Abduction: With the patient abducting the thigh as far as possible (Figure 75), follow the range of motion with the goniometer arm. Record the angle that subtends the arc of motion.

• Adduction: Starting from the neutral position with the patient swinging the leg across the body as far as possible (Figure 76), follow the range of motion with the goniometer arm. Record the angle that subtends the arc of motion.

• Consult the Abnormal Motion Section of Table 39 to determine the impairment of the lower extremity.

Example: 20° abduction from neutral position is equivalent to 8% impairment of the lower extremity.

• *Add* the lower extremity impairment values contributed by abduction and adduction. Their sum represents impairment of the lower extremity that is contributed by abnormal abduction and adduction of the hip.

Ankylosis
• Place the goniometer base as if measuring the neutral position (Figure 74). Measure the deviation from the neutral position with the goniometer arm and record the reading.

• Consult the Ankylosis Section of Table 39 to determine the impairment of the lower extremity.

Example: A hip joint with ankylosis at 20° abduction is equivalent to 85% impairment of the lower extremity.

Hip Joint—Rotation
Abnormal Motion
• Place the patient in the neutral position (Figure 77).

Table 38. Impairment Due to Amputation, Abnormal Motion and Ankylosis of the Hip Joint—Backward Flexion

Amputation	% Impairment of Lower Extremity
At Joint	100

Abnormal Motion
Average range of *Forward Flexion-Backward Extension* is 130°
Value to total range of joint motion is 33%

Backward extension from neutral (0°) to:	Degrees of Joint Motion Lost	Retained	% Impairment of Lower Extremity
0°	30°	0°	5
10°	20°	10°	4
20°	10°	20°	2
30°	0°	30°	0

Ankylosis

Joint ankylosed at:	% Impairment of Lower Extremity
0° (neutral position)	70
10°	80
20°	90
30° (full backward ext.)	100

Table 39. Impairment Due to Amputation, Abnormal Motion and Ankylosis of the Hip Joint—Abduction-Adduction

Amputation	% Impairment of Lower Extremity
At Joint	100

Abnormal Motion
Average range of *Abduction-Adduction* is 60°
Value to total range of joint motion is 33%

Abduction from neutral position (0°) to:	Degrees of Joint Motion Lost	Retained	% Impairment of Lower Extremity
0°	40°	0°	16
10°	30°	10°	12
20°	20°	20°	8
30°	10°	30°	4
40°	0°	40°	0

Adduction from neutral position (0°) to:			
0°	20°	0°	8
10°	10°	10°	4
20°	0°	20°	0

Ankylosis

Joint ankylosed at:	% Impairment of Lower Extremity
* 0° (neutral position)	70
10°	78
20°	85
30°	93
40° (full abduction)	100

Joint ankylosed at:	
* 0° (neutral position)	70
10°	85
20° (full adduction)	100

*position of function

- Center the goniometer over the middle of the heel (Figure 77). Record the goniometer reading with the goniometer arm lying between the second and third toes. Consider 90° as the neutral point.

- External rotation: With the patient externally rotating the hip as far as possible (Figure 78), follow the range of motion with the goniometer arm. Record the angle that subtends the arc of motion.

- Internal rotation: Starting from the neutral position with the patient internally rotating the hip as far as possible (Figure 78), follow the range of motion with the goniometer arm. Record the angle that subtends the arc of motion.

- Consult the Abnormal Motion Section of Table 40 to determine the impairment of the lower extremity.

Table 40. Impairment Due to Amputation, Abnormal Motion and Ankylosis of the Hip Joint—Rotation

Amputation	% Impairment of Lower Extremity
At Joint	100

Abnormal Motion
Average range of *Rotation* is 90°
Value to total range of joint motion is 33%

Internal Rotation from neutral position (0°) to:	Degrees of Joint Motion Lost	Retained	% Impairment of Lower Extremity
0°	40°	0°	10
10°	30°	10°	8
20°	20°	20°	5
30°	10°	30°	3
40°	0°	40°	0

External Rotation from neutral position (0°) to:			
0°	50°	0°	13
10°	40°	10°	10
20°	30°	20°	8
30°	20°	30°	5
40°	10°	40°	3
50°	0°	50°	0

Ankylosis

Joint ankylosed at:	% Impairment of Lower Extremity
* 0° (neutral position)	70
10°	78
20°	85
30°	93
40° (full int. rotation)	100

Joint ankylosed at:	
* 0° (neutral position)	70
10°	76
20°	82
30°	88
40°	94
50° (full ext. rotation)	100

*position of function

Figures 74, 75, 76. Neutral Position, Abduction and Adduction of Right Hip

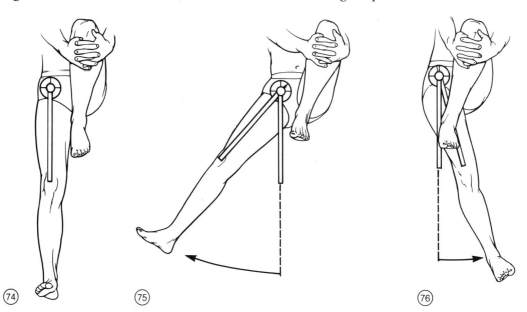

Ⓐ74   Ⓐ75   Ⓐ76

Example: 20° active external rotation from neutral position (0°) is equivalent to 8% impairment of the lower extremity.

• *Add* the impairment values contributed by internal and external rotation. Their sum is the impairment of the lower extremity contributed by rotation of the hip.

Ankylosis

• Place the goniometer base as if measuring the neutral position (Figure 77). Measure the deviation from neutral position with the goniometer arm and record the reading.

• Consult the Ankylosis Section of Table 40 to determine the impairment of the lower extremity.

Example: A hip joint with ankylosis at 20° internal rotation is equivalent to 85% impairment of the lower extremity.

Figure 77. Placement of Foot for Neutral Position of Hip Rotation

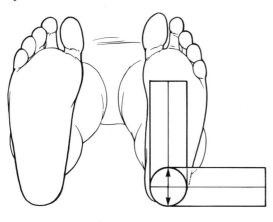

Hip Joint—Two or More Ranges of Motion Abnormal Motion

Measure separately and record the impairment of the lower extremity contributed by each range of motion. *Add* the impairment values contributed by ranges of motion. Their sum is the impairment of the lower extremity contributed by the hip joint.

Example: Description	% **Impairment of** **Lower Extremity**
10° active forward flexion	16
10° active backward extension	4
10° active abduction	12
10° active adduction	4
(16% +4% + 12% +4% = 36%)	36

Ankylosis

Measure separately and record the impairment of the lower extremity contributed by ankylosis in each position. The largest impairment due to ankylosis is the impairment of the lower extremity contributed by the hip joint.

Example: Description	% **Impairment of** **Lower Extremity**
Ankylosis at 25° forward flexion	50
Ankylosis at 20° internal rotation	85

The largest impairment value is 85%; therefore, the impairment rating is 85%.

Table 41 lists impairment values due to other disorders of the hip joint.

3.2e Lower Extremity—Involvement of Multiple Units

Measure separately and record the impairment of the lower extremity contributed by each unit (foot, ankle and subtalar joints, knee joint, and hip joint). Then, combine the impairment values using the Combined Values Chart.

Example:		
Description	% **Impairment of** **Lower Extremity**	
Foot impaired at 57%	40	(Table 32)
Hind foot impaired	30	
Knee impaired	20	
(40% combined with 30% = 58%; 58% combined with 20% = 66%)	66	

Finally, consult Table 42 to determine the impairment of the whole person that is contributed by the lower extremity.

Impairment values for amputations of various parts of the lower extremity are found in Table 43.

3.2f Impairment of the Lower Extremity Due to Peripheral Nervous System Disorders

Table 44 shows the site of origin and function of the peripheral nerves to the lower extremity. Figure 79 shows the sensory nerves and their roots of origin. The principles and methods of evaluation discussed in Section 3.1i (page 36) for the upper extremity apply to the lower extremity as well.

Figure 78. Movement of Foot as Measure of Internal and External Rotation of Hip

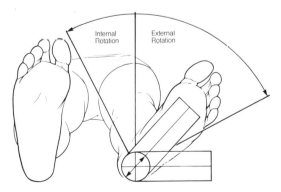

Table 41. Impairment of the Lower Extremity Due to Other Disorders of the Hip Joint

Disorder	% Impairment of Lower Extremity*
1. Replacement Arthroplasty (in optimum position)	20
2. Non-union of hip fracture	30
3. Avascular necrosis of the hip	10-30
4. Loose hip prosthesis	40

*These ratings should be combined with the ratings for loss of motion to determine impairments of the lower extremity (Tables 37-40), using the Combined Values Chart.

Table 42. Relationship of Impairment of the Lower Extremity to Impairment of the Whole Person

% Impairment of		% Impairment of		% Impairment of	
Lower Extremity	Whole Person	Lower Extremity	Whole Person	Lower Extremity	Whole Person
0 = 0		34 = 14		68 = 27	
1 = 0		35 = 14		69 = 28	
2 = 1		36 = 14		70 = 28	
3 = 1		37 = 15		71 = 28	
4 = 2		38 = 15		72 = 29	
5 = 2		39 = 16		73 = 29	
6 = 2		40 = 16		74 = 30	
7 = 3		41 = 16		75 = 30	
8 = 3		42 = 17		76 = 30	
9 = 4		43 = 17		77 = 31	
10 = 4		44 = 18		78 = 31	
11 = 4		45 = 18		79 = 32	
12 = 5		46 = 18		80 = 32	
13 = 5		47 = 19		81 = 32	
14 = 6		48 = 19		82 = 33	
15 = 6		49 = 20		83 = 33	
16 = 6		50 = 20		84 = 34	
17 = 7		51 = 20		85 = 34	
18 = 7		52 = 21		86 = 34	
19 = 8		53 = 21		87 = 35	
20 = 8		54 = 22		88 = 35	
21 = 8		55 = 22		89 = 36	
22 = 9		56 = 22		90 = 36	
23 = 9		57 = 23		91 = 36	
24 = 10		58 = 23		92 = 37	
25 = 10		59 = 24		93 = 37	
26 = 10		60 = 24		94 = 38	
27 = 11		61 = 24		95 = 38	
28 = 11		62 = 25		96 = 38	
29 – 12		63 = 25		97 = 39	
30 = 12		64 = 26		98 = 39	
31 = 12		65 = 26		99 = 40	
32 = 13		66 = 26		100 = 40	
33 = 13		67 = 27			

Note: In case of shortening due to overriding or malalignment or fracture deformities, but not to include flexion or extension deformities, combine the following values with other functional sequelae, using the Combined Values Chart.

> 0-½ inch =   5% of lower extremity
> ½-1 inch = 10% of lower extremity
> 1-1½ inch = 15% of lower extremity
> 1½-2 inch = 20% of lower extremity

Note: Impairment of whole person contributed by lower extremity may be rounded to the nearest 5 percent only when it is the *sole* impairment involved.

Figure 79. Sensory Nerves of the Lower Extremity and their Roots of Origin

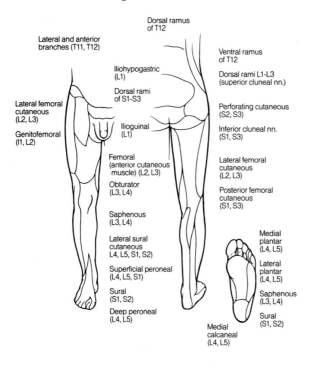

Note: Restrictions of motion and ankyloses may result from peripheral spinal nerve impairments. Consideration was given to such impairments when the percentage values set forth in this section were derived. Therefore, if an impairment results strictly from a peripheral nerve lesion, the evaluator *should not* apply the impairment values from both Sections 3.2a through 3.2d and this section, because this would result in a duplication and a multiplying of the impairment rating. However, when restricted motion or ankylosis exists but cannot be attributed to sensory involvement or muscle weakness, then values from Sections 3.2a through 3.2d may be combined with values of this section using the Combined Values Chart.

It is necessary for the physician to establish as accurately as possible the anatomic distribution of sensory and/or motor loss and verify that the distribution relates to a specific peripheral nerve or nerves before determining the percentage of permanent impairment. The diagnosis is based firmly on the patient's signs and symptoms. With a carefully obtained history, a thorough medical and neurological examination, and appropriate laboratory aids, the physician should characterize the pain, discomfort, and loss of sensation occurring in the areas innervated by the affected nerve, and also the degree of muscle strength that has been lost.

Pain: The pain associated with peripheral spinal nerve impairment, and particularly with that of the sciatic and tibial nerves, sometimes has a constant burning quality. This pain is described as a major or minor causalgia in accordance with its severity, and it is evaluated on the same percentage basis as are other types of pain. Major causalgia that persists despite appropriate treatment can result in loss of function of the affected extremity and impairment that is as great as 100%.

In evaluating pain that is associated with peripheral spinal nerve disorders, the physician should consider: (1) how the pain interferes with the individual's performance of the activities of daily living; (2) to what extent the pain follows the defined anatomical pathways of the root (dermatome), plexus, or peripheral nerve; and (3) to what extent the description of the pain indicates that it is caused by the peripheral spinal nerve impairment. That is, the pain should correspond to other kinds of disturbances of the involved nerve or nerve root.

Complaints of pain that cannot be substantiated as above are not considered within the scope of this

Table 43. Impairment of the Digits, Foot, Lower Extremity and Whole Person Due to Amputations

	% Impairment of			
	Digit	Foot	Lower Extremity	Whole Person
Hemipelvectomy				50
Disarticulation at hip joint			100	40
Amputation above knee joint with short thigh stump (3" or less below tuberosity of ischium)			100	40
Amputation above knee joint with functional stump			90	36
Disarticulation at knee joint			90	36
Gritti-Stokes amputation			90	36
Amputation below knee joint with short stump (3" or less below intercondylar notch)			90	36
Amputation below knee with functional stump			70	28
Amputation at ankle (Syme)		100	70	28
Partial amputation of foot (Chopart's)		75	53	21
Mid-metatarsal amputation		50	35	14
Amputation of all toes at metatarsophalangeal joints		30	21	8
Amputation of Great Toe With resection of metatarsal bone		30	21	8
At metatarsophalangeal joint	100	18	13	5
At interphalangeal joint	75	14	10	4
Amputation of Lesser Toe (2nd-5th) With resection of metatarsal bone		5	4	2.
At metatarsophalangeal joint	100	3	2	1
At proximal interphalangeal joint	80	2	1	0
At distal interphalangeal joint	45	1	1	0

Table 44. Origins and Functions of the Peripheral Nerves to the Lower Extremity

Plexus and Nerve Root Origins	Nerves of Plexus	Primary Branches	Secondary Branches	Function
	Iliohypogastric			Sensory to skin over hypogastric and lateral gluteal regions
	Ilioinguinal			Sensory to skin over upper medial aspect of thigh and genitalia
	Genitofemoral	External spermatic		Sensory to skin over scrotum and adjacent thigh Motor to Cremaster
		Lumboinguinal		Sensory to skin over upper anterior aspect of thigh
	Lateral femoral cutaneous			Sensory to skin over entire lateral aspect of thigh
	Obturator			Motor to Adductor longus, brevis and magnus. Obtutrator externis, Gracilis
	Muscular branches	Unnamed		Motor to Psoas major and minor, Quadratus femoris, Gemellus inferior and superior, Piriformis, and Obturator internus
	Femoral	Anterior femoral cutaneous		Sensory to skin over anterior and medial aspects of thigh and knee
		Saphenous		Sensory to skin over medial and anterior aspects of leg and dorsum of foot to base of first metatarsal
		Unnamed		Motor to Iliacus, Pectineus, Sartorius, Quadriceps femoris
	Superior gluteal			Motor to Gluteus minimus and medius, Tensor fascie latae
	Inferior gluteal			Motor to Gluteus maximus
Lumbosacral Thoracic 12, Lumbar 1 to 5 and Sacral 1 to 4)	Posterior femoral cutaneous			Sensory to skin over inferior aspect of buttock, entire posterior aspect of thigh, politeal space, perineum, external genitalia
	Sciatic	Unnamed		Motor to Hamstrings (Biceps femoris, Semitendinosus, Semimembranosus): Adductor magus
		Tibial	Unnamed	Motor to Gastrocnemius, Plantaris, Soleus, Popliteus, Tibialis posterior, Flexor digitorum longus, Flexor hallucis longus
			Sural	Sensory to skin over posterolateral aspect of leg and lateral aspect of foot and heel
			Medial calcaneal	Sensory to skin over heel and medial aspect of sole
			Medial plantar	Sensory to skin over medial aspect sole, great toe, 2nd, 3rd and medial aspects of 4th toe. Motor to Abductor hallucis, Flexor digitorum brevis, Flexor hallucis brevis, 1st Lumbrical
			Lateral plantar	Sensory to skin over lateral aspect of sole and 5th and lateral half of 4th toes. Motor to Quadratus plantae, Abductor digiti quinti, Flexor digiti quinti brevis, all Interossei, 2nd, 3rd, and 4th Lumbricals, Adductor hallucis
		Common peroneal	Unnamed	Sensory to skin over upper 1/3 of lateral aspect of leg below knee
			Superficial peroneal	Sensory to skin over anterolateral aspect of leg and dorsum of foot and toes except for area between great and 2nd toes. Motor to Peroneus longus and brevis
			Deep peroneal	Sensory to skin on dorsum of foot between great toe and 2nd toe. Motor to Tibialis anterior, Extensor digitorum longus and brevis. Peroneus tertius, Extensor hallucis longus, 1st and 2nd Interossei dorsalis
	Pudendal (plexus)	Unnamed		Motor to Levator ani, Coccygeus, and Sphincter ani externus
		Inferior hemorrhoidal		Sensory to skin of genitalia and anus. Motor to Sphincter ani externus
		Perineal		Sensory to skin of scrotum (Labium majus). Motor to Transversus perinei superficialis and profundus, Bulbocavernosus, Ischiocavernosus, Sphincter urethrea membranacae
		Dorsal n. of penis (clitoris)		Sensory to penis (clitoris)
Coccygeal (Sacral 4, 5 and Coccygeal 1)	Anococcygeal			Sensory to skin in the region of the coccyx

Figure 80. Lumbosacral Plexus

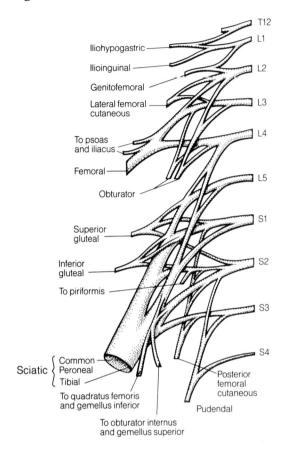

section (for a discussion of categories of pain and their characterization, see Appendix B). The examiner must determine whether the sensory or motor deficit is due to involvement of one or more nerve roots or of one or more peripheral nerves in order to use the appropriate table. Table 45 relates to nerve roots, Table 46 relates to the lumbosacral plexus, and Table 47 relates to the peripheral nerves affecting the lower extremity.

A grading scheme and procedure for determining impairment of a body part that is affected by pain, discomfort, or loss of sensation are found in Tables 10a and 10b, respectively.

Strength: Involvement of peripheral spinal nerves or nerve roots may lead to paralysis or to weakness of the muscles supplied by them, as well as to characteristic sensory changes. In the case of weakness, the patient often will attempt to substitute stronger muscles to accomplish the desired motion. Thus, the physician should have an understanding of the muscles that are involved in the performance of the various movements of the body and its parts.

Muscle testing, including tests for strength, duration, repetition of contraction, and function, aids evaluation of the functions of specific nerves. Muscle testing is based on the principle of gravity and resistance, that is, the ability to raise a segment of the body through its range of motion against gravity and to hold the segment at the end of its range of motion against

Figure 81. Motor Innervation of the Lower Extremity

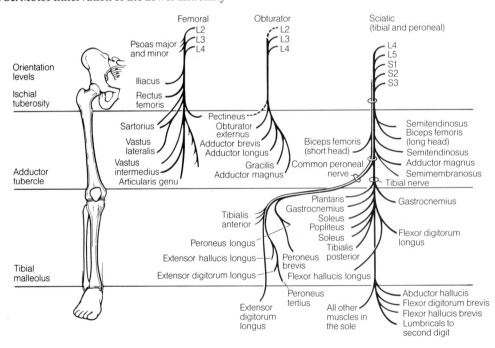

resistance. In interpreting muscle testing, comparable muscle functions on both sides of the body should be considered.

A grading scheme and procedure for determining impairment of a body part that is affected by loss of strength are found in Tables 11a and 11b, respectively.

Example: An injury of a patient's right knee resulted in surgery and prolonged therapy. Following maximum medical rehabilitation, the examining physician found that the patient could extend his leg fully against gravity and some resistance.

1. Motion involved is extension of the knee.

2. Muscle performing motion is quadriceps femoris; see Table 44.

3. Maximum loss of nerve due to loss of strength of femoral nerve is 30%; see Table 47.

4. Gradation of loss of strength is 5% to 20%; see Table 11.

5. Therefore, impairment of the lower extremity is 20% x 30%, or 6%.

After the individual values for loss of function due to sensory deficit, pain, or discomfort, and loss of function due to loss of strength have been determined, the impairment to the part of the body or to the whole person is calculated by combining the values using the Combined Values Chart.

Determination of impairment: The order in which permanent impairment of the peripheral spinal nerves will be discussed is (1) the spinal nerve roots; (2) the lumbosacral plexus; and (3) the named spinal nerves.

The Spinal Nerve Roots

The roots of the spinal nerves can be impaired by various diseases or by injuries that produce partial or complete, and unilateral or bilateral, effects. The degree of permanent impairment resulting from a spinal nerve root dysfunction would be reflected in the loss of function of the named spinal nerves having fibers from the specific nerve root. Since the named spinal nerves have fibers from more than one root, a dysfunction affecting two or more roots that supply fibers to the same nerves usually will be more impairing than a combination of the individual root impairment values (see section on lumbosacral plexus).

Table 45 provides values for the spinal nerve roots that are most frequently involved in the permanent impairment of the lower extremity. The values given are for unilateral involvement only. Where there is bilateral involvement, the values should be combined, using the Combined Values Chart at the end of the book.

Values for impairment of a specific spinal nerve root that is not mentioned should be determined by

taking into consideration the values that are suggested for a nerve having fibers from the specific nerve root. The reader should refer to the "The Named Spinal Nerves."

The Lumbosacral Plexus

Impairment due to lumbosacral plexus injury or disease can be determined by evaluating the various functions that are lost. The major nerves of the lower extremity and of the pelvic girdle are derived from the lumbosacral plexus (Figure 80). Thus, that plexus involves not only the lower extremity, but also bowel, bladder, and reproductive functions and trunk stabilization. Percentages for unilateral lumbosacral impairments are given in Table 46.

The Named Spinal Nerves

The named spinal nerves most frequently associated with impairments of the lower extremity are found in Table 47. The absence of some of the named spinal nerves

Table 45. Unilateral Spinal Nerve Root Impairment Affecting the Lower Extremity

Nerve Root Impaired	Maximum % Loss of Function Due to Sensory Deficit, Pain or Discomfort	Maximum % Loss of Function Due to Loss of Strength	% Impairment of Lower Extremity*
L-3	5	20	0-24
L-4	5	34	0-37
L-5	5	37	0-40
S-1	5	20	0-24

*See Tables 10 and 11 for grading schemes for deriving the percent impairment of the upper or lower extremity due to sensory deficit or loss of strength. See Table 42 for converting lower extremity impairments to whole person impairment. Conversion to whole person impairment should be made *only* when all impairments involving the upper extremity have been combined.

Table 46. Unilateral Lumbosacral Plexus Impairment

	Maximum % Loss of Function Due to Sensory Deficit, Pain or Discomfort	Maximum % Loss of Function Due to Loss of Strength	% Impairment Whole Person
Lumbosacral Plexus	40	50	0-70

*See Tables 10 and 11 for grading schemes for deriving the percent impairment of the upper extremity due to sensory deficit or loss of strength. See Table 42 for converting impairment of the lower extremity to impairment of the whole person. Conversion to whole person impairment should be made *only* when all impairments involving the one upper extremity have been combined.

Table 47. Specific Unilateral Spinal Nerve Impairment Affecting the Lower Extremity

Nerve	Maximum % Loss of Function Due to Sensory Deficit, Pain or Discomfort	Maximum % Loss of Function Due to Loss of Strength	% Impairment of Lower Extremity*
Femoral (anterior crural)	5	35	0-38
Femoral (anterior crural) (below iliacus nerve)	5	30	0-34
Genitofemoral (genito crural)	5	0	0- 5
Inferior gluteal	0	25	0-25
Lateral femoral cutaneous	10	0	0-10
N. to obturator interus muscle N. to piriformis muscle	0	10	0-10
N. to quadratus femoris muscle N. to superior gemellus muscle Obturator	0	10	0-10
Posterior cutaneous of thigh	5	0	0- 5
Superior gluteal	0	20	0-20
Sciatic (above hamstring innervation)	25	75	0-81
Common peroneal (lateral, or external popliteal)	5	35	0-38
Deep (above midshin)	0	25	0-25
Deep (below midshin) anterior tibial	0	5	0- 5
Superficial	5	10	0-14
Tibial nerve (medial, or internal popliteal)			
Above knee	15	35	0-45
Posterior tibial (midcalf and knee)	15	25	0-33
Below midcalf	15	15	0-28
Lateral plantar branch	5	5	0-10
Medial plantar branch	5	5	0-10
Sural (external saphenous)	5	0	0- 5

*See Tables 10 and 11 for grading schemes for determing impairment of the lower extremity due to sensory deficit or loss of strength.

See Table 42 for converting impairment of lower extremity to impairment of whole person. Note: Conversion to whole person impairment should be made *only* when all impairments involving the one lower extremity have been completed.

and their impairment values indicates that impairment associated with those particular nerves seldom occurs or is considered to be of little significance.

The percentages are expressed in terms of unilateral involvement. When there is bilateral involvement, the unilateral impairments should be determined separately and each converted to whole person impairment. Finally, the unilateral values are combined by using the Combined Values Chart.

Figure 81 is a schematic diagram of the major peripheral motor nerves of the lower extremities.

Example: A patient suffered a simple fracture of the lower third of the femur with involvement of the sciatic nerve. After maximal medical rehabilitation, he still has some inability to extend his toes or dorsi-flex his foot, unless gravity is eliminated. He can plantar-flex against gravity and against some resistance. These losses of strength are determined to be equivalent to a 60% loss of strength due to involvement of the deep common peroneal nerve, and a 20% loss of strength due to involvement of the tibial nerve. There is also complete sensory loss over the posterolateral aspect of the leg and over the lateral aspect of the foot and heel, which is determined to be equivalent to a 100% loss of sensation due to sural nerve involvement. The evaluation of impairment would be determined as follows:

Description	% Impairment of Lower Extremity	Whole Person
Loss of function due to involvement of		
(a) deep common peroneal nerve (60% gradation in loss of strength x 25%, which is the maximum value for loss of function = 15%)	15	
(b) tibial nerve (20% gradation in loss of strength x 35%, which is the maximum loss of function = 7%)	7	
Loss of function of lower extremity due to loss of strength (15% combined with 7% = 21%)	21	
Loss of function of lower extremity due to sensory deficit from sural nerve involvement (100% x 5%)	5	
Impairment of lower extremity (21% combined with 5% = 25%)	25	
Impairment of whole person (Table 42)		10

Note: If, as a result of the fracture and not of the sciatic nerve injury, a permanent ankylosis of the knee were to occur, the impairment value for ankylosis, as set forth in Section 3.2c, would be combined with the above peripheral spinal nerve impairment value.

3.2g Impairment Due to Vascular Disorders of the Lower Extremity

Table 48 provides a classification of impairments due to peripheral vascular disease. When amputation due to peripheral vascular disease is involved, the impairment due to amputation should be evaluated according to Section 3.2a, 3.2b, 3.2c, or 3.2d, and combined with the appropriate value in Table 48, using the Combined Values Chart. Note that the values in Table 48 relate to impairment of the lower extremity.

3.3 The Spine

3.3a General Principles of Measurement

Because small, inaccessible spinal joints do not readily lend themselves to external visual observation required by goniometric measurement, standard goniometric techniques for measuring spinal movement can be highly inaccurate. Furthermore, the mobility of spinal segments is confounded by motion above and below the points of measurement. For example, forward hunching of the shoulders may increase the perceived degree of cervical flexion, unless the degrees of forward flexion of the shoulders is also measured. Hence, regional spinal motion is a *compound* motion, and it is essential to measure simultaneously motion of both the upper and lower extremes of that region. For this reason, measurement techniques using *inclinometers* are necessary to obtain reliable spinal mobility measurements.

Pain, fear, acute spasm, or neuromuscular inhibition may temporarily decrease spinal movement. Acute spasm is a phenomenon induced by recent overload and is a *contraindication* to the assessment of impairment of spinal mobility at that point in time. Impairment evaluation should be performed when a person's condition has become static and well-stabilized following completion of all necessary passive, surgical, and rehabilitative treatment, thus precluding measurement when acute processes remain active. If acute spasm is observed by the examiner, it should be noted in the

report and the mobility measurements recorded for comparison purposes only. The patient must be re-examined in a few days or weeks when spasm has resolved, in order to obtain a valid mobility measurement.

Pain, fear of injury, or neuromuscular inhibition may also limit mobility by diminishing effort. Such limitations provide inaccurately low and inconsistent mobility measurements, leading to improperly inflated impairment values. Reproducibility of abnormal motion is currently the only known way to validate optimum effort. The examiner must take at least three consecutive mobility measurements, which must fall within +/−10% or 5° (whichever is greater) of each other to be considered consistent. Measurements may be repeated up to six times until consecutive measurements fall within this guideline. However, if inconsistency persists, the measurements are invalid and that portion of the examination is then disqualified.

Principles for Calculating Impairment

Evaluation of impairment of the spine involves both diagnosis-related factors (i.e., structural abnormalities), and musculoskeletal/neurological factors that require physiologic measurements. These sections provide

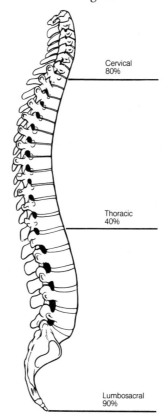

Figure 82. The Whole Spine Divided into Regions Indicating the Impairment of the Spine Represented by Total Impairment of One Region

Cervical
80%

Thoracic
40%

Lumbosacral
90%

guidance in both areas: first, a comprehensive diagnosis-based table (Table 49) is presented. Second, the technique for performing range of motion measurements of the spine using inclinometers is described. In addition, the evaluator should use the appropriate sections of the evaluation of the upper and lower extremities (Sections 3.1i, and 3.2f) for assessment of radiculopathies associated with spine impairment. (As new technology permits, valid, reproducible, and relevant measurement of other elements of human performance, such as isolated trunk strength, lifting, and task performance capabilities will be included in future editions of the *Guides*.)

The spine consists of three major regions: cervical, thoracic, and lumbar. Each region taken alone may result in a maximum percentage impairment of the whole spine (Figure 82) as follows: cervical = 80%, thoracic = 40%, and lumbar = 90%. The spine as a whole is considered equivalent to the whole person for purposes of impairment evaluation. For the sake of simplicity, all impairments in this section have already been adjusted for each regional percentage, permitting their expression as a percent impairment of the whole person.

In order to calculate total impairment of the whole person due to spine impairment:

A. Select the primarily impaired region (cervical, thoracic, lumbar);

1. If applicable, use Table 49 to obtain a diagnosis-based percentage of impairment.

2. Test the regional range of motion (Section 3.3c, 3.3d or 3.3e) and obtain the percentage of impairment due to abnormal motion or ankylosis for each specific movement, using dual- or single-inclinometer methods.

3. Perform at least three measurements of each range of motion, and calculate the permitted variability (+/-10% or 5°) based on either the *maximum* or *median* motion values. That is, check whether all three measurements fall within reproducibility guidelines by varying less than those amounts from either the maximum or median value.

4. If consistency requirements are *not* met, perform additional tests up to a maximum of six until reproducibility criteria are satisfied. If testing remains inconsistent after six measurements, consider the test invalid and re-examine at a later date.

5. Use the *maximum* range of motion and find the percentage of impairment in the appropriate tables.

Table 48. Impairment of the Lower Extremity Due to Peripheral Vascular Disease

Class 1 (0-5% Impairment)	Class 2 (10-35% Impairment)	Class 3 (40-65% Impairment)	Class 4 (70-85% Impairment)	Class 5 (90-100% Impairment)
The patient experiences neither claudication nor pain at rest;	The patient experiences intermittent claudication on walking at least 100 yards at an average pace;	The patient experiences intermittent claudication on walking as few as 25 yards and no more than 100 yards at average pace;	The patient experiences intermittent claudication on walking less than 25 yards, or the patient experiences intermittent pain at rest;	The patient experiences severe and constant pain at rest;
and	**or**	**or**	**or**	**or**
The patient experiences only transient edema;	There is persistent edema of a moderate degree, incompletely controlled by elastic supports;	There is marked edema that is only partially controlled by elastic supports;	The patient has marked edema that cannot be controlled by elastic supports;	There is vascular damage as evidenced by signs such as amputations at or above the ankles of two extremities, or amputation of all digits of two or more extremities, with evidence of persistent vascular disease or of persistent, widespread, or deep ulceration involving two or more extremities.
and	**or**	**or**	**or**	
On physical examination, not more than the following findings are present: loss of pulses; minimal loss of subcutaneous tissue; calcification of arteries as detected by radiographic examination; asymptomatic dilation of arteries or of veins, not requiring surgery and not resulting in curtailment of activity.	There is vascular damage as evidenced by a sign, such as that of a healed, painless stump of an amputated digit showing evidence of persistent vascular disease, or of a healed ulcer.	There is vascular damage as evidenced by a sign such as healed amputation of two or more digits of one extremity, with evidence of persisting vascular disease or superficial ulceration.	There is vascular damage as evidenced by signs such as an amputation at or above an ankle, or amputation of two or more digits of two extremities with evidence of persistent vascular disease, or persistent widespread or deep ulceration involving one extremity.	

Table 49. Impairments Due to Specific Disorders of the Spine

Disorder	% Impairment of Whole Person		
	Cerv	Thor	Lumb
I. Fractures			
A. Compression of one vertebral body			
0%-25%	4	2	5
26%-50%	6	3	7
>50%	10	5	12
B. Fracture of posterior elements (pedicles, laminae, articular processes, or transverse processes)	4	2	5
Note: Impairments due to compression of the vertebral body and to fractures of the posterior elements are combined using the Combined Values Chart.			
Note: When two or more vertebrae are compressed or fractured, combine all impairment values.			
C. Reduced dislocation of one vertebra	5	3	6
Note: If two or more vertebrae are dislocated and reduced, combine the impairment values using the Combined Values Chart.			
Note: An unreduced dislocation causes temporary impairment until it is reduced; then the physician should evaluate permanent impairment on the basis of the subject's condition with the reduced dislocation. If no reduction is possible, then the physician should evaluate impairment on the basis of restricted motion and concomitant neurological findings in the spinal region involved, according to the criteria in this Chapter and in Chapter 4.			
II. Intervertebral disc or other soft tissue lesions			
A. Unoperated, with no residuals	0	0	0
B. Unoperated with medically documented injury and a minimum of six months of medically documented pain, recurrent muscle spasm or rigidity associated with none-to-minimal degenerative changes on structural tests	4	2	5
C. Unoperated, with medically documented injury and a minimum of six months of medically documented pain, recurrent muscle spasm, or rigidity associated with moderate to severe degenerative changes on structural tests, including unoperated herniated nucleus pulposus, with or without radiculopathy	6	3	7
D. Surgically treated disc lesion, with no residuals	7	4	8
E. Surgically treated disc lesion, with residual symptoms	9	5	10
F. Multiple operative levels, with or without residual symptomatology	*Add 1%/level*		
G. Multiple operations ("failed back surgery") with or without residual symptoms:			
1. Second operation	*Add 2%*		
2. Third or subsequent surgery	*Add 1%/operation*		
III. Spondylolysis and spondylolisthesis, unoperated			
A. Spondylolysis or Grade I (1%-25% slippage) or Grade II (26%-50% slippage) spondylolisthesis, accompanied by medically documented injury and a minimum of six months of medically documented pain, recurrent muscle spasm, or rigidity	7	4	8
B. Grade III (51%-75% slippage) or Grade IV (76%-100% slippage) spondylolisthesis, accompanied by medically documented injury and a minimum of six months of medically documented pain, recurrent muscle spasm, or rigidity	9	5	10
IV. Spinal stenosis, segmental instability, or spondylolisthesis, operated			
A. Single level operation, with no residuals	8	4	9
B. Single level operation, with residual symptoms	10	5	12
C. Multiple levels operated, with residual symptoms	*Add 1%/level*		
D. Multiple operations ("failed back surgery") with residual symptoms:			
1. Second operation	*Add 2%*		
2. Third or subsequent surgery	*Add 1%/operation*		

Note: List impairments separately for cervical, thoracic, and lumbar regions (Figures 83a-c).

Note: All impairment ratings above should be combined with the appropriate values of residuals, such as:

1. Ankylosis (fusion) in the spinal area or extremities

2. Abnormal motion in the spinal area (i.e., objectively measured rigidity) or extremities

3. Spinal cord and spinal nerve root injuries, with neurologic impairment (see Upper Extremity and Lower Extremity sections of Chapter 3 and Peripheral Nervous System section of Chapter 4)

4. Any combination of the above using the Combined Values Chart.

6. *Add* all range of motion impairment values for the one region; if the region is ankylosed, use the largest ankylosis impairment value.

7. To obtain the impairment of the whole person due to the impairment of the region of the spine, use the Combined Values Chart to combine the diagnosis-based impairment(s) with the impairment due to limited range of motion or ankylosis.

B. *Repeat the above steps for secondarily impaired spinal regions (cervical, thoracic, lumbar), if applicable.*

C. *Combine all regional spine impairments into a single impairment of the whole person using the Combined Values Chart.*

D. *Identify impairments due to neurological deficits (Sections 3.1i and 3.2f) including radiculopathy and peripheral nerve injury, if applicable.* Be sure to equate these to *impairment of the whole person.*

E. *Combine all radicular and peripheral nerve injury impairments with the impairment of the whole person due to impairments of the spine.*

Note: Use the forms in Figures 83a-c to note ranges of motion, and the form in Figure 84 to summarize the ratings of impairment. These forms may be reproduced without permission from the AMA.

Note: For the purpose of impairment evaluation, ankylosis is defined as either: (a) complete absence of motion, or (b) planar restriction of motion preventing the subject from reaching the neutral position of motion in that plane. Using an impairment rating for ankylosis *excludes* the simultaneous use of the abnormal motion measurements from the same table. For example, an individual with a cervical flexion ankylosis angle of 40° may either: (a) have a fixed head position at 40° flexion, or (b) have sagittal range of motion from a minimum of 40° to a maximum of 60° flexion only (i.e., the person is unable to extend beyond 40° flexion). In either case, the impairment is 30% of the whole person.

Use Table 50 if radiographic methods are used to determine impairment due to ankylosis.

3.3b Impairments Due to Specific Disorders of the Spine

Consult Table 49 for the rating of impairments due to specific disorders of the spine.

3.3c Impairments Due to Range of Motion Abnormalities— Cervical Region

Flexion and Extension
Measurement of cervical flexion/extension using 2-inclinometer method

1. Locate and place a skin mark over the T1 spinous process. Place the first inclinometer aligned in the sagittal plane over the T1 spinous process while holding the second inclinometer over the occiput with the subject in the seated position (Figure 85a). The head should be in neutral position while the inclinometers are "zeroed out."

2. Ask the subject to flex maximally and record both angles. Subtract the T1 inclination from occipital inclination to obtain the *cervical flexion angle* (Figure 85b). Return the head to the neutral position so that both inclinometers read "0" again.

3. Instruct the subject to extend the neck as far as possible, again recording both inclinometer angles. Subtract the T1 inclination from the occipital inclination angle to obtain the *cervical extension angle* (Figure 85c). Again ask the subject to return the head to the neutral position.

Note: Full cervical extension may interfere with the customary placement of the inclinometers; the examiner will find the head striking the T1 inclinometer. In this situation the inclinometer at T1 should simply be moved laterally to sit in the sagittal plane over an alternative high thoracic measuring point, such as the spine of the scapula (Figure 85d). Extension should then be measured in the customary 2-inclinometer method with the thoracic inclinometer "zeroed out" with the head in the neutral position. Since it is only the difference between the upper and lower inclinometers that is of importance (rather than the absolute value of the lower inclinometer), this choice of placement will not affect the overall mobility or consistency factors in any significant way.

4. Repeat the procedure three times. Only the *cervical flexion angle* and *extension angle* need be consistently measured to within +/-10% or 5°, whichever is greater. The final measurement for impairment evaluation is the greatest angle measured.

5. Consult the Abnormal Motion Section of Table 51 to determine the impairment of the whole person.

Figure 83a. Cervical Range of Motion

Movement	Description	Range						
Cervical Flexion	Occipital ROM							
	T1 ROM							
	Cervical flexion angle							
	±10% or 5°?	Yes	No					
	Maximum cervical flexion angle							
	% Impairment							
Cervical Extension	Occipital ROM							
	T1 ROM							
	Cervical extension angle							
	±10% or 5°?	Yes	No					
	Maximum cervical extension angle							
	% Impairment							
Cervical Ankylosis in Flexion/Extension	Position		(Excludes any impairment for abnormal flexion/extension motion)					
	% Impairment							
Cervical Right Lateral Flexion	Occipital ROM							
	T1 ROM							
	Cervical right lat flexion angle							
	±10% or 5°?	Yes	No					
	Maximum cervical right lat flexion angle							
	% Impairment							
Cervical Left Lateral Flexion	Occipital ROM							
	T1 ROM							
	Cervical left lat flexion angle							
	±10% or 5°?	Yes	No					
	Maximum cervical left lat flexion angle							
	% Impairment							
Cervical Ankylosis in Lateral Flexion	Position		(Excludes any impairment for abnormal flexion/extension motion)					
	% Impairment							
Cervical Right Rotation	Cervical right rotation angle							
	±10% or 5°?	Yes	No					
	Maximum cervical right rotation angle							
	% Impairment							
Cervical Left Rotation	Cervical left rotation angle							
	±10% or 5°?	Yes	No					
	Maximum cervical left rotation angle							
	% Impairment							
Cervical Ankylosis in Rotation	Position		(Excludes any impairment for abnormal flexion/extension motion)					
	% Impairment							

Total Cervical Range of Motion Impairment
(*add* all ROM impairments if no ankylosis;
use largest ankylosis impairment value if ankylosis is present)

Figure 83b. Thoracic Range of Motion

Movement	Description	Range					
Angle of Minimum Kyphosis (Thoracic Ankylosis in Extension)	T1 reading		XXXX	XXXX	XXXX	XXXX	XXXX
	T12 reading		XXXX	XXXX	XXXX	XXXX	XXXX
	Angle of minimum kyphosis		XXXX	XXXX	XXXX	XXXX	XXXX
	% Impairment due to thoracic ankylosis	(Use larger of either ankylosis or flexion impairment)					
Thoracic Flexion	T1 ROM						
	T12 ROM						
	Thoracic flexion angle						
	± 10% or 5°?	Yes	No				
	Maximum thoracic flexion angle						
	% Impairment						
Thoracic Right Rotation	T1 ROM						
	T12 ROM						
	Thoracic right rotation angle						
	± 10% or 5°?	Yes	No				
	Maximum thoracic right rotation angle						
	% Impairment						
Thoracic Left Rotation	T1 ROM						
	T12 ROM						
	Thoracic left rotation angle						
	± 10% or 5°?	Yes	No				
	Maximum thoracic left rotation angle						
	% Impairment						
Thoracic Ankylosis in Rotation	Position						
	% Impairment	(Excludes any impairment for abnormal flexion/extension motion)					

Total Thoracic Range of Motion Impairment
(*add* all ROM impairments if no ankylosis is present;
use larger ankylosis impairment value if ankylosis is present)

Figure 83c. Lumbar Range of Motion

Movement	Description	Range						
Lumbar Flexion	T12 ROM							
	Sacral ROM							
	True lumbar flexion angle							
	±10% or 5°?	Yes	No					
	Maximum true lumbar flexion angle							
	% Impairment							
Lumbar Extension	T12 ROM							
	Sacral ROM							
	True lumbar extension angle							
	±10% or 5°?	Yes	No					
	Maximum true lumbar extension angle			(add Sacral flexion and extension ROM and compare to tightest Straight Leg Raising Angle)				
	% Impairment							
Straight Leg Raising, Right	Right SLR							
	±10% or 5°?	Yes	No	(if tightest SLR ROM exceeds sum of Sacral flexion and extension by more than 10%, Lumbar ROM test is invalid)				
	Maximum SLR Right							
Straight Leg Raising, Left	Left SLR							
	±10% or 5°?	Yes	No	(if tightest SLR ROM exceeds sum of Sacral flexion and extension by more than 10%, Lumbar ROM test is invalid)				
	Maximum SLR Left							
Lumbar Right Lateral Flexion	T12 ROM							
	Sacral ROM							
	Lumbar right lat flexion angle							
	±10% or 5°?	Yes	No					
	Maximum lumbar right lat flexion angle							
	% Impairment							
Lumbar Left Lateral Flexion	T12 ROM							
	Sacral ROM							
	Lumbar left lat flexion angle							
	±10% or 5°?	Yes	No					
	Maximum lumbar left lat flexion angle							
	% Impairment							
Lumbar Ankylosis in Lateral Flexion	Position			(Excludes any impairment for abnormal flexion/extension motion)				
	% Impairment							

Total Lumbar Range of Motion Impairment
(*add* all ROM impairments if no ankylosis;
use ankylosis impairment value if ankylosis is present)

Figure 84. Spine Impairment Summary

Impairment		Cervical	Thoracic	Lumbar
1. Due to Specific Disorders (Table 49)				
2. Range of Motion				
3. Neurological (From Chapter 4)	Pain, discomfort, or loss of sensation		XXXXXXXXXXXXXX	
	Loss of Strength		XXXXXXXXXXXXXX	
4. Other				
5. Regional Impairment Total (Combine impairments in each column using the Combined Values Chart)				
6. Spine Impairment Total (Combine all regional totals using the Combined Values Chart)				

Measurement of cervical spine flexion/extension using single inclinometer method

(for automated devices capable of calculating compound joint motions)

1. Locate and place a skin mark over the T1 spinous process. With subject in the seated position, place the inclinometer aligned in the sagittal plane over the skin mark and set the first "0" reading (Figure 86a, position 1). Move the inclinometer to the occiput and set the second "0" reading (Figure 86a, position 2).

2. Ask the subject to flex the head maximally and record the occipital flexion angle (Figure 86b, position 3). Move the inclinometer to the T1 skin mark duplicating the original inclinometer position and record the angle while the subject maintains the flexed position (Figure 86b, position 4). Then ask the subject to return to the neutral head position and obtain the calculated *cervical flexion angle.*

3. After recording the "0" readings first at T1, then over the occiput, ask the subject to produce a full cervical extension and rerecord the angles at the occiput and T1 sequentially to obtain calculated *cervical extension angle.*

Note: When extension is near normal, placement of the inclinometer at T1 in maximal extension may be impossible, and the examiner must place a skin mark over the scapular spine. The "0" reference points are measured initially at the scapular spine, then at the occiput in neutral position. The third data point is recorded as the inclinometer remains on the occiput while the cervical spine is fully extended. The 4th point is recorded again over the scapular spine.

4. Repeat the procedure three times. Only the *cervical flexion angle* and *extension angle* need be consistently measured within +/-10% or 5°, whichever is greater. The final measurement for impairment evaluation is the greatest angle measured.

5. Consult the Abnormal Motion Section of Table 51 to determine the impairment of the whole person.

Example: Occipital flexion measurements of 60°, 40°, and 45°, respectively, are matched with T1 flexion measurements of 20°, 5°, and 5°, respectively. This provides cervical flexion angle measurements of 40°, 35°, and 40°, respectively. Reproducibility falls within the criteria for validity since the difference between the three measures is within +/-5°. The largest flexion angle is 40° and the impairment due to abnormal motion is 2%. (See Table 51.)

Figure 85. 2-inclinometer Measurement Technique for Cervical Flexion/Extension
(a) The subject is sitting with the head in the neutral position, with inclinometers over the occiput and T1

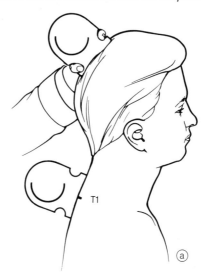

Table 50. Impairment of Cervical, Thoracic and Lumbar Regions Due to Ankylosis, Determined by Radiographic Methods

Favorable (neutral) Position	% Impairment of Whole Person	Unfavorable Position	% Impairment of Whole Person
Any 2 cervical	2	Any 2 cervical	4
Any 3 cervical	5	Any 3 cervical	10
Any 4 cervical	7	Any 4 cervical	14
Any 5 cervical	9	Any 5 cervical	18
Any 6 cervical	12	Any 6 cervical	24
Any 7 cervical	14	Any 7 cervical	28
C7 and T1	2	C7 and T1	4
Any 2 thoracic	1	Any 2 thoracic	2
Any 3 thoracic	2	Any 3 thoracic	4
Any 4 thoracic	3	Any 4 thoracic	5
Any 5 thoracic	4	Any 5 thoracic	7
Any 6 thoracic	5	Any 6 thoracic	9
Any 7 thoracic	5	Any 7 thoracic	11
Any 8 thoracic	6	Any 8 thoracic	13
Any 9 thoracic	7	Any 9 thoracic	15
Any 10 thoracic	8	Any 10 thoracic	16
Any 11 thoracic	9	Any 11 thoracic	18
Any 12 thoracic	12	Any 12 thoracic	20
T12 and L1	3	T12 and L1	6
Any 2 lumbar	3	Any 2 lumbar	6
Any 3 lumbar	6	Any 3 lumbar	12
Any 4 lumbar	9	Any 4 lumbar	18
Any 5 lumbar	12	Any 5 lumbar	24
C1-C7	14	C1-C7	28
T1-T12	10	T1-T12	20
L1-L5	12	L1-L5	24
C1-T12	23	C1-T12	28
T1-L5	21	T1-L5	39
C1-L5	32	C1-L5	56

Example: Occipital flexion is recorded at 20°, 30°, and 40°, respectively, while T1 motion is recorded at 20°, 10°, and 5°, respectively. This produces cervical flexion angles of 0°, 20°, and 35°, falling outside validity criteria. Repeated gross (occipital) measures were 50°, 40°, and 25°, respectively, while T1 measurements were 5°, 10°, and 10°, respectively, providing a flexion angle of 45°, 30°, and 15°. Persistent inconsistency provides evidence of suboptimal patient effort, invalidating the test. Impairment based on abnormal motion is deferred to a later date when valid measurements can be obtained. Complete the examination combining impairments on the forms (Figures 83a and 84) *excluding* impairment for cervical flexion/extension.

Ankylosis

1. Note whether there is no motion of the cervical spine whatsoever in the sagittal plane, or simply whether the spine is not able either to flex or extend beyond the neutral point. Determine if the ankylosis is in flexion or extension. If some motion is possible in the sagittal plane, ask the subject to hold the position *closest to the neutral point.*

2. Place an inclinometer base against a vertical surface to measure the neutral "0" position. Place the inclinometer in the sagittal plane at the upper aspect of the cervical spine along the long axis of the cervical spine with head in the position as described above.

3. Place the inclinometer at T1 and record the T1 angle. Subtract the T1 angle from the upper cervical angle to obtain the *ankylosis angle* in either flexion or extension.

4. Consult the Ankylosis Section of Table 51 to determine the impairment of the whole person.

Example: A cervical region with ankylosis at 25° extension is equivalent to 20% impairment of the whole person.
    Consult Table 50 if radiographic methods are chosen to determine impairment due to ankylosis.

Cervical Region—Lateral Flexion
Measurement of cervical spine lateral flexion using 2-inclinometer method

1. Locate and place a skin mark over the T1 spinous process. With the subject in the seated position, place the first inclinometer aligned in the coronal plane over the T1 spinous process while holding the second over the occiput (Figure 87a). The head should be in the neutral position while the inclinometers are "zeroed out."

2. Ask the subject to incline the head maximally to the right and record both angles (Figure 87b). Subtract the

T1 inclination from the occipital inclination for the *cervical right lateral flexion angle.* Return the head to the neutral position so that both inclinometers read "0" again.

3. Instruct the subject to incline the head maximally to the left as far as possible, again recording both inclinometer angles and subtracting the T1 angle from the occipital inclinometer angle to obtain the *cervical left lateral flexion angle* (Figure 87c). Again ask the subject to return the head to the neutral position.

4. Repeat the procedure three times. Only the *left and right lateral flexion angles* need be consistently measured to with +/-10% or 5°, whichever is greater. The final measurement for impairment evaluation is the greatest angle measured.

5. Consult the Abnormal Motion Section of Table 52 to determine the impairment of the whole person.

Measurement of cervical spine lateral flexion using the single inclinometer method
(for automated devices capable of calculating compound joint motions)

1. With the subject in the seated position, locate and place a skin mark over the T1 spinous process (Figure 88a, position 1). Place the inclinometer aligned in the coronal plane over the skin mark and set the first "0"

Figure 85. 2-inclinometer Measurement Technique for Cervical Flexion/Extension
(b) With the subject in full flexion position, subtract the angle at the lower inclinometer from the upper inclinometer to obtain the cervical flexion angle

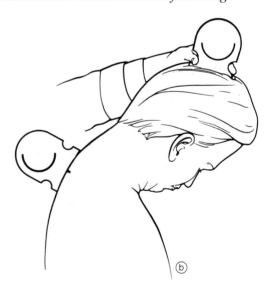

reading. Move the inclinometer to the occiput and set the second "0" reading (Figure 88a, position 2).

2. Ask the subject to incline the head maximally to the right and record the occipital flexion angle (Figure 88b, position 3). Move the inclinometer to the T1 skin mark duplicating the original inclinometer position and record the angle (Figure 88b, position 4). Then ask the subject to resume the neutral head position, rerecord the "0" reading at T1 and calculate the *cervical right lateral flexion angle.*

3. Record the "0" readings at T1, then over the occiput, asking the subject to incline the head maximally to the left, and rerecord the angles at the occiput and T1 sequentially to obtain the calculated *cervical left lateral flexion angle.*

4. Repeat the procedure three times. Only the *left and right lateral flexion angles* need be consistently measured to within +/-10% or 5°, whichever is greater. The final measurement for impairment evaluation is the greatest angle measured.

5. Consult the Abnormal Motion Section of Table 52 to determine the impairment of the whole person.

Example: Occipital right lateral flexion measures 20°, 35°, 35°, and 40°, respectively. T1 right lateral flexion

Table 51. Impairment Due to Abnormal Motion and Ankylosis of the Cervical Region—Flexion/Extension

Abnormal Motion
Average range of *Flexion-Extension* is 135°.
Value to total range of cervical motion is 40%.

Flexion from neutral position (0°) to:	Degrees of Cervical Motion Lost	Retained	% Impairment of Whole Person
0°	60°	0°	6
20°	40°	20°	4
40°	20°	40°	2
60°	0°	60°+	0

Extension from neutral position (0°) to:	Degrees of Cervical Motion Lost	Retained	% Impairment of Whole Person
0°	75°	0°	6
25°	50°	25°	4
50°	25°	50°	2
75°	0°	75°+	0

Ankylosis

Region ankylosed at:	% Impairment of Whole Person
0° (neutral position)	12
20°	20
40°	30
60° (full flexion)	40

Region ankylosed at:	% Impairment of Whole Person
0° (neutral position)	12
25°	20
50°	30
75° (full extension)	40

Figure 85. 2-inclinometer Measurement Technique for Cervical Flexion/Extension
(c) Subtract the T1 inclinometer angle from the occipital angle to obtain the extension angle

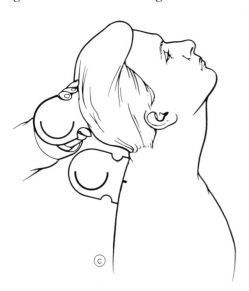

Figure 85. 2-inclinometer Measurement Technique for Cervical Flexion/Extension
(d) Alternative placement of lower inclinometer when extension motion is so great as to displace inclinometer over T1. Use skin mark for placement over the scapular spine

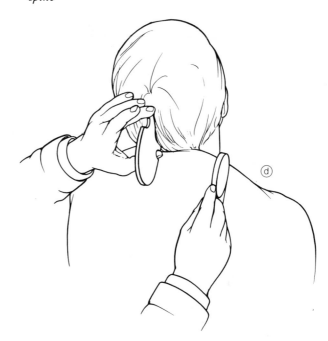

Figure 86. Single-inclinometer Measurement Technique for Cervical Flexion/Extension

(a) Obtain "0" readings first at T1 (position 1) and then over the occiput (position 2)

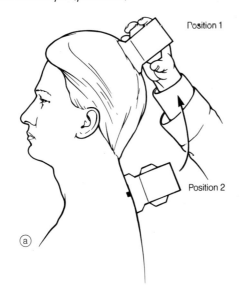

Figure 86. Single-inclinometer Measurement Technique for Cervical Flexion/Extension

(b) Flex the spine, first obtaining the occipital angle (position 3) and then the T1 angle (position 4)

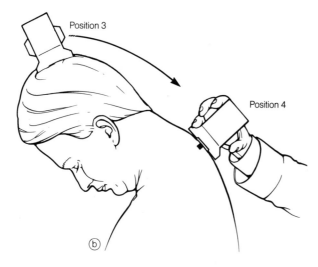

measures 15°, 5°, 10°, and 10°, respectively. Cervical right lateral flexion angle measures 5°, 30°, 25°, and 30°, respectively. The first measurement was thrown out as an invalid measure, necessitating a fourth measurement, but the succeeding three consecutive measures fulfilled validation criteria. The best right lateral flexion angle is 30°, and the impairment is 1%.

6. *Add* the impairment values contributed by left lateral flexion and right lateral flexion. Their sum represents the impairment of the whole person that is contributed by abnormal lateral flexion of the cervical region.

Ankylosis

1. Determine if the subject has no cervical coronal motion whatsoever, or is simply unable to attain the neutral position. If the patient has some motion, ask him or her to maintain the position *closest to neutral.*

2. Place the inclinometer base against a horizontal surface (desk or table top) to obtain the neutral "0" coronal plane position. Place the inclinometer at the upper edge of the cervical spine aligned perpendicular to the long axis of the cervical spine and record deviation from neutral.

3. Align the inclinometer perpendicular to T1 in the coronal plane to measure the deviation of the shoulder/thoracic spine. Subtract T1 measurement from the shoulder/thoracic measurement to obtain the *ankylosis angle.*

4. Consult the Ankylosis Section of Table 52 for the cervical region to determine the impairment of the whole person.

Example: A cervical region with ankylosis angle of 30° right lateral flexion is equivalent to a 30% impairment of the whole person.

Cervical Region—Rotation

Because the technique stabilizes the shoulders in the supine position, for measurement of rotation only a single inclinometer is needed. In effect, this is a simple, not a compound, joint mobility measurement.

Measurement of cervical rotation

1. Have the subject recline in the supine position on a flat examination table with shoulders exposed to permit direct observation of excessive shoulder rotation. Stand at the head of the table and place the inclinometer in the coronal plane with the base near the back of

the head approximately in line with the cervico-occipital junction. Record the neutral "0" position with the subject's nose pointing to the ceiling (Figure 89a).

2. Ask the subject to rotate the head maximally to the right and record the *cervical right rotation angle* (Figure 89b).

3. Ask the subject to rotate the head maximally to the left and record the *cervical left rotation angle.*

4. Repeat the procedure three times. Only the *right and left cervical rotation angles* need be consistently measured to within +/-10% or 5°, whichever is greater. The final measurement for impairment evaluation is the greatest angle measured.

5. Consult the Abnormal Motion Section of Table 53 to determine the impairment of the whole person.

Example: Left rotation is recorded at 15°, 35°, 40°, and 35°, respectively. The invalid initial measurement is thrown out, necessitating a fourth measurement that meets validation criteria. The best measurement of 40° corresponds to an impairment rating due to abnormal left cervical rotation of 2%.

6. *Add* the impairment values contributed by left rotation and right rotation. Their sum is the impairment of the whole person that is contributed by abnormal rotation of the cervical region.

Ankylosis

1. Determine if the subject has no cervical axial motion whatsoever, or is simply unable to attain the neutral position. If the patient has some motion, ask him or her to maintain the position *closest to neutral.*

2. Place the base of the inclinometer on a horizontal flat surface (desk or table top) to obtain the neutral "0" position. With the subject in the supine position, place the base of the inclinometer at the base of the head in a position identical to that used for measuring cervical rotation, but in line with the patient's nose. Record the rotational ankylosis angle.

3. Consult the Ankylosis Section of Table 53 to determine the impairment of the whole person.

Example: A cervical region with ankylosis at 20° right rotation is equivalent to an impairment of 20% of the whole person.

Consult Table 50 if radiographic methods are chosen to determine impairment due to ankylosis.

Table 52. Impairment Due to Abnormal Motion and Ankylosis of the Cervical Region—Lateral Flexion

Abnormal Motion
Average range of *Lateral Flexion* is 90°.
Value to total range of cervical motion is 25%.

Right lateral flexion from neutral position (0°) to:	Degrees of Cervical Motion Lost	Degrees of Cervical Motion Retained	% Impairment of Whole Person
0°	45°	0°	4
15°	30°	15°	2
30°	15°	30°	1
45°	0°	45°+	0

Left lateral flexion from neutral position (0°) to:			
0°	45°	0°	4
15°	30°	15°	2
30°	15°	30°	1
45°	0°	45°+	0

Ankylosis

Region ankylosed at:	% Impairment of Whole Person
0° (neutral position)	8
15°	20
30°	30
45° (full right/left lateral flexion)	40

Table 53. Impairment Due to Abnormal Motion and Ankylosis of the Cervical Region—Rotation

Abnormal Motion
Average range of *Rotation* is 160°.
Value to total range of cervical motion is 35%.

Right rotation from neutral position (0°) to:	Degrees of Cervical Motion Lost	Degrees of Cervical Motion Retained	% Impairment of Whole Person
0°	80°	0°	6
20°	60°	20°	4
40°	40°	40°	2
60°	20°	60°	1
80°	0°	80°+	0

Left rotation from neutral position (0°) to:			
0°	80°	0°	6
20°	60°	20°	4
40°	40°	40°	2
60°	20°	60°	1
80°	0°	80°+	0

Ankylosis

Region ankylosed at:	% Impairment of Whole Person
0° (neutral position)	12
20°	20
40°	30
60°	40
80° (full right/left rotation)	50

3.3d Impairments Due to Range of Motion Abnormalities— Thoracic Region

Flexion and Extension

Thoracic flexion/extension is a relatively limited motion with a degree of extension significantly determined by the subject's posture and the degree of fixed kyphosis in the thoracic spine. For this reason, in this region of the spine it is more convenient to substitute a slightly different concept for measurement of flexion/extension. Instead of extension, the subject is measured in the "military brace" posture to obtain the *angle of minimum kyphosis*. Following this, the *angle of thoracic flexion* is obtained by fully flexing the thoracic spine from the "military brace" position. The angle of minimum kyphosis is actually a measure of ankylosis, and impairment resulting from this angle should be found in the Ankylosis Section of Table 54.

Measurement of thoracic flexion/extension using 2-inclinometer method

1. Locate and place a skin mark over the T1 and T12 spinous processes. Place both inclinometers against a

---

Figure 87. 2-inclinometer Measurement Technique for Cervical Lateral Flexion *(a) The subject is sitting with head in the neutral position, and the inclinometers are over the occiput and T1 (b) Full right lateral flexion position (c) Subtract the angle to obtain the left lateral flexion angle*

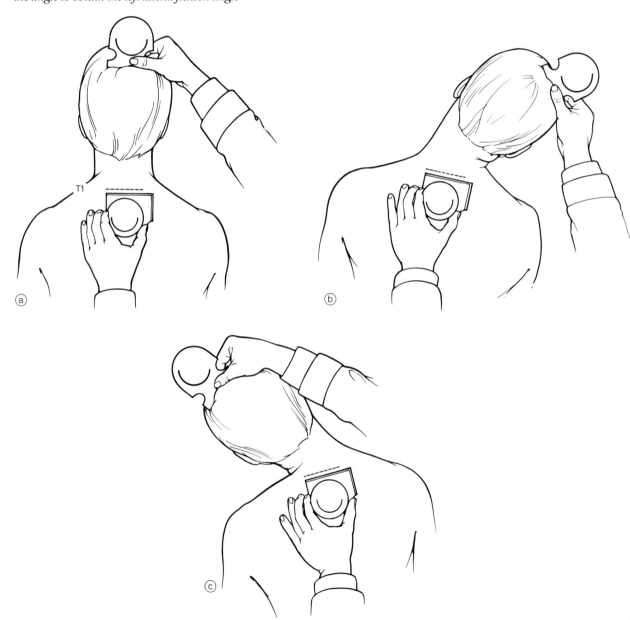

true vertical surface, such as a wall, and record the neutral "0" position. Place the inclinometers over T1 and T12 spinous processes while instructing the subject to maintain the maximally extended "military brace," straight posture position (Figures 90a or b). Subtract the T12 inclinometer reading from the T1 inclinometer reading to obtain *angle of minimum kyphosis*. Find the impairment level in the Ankylosis Section of Table 54.

2. Next, "zero out" the inclinometers to the neutral "0" position with subject in the erect "military brace" posture. Then ask the subject to place the hands on the hips and flex fully by curving the thoracic spine. Bending at the hips is permitted. Subtract the T12 inclinometer reading from the T1 inclinometer reading to obtain the *angle of thoracic flexion* (Figures 90c or d).

3. A reproducibility test is best facilitated in the sitting position. Seat the subject on a stool and ask the subject to flex maximally the thoracic spine from the "military brace" position after recording the neutral "0" position with the subject sitting erect on the stool. The seated *angle of thoracic flexion* should be identical to the angle obtained in the erect position. Repeat either the sitting or standing test to obtain three values that are within +/-10% or 5°, whichever is greater. If the validity characteristics of the three tests are insufficient, simply repeat alternating tests (sitting or standing) to obtain up to six measurements.

4. Consult the Abnormal Motion Section of Table 54 to determine the impairment of the whole person.

Measurement of thoracic spine flexion/extension using single inclinometer method
(for automated devices capable of calculating compound joint motions)

1. Utilize either the standing or sitting methods as described under the 2-inclinometer method. Obtain the neutral reading "0" on a vertical surface such as a wall. With the subject in the erect "military brace" position place the inclinometer at T1 and record, followed by an inclinometer reading at T12. Subtract one measurement from another to obtain the *angle of minimum kyphosis*.

2. With the subject in either the standing or sitting position, with the subject in the erect "military brace" posture and the inclinometer over the T12 skin mark, record the position, then move the inclinometer to the T1 skin mark and record the position.

3. Ask the subject to flex maximally by curving the thoracic spine with the inclinometer maintained over T1, and record the position. Facilitate maximum movement

Figure 88. Single-inclinometer Measurement Technique for Cervical Lateral Flexion
(a) Obtain "0" readings first at T1 (position 1) and then over the occiput (position 2)
(b) Flex the spine, first obtaining the occipital (position 3) and then the T1 (position 4) angles

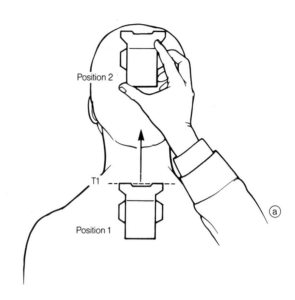

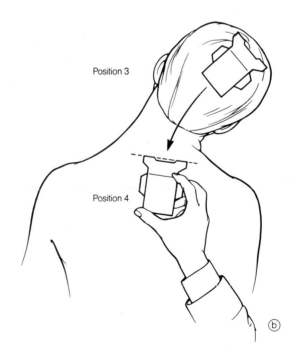

Figure 89. Measurement of Cervical Rotation
(a) The subject is in the supine position with the incli-nometer held in the coronal plane in the neutral position (b) The head is rotated to the right with the inclinometer indicating the right rotation angle. Be certain the shoul-ders remain horizontally aligned on the table

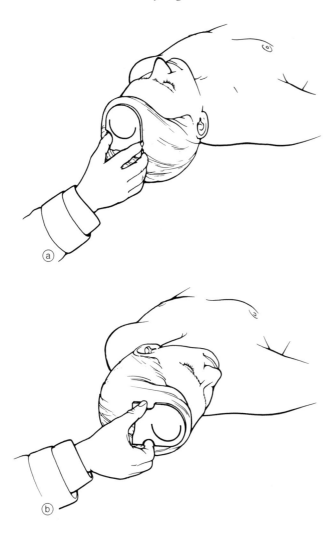

by asking the subject to place the hands on the hips if in the standing position or to drop the head between the knees if in the sitting position. Then move and record the position at the T12 skin mark, calculating the *angle of thoracic flexion.*

4. Alternately repeat the standing and sitting techniques to obtain at least three measurements of the *angle of thoracic flexion* that are within +/-10% or 5°, which-ever is greater.

5. Consult the Abnormal Motion Section of Table 54 to determine the impairment of the whole person.

Ankylosis
In thoracic flexion/extension, *the angle of minimum kyphosis* is actually the ankylosis angle. Excessive kypho-sis or thoracic lordosis may produce an impairment, as noted in Table 54.

Example: A subject with ankylosing spondylitis attempts to extend his thoracic spine fully, but demonstrates an angle of minimum kyphosis of 45°. On attempting max-imum flexion, T1 readings of 80°, 90°, and 100° are recorded, respectively, while T12 flexion angles of 25°, 30°, and 40° are recorded, respectively. The maximum true thoracic flexion is 55°, 60°, and 60°, respectively. The *angle of thoracic flexion,* which is derived by sub-tracting the angle of minimum kyphosis for each trial is 10°, 15°, and 15°, respectively. These meet validity cri-teria. According to Table 54 the impairment due to ankylosis (angle of minimum kyphosis) is 5% of the whole person, while the impairment due to abnormal motion of 15° is 2%. The total impairment is the *greater* of the ankylosis or abnormal motion percentages, or in this instance, 5%.

Consult Table 50 if radiographic methods are chosen to determine impairment due to ankylosis.

Thoracic Region—Rotation
**Measurement of thoracic rotation using
2-inclinometer method**
1. The subject may be seated or standing (whichever is more comfortable) in a forward flexed position with the thoracic spine in as horizontal a position as can be achieved. Locate and place a skin mark over the T1 and T12 spinous processes. Place the first inclinometer, aligned in the axial and vertical planes, over the T1 spinous process while holding the second over the T12 spinous process. The trunk should be in the neutral rotational position while the inclinometers are "zeroed out" (Figure 91a).

2. Ask the subject to rotate the trunk maximally to the right and record both angles. Subtract the T12 inclination from the T1 inclination for the *thoracic right rotation angle* (Figure 91b). Return the trunk to the neutral position so that both inclinometers read "0" again.

3. Instruct the subject to rotate the trunk maximally to the left as far as possible, again recording both inclinometer angles and subtracting the T12 angle from the T1 inclinometer angle to obtain the *thoracic left rotation angle* (Figure 91c).

4. Repeat the procedure three times. Only the *left and right rotation angles* need be consistently measured to within +/-10% or 5°, whichever is greater. The final measurement for impairment evaluation is the greatest angle measured.

5. Consult the Abnormal Motion Section of Table 55 to determine the impairment of the whole person.

Figure 90. 2-inclinometer Measurement Technique for Obtaining Angle of Minimum Kyphosis. *(a) Standing and (b) sitting techniques, with the inclinometers at T1 and T12 and with the subject in the erect "military brace" posture to obtain <u>angle of minimum kyphosis</u>. (c) Standing and (d) sitting techniques with inclinometers over T1 and T12 and with thoracic spine maximally flexed to obtain <u>angle of thoracic flexion</u>.*

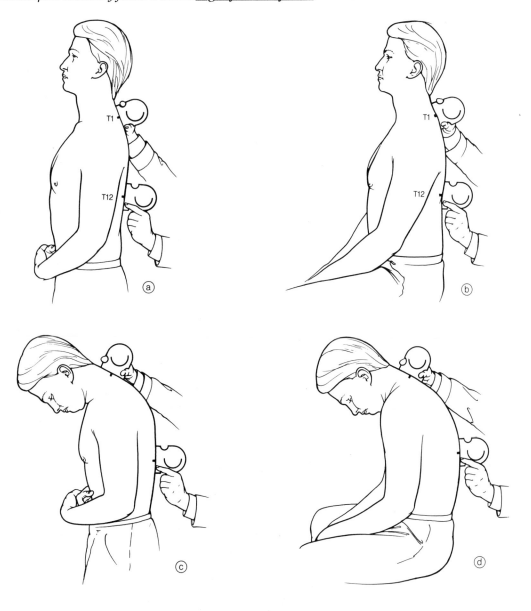

Measurement of thoracic spine rotation using single inclinometer method
(for automated devices capable of calculating compound joint motions)

1. The subject may be seated or standing (whichever is more comfortable) in a forward flexed position with the thoracic spine in as horizontal a position as can be achieved. Locate and place a skin mark over the T1 and the T12 spinous processes. Place the inclinometer aligned in the axial and vertical planes, over the T12 spinous process and set the first "0" reading. Move the inclinometer to T1 and set the second "0" reading.

2. Ask the subject to rotate the trunk maximally to the right and record the Tl rotation angle. Move the inclinometer to the T12 skin mark duplicating the original inclinometer position and record the angle. Then ask the subject to resume the neutral trunk position and rerecord the "0" reading. Calculate the *thoracic right rotation angle.*

Figure 91. 2-inclinometer measurement technique for thoracic rotation *(a) The subject may be standing or sitting in a forward flexed position with the spine as parallel to the floor as possible to permit the inclinometers to be aligned in vertical plane (b) In the full right rotation position, subtract the angle at the lower inclinometer (T12) from the angle at the upper inclinometer (T1) to obtain the thoracic right rotation angle (c) Subtract T12 inclinometer angle from the T1 angle to obtain left rotation angle*

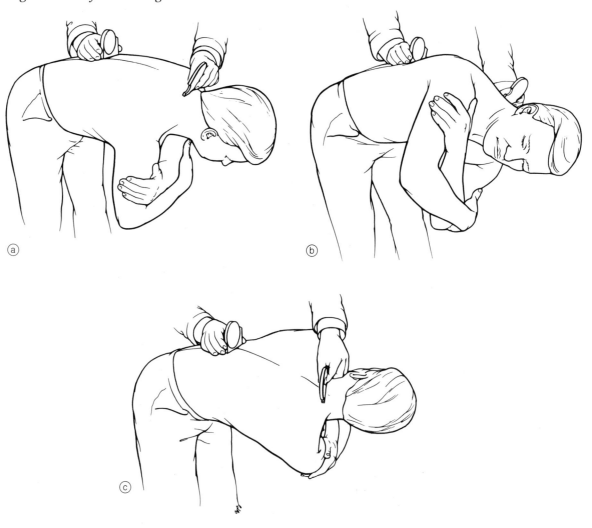

3. Record the "0" readings first at T12 then at T1; ask the subject to produce full thoracic left rotation and rerecord angles at T1 and T12 sequentially to obtain the calculated *thoracic left rotation angle.*

4. Repeat the procedures three times. Only the *thoracic right and left rotation angles* need be consistently measured to within +/-10% or 5°, whichever is greater.

5. Consult the Abnormal Motion Section of Table 55 to determine the impairment of the whole person.

Example: T1 rotation to the right measures 15°, 25°, and 15°, respectively. T12 rotation measures 5°, 15°, and 5°, respectively. The right rotation angle is 10°, and the impairment is 2%.

Ankylosis

Rotational ankylosis in the thoracic spine is generally a component of a scoliosis deformity, and creates only limited impairment. Utilize the same posture used for measuring abnormal motion in the thoracic spine, and ask the subject to achieve maximum correction of the rotatory deformity. Then, subtract the T12 rotation angle from the T1 rotation angle, which gives the ankylosis angle. Refer to the Ankylosis Section of Table 55 to determine impairment.

3.3e Impairments Due to Range of Motion Abnormalities— Lumbosacral Region

Flexion and Extension
Abnormal Motion

1. An additional "effort factor" is available to check lumbar spine flexion. This is particularly useful because perceived lumbar flexion is actually a compound movement of both the lumbar spine and the hips (measured at the sacrum), in which hip flexion normally accounts for at least 50% of total flexion. A comparison of hip flexion to straight leg raising on the tightest side offers a validation measure independent of reproducibility. The test is invalid and must be repeated if the following validity criterion is *not* met:

Tightest straight leg raising (SLR)—(hip flexion + hip extension) ≤ 10°

If repeat flexion measurements that are otherwise reproducible are consistently associated with an abnormal hip/SLR motion pattern, the measurements are not valid.

Table 54. Impairment Due to Abnormal Motion and Ankylosis of the Thoracic Region—Flexion/Extension

Abnormal Motion
Average range of *Flexion/Extension* is 50°.
Value to total range of thoracic motion is 60%.

Flexion from erect position (angle of thoracic flexion) to:	Degrees of Thoracic Motion Lost	Degrees of Thoracic Motion Retained	% Impairment of Whole Person
0°	50°	0°	4
15°	35°	15°	2
30°	20°	30°	1
50°	0°	50°	0

Ankylosis

Range of Angle of Minimum Kyphosis	% Impairment of Whole Person
−30° to 0° (Extension-Thoracic Lordosis)	20
0° to 40° (Neutral)	0
40° to 60°	5
60° to 90°	20
Above 90°	40

Table 55. Impairment Due to Abnormal Motion and Ankylosis of the Thoracic Region—Rotation

Abnormal Motion
Average range of *Rotation* is 60°.
Value to total range of thoracic motion is 40%.

Right Rotation from neutral position (0°) to:	Degrees of Thoracic Motion Lost	Degrees of Thoracic Motion Retained	% Impairment of Whole Person
0°	30°	0°	3
10°	20°	10°	2
20°	10°	20°	1
30°	0°	30°	0

Left Rotation from neutral position (0°) to:			
0°	30°+	0°	3
10°	20°	10°	2
20°	10°	20°	1
30°	0°	30°	0

Ankylosis

Region ankylosed at:	% Impairment of Whole Person
0° (neutral position)	6
15°	10
25°	20
35°+ (full thoracic right/left rotation)	30

2. There is a normal relationship between true lumbar flexion and hip flexion, in which true lumbar flexion represents the higher percentage of gross flexion during early forward bending, whereas hip motion represents the higher percentage of terminal forward mobility (Figure 92). Suboptimal effort on repeated tests may still show a "normal" pattern to the spine/hip ratio consistent with Figure 92. Even if this "normal" pattern is seen, the persistence of suboptimal effort of spine motion should result in the examiner deferring the examination to a later date when valid measurements can be obtained (unless the visualized true spine motion is high enough to warrant a 0% impairment).

Measurement of lumbosacral flexion/extension using 2-inclinometer method

1. Locate and place skin marks over the T12 spinous process and the sacrum. Place the first inclinometer aligned in the sagittal plane over the T12 spinous

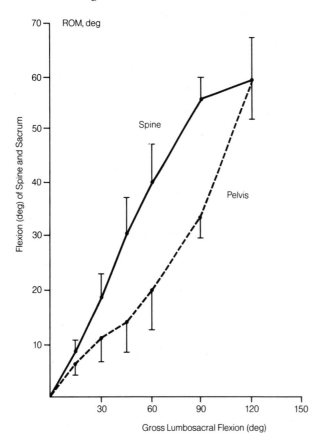

Figure 92. Relationship of Spine Flexion to Sacral (Hip) Flexion During Gross Lumbosacral Flexion

Adapted from Mayer TG, Tencer AF, Kristoferson S, Mooney V: Use of non-invasive techniques for quantification of spinal range-of-motion in normal subjects and chronic low back dysfunction patients. Spine 1984; 9:588-595. Reprinted with permission. Copyright © 1984, JB Lippincott, Philadephia.

process while holding the second over the sacrum. It is generally convenient to place the sacral mark at or near the sacral midpoint, since if the mark is placed too high on the sacral convexity, the inclinometer may be displaced when performing the measurement of extension. The subject should be in the standing position, with knees straight, with weight balanced on both feet, with hands on hips for support if necessary to permit greater motion. The trunk should be in the neutral position while the inclinometers are "zeroed out" (Figure 93a).

2. Ask the subject to flex maximally and record both angles. Subtract the sacral (hip) inclination from the T12 inclination for the *true lumbar flexion angle.* Return the trunk to the neutral position so that both inclinometers read "0" again (Figure 93b).

3. Instruct the subject to extend the trunk as far as possible, again recording both inclinometer angles and subtracting the sacral (hip) angle from the T12 inclinometer angle to obtain the *true lumbar extension angle* (Figure 93c). Again ask the subject to return the trunk to the neutral position.

4. Record the straight leg raising (SLR) angle by placing the inclinometer on each tibial spine with both knees extended, and compare the tightest SLR to sacral (hip) motion (flexion + extension). If the SLR exceeds total sacral (hip) motion by more than 10°, the test is invalid and should be repeated (Figure 93d).

5. Consult the Abnormal Motion Section of Table 56 to determine the impairment of the whole person.

Measurement of lumbosacral spine flexion/ extension using single inclinometer method
(for automated devices capable of calculating compound joint motions)

1. Locate and place skin marks over the T12 spinous process and the sacrum. It is generally convenient to place the sacral mark at or near the sacral midpoint, since if the mark is placed too high on the sacral convexity, the inclinometer may be displaced when performing the measurement of extension. Place the inclinometer aligned in the sagittal plane, with the subject in the standing position, with knees straight, with weight balanced on both feet, and with hands on hips for support if necessary to permit greater motion. Place the inclinometer over the T12 skin mark and set the first "0" reading. Move the inclinometer to the sacrum and set the second "0" reading.

2. Ask the subject to flex the trunk maximally and record the sacral (hip) flexion angle. Move the inclinometer to the T12 skin mark duplicating the original inclinometer position and record the angle. Then ask the subject to resume the neutral trunk position, rerecord the "0" readings and calculate the *true lumbar flexion angle*.

3. Record the "0" readings first at T12 then over the sacrum, then ask the subject to produce full lumbosacral extension and rerecord the angles at the sacrum (hip) and T12 sequentially to obtain the calculated *true lumbar extension angle*.

4. Record the straight leg raising angle (SLR) by placing the inclinometer on each tibial spine with both knees extended, and compare the tightest SLR to sacral (hip) motion (flexion + extension). If the SLR exceeds total sacral (hip) motion by more than 10°, the test is invalid and should be repeated.

5. Consult the Abnormal Motion Section of Table 56 to determine the impairment of the whole person.

Example: T12 flexion measurements of 50° and 90° are matched with sacral (hip) flexion measurements of 25° and 65°, respectively. Sacral (hip) extension angles are 10° and 10°, respectively, while the tightest SLR is measured at 70° and 75°, respectively.

   In the first test, there is total sacral (hip) motion of 25° + 10° = 35°, compared to a straight leg raise of 70°, which fails the validation criterion of SLR (total sacral (hip) motion is exceeded by more than 10°). In the second test, however there is total sacral (hip) motion of 65° + 10° = 75°, exactly identical to the SLR of 75° on the second test, producing a valid test. In this case, the true lumbar motion is 25° (90°−65°) and the impairment rating, according to Table 56, is 7% (sacral flexion angle = 45°+, true lumbar flexion angle = 15-30°).

Ankylosis

Ankylosis in the lumbosacral spine has significance only if immobility occurs in *both* the hips and the lumbar spine region, so that that neutral position cannot be attained in the sagittal plane. This is a very rare event. Isolated fusions of either a hip or two to three spinal levels place additional stresses on adjacent segments, but do not lead to biomechanical failure of the functional unit. Thus, impairments related to fusion of part of the lumbar/hip motion complex are treated only under the Abnormal Motion Section of Table 56.

Lumbosacral Region—Lateral Flexion
Abnormal Motion
Measurement of lumbosacral lateral flexion using 2-inclinometer method

1. With the subject standing erect with knees straight, locate and place a skin mark over the T12 spinous

Table 56. Impairment Due to Abnormal Motion* of the Lumbosacral Region—Flexion/Extension *(Use only if the sum of hip flexion plus hip extension angles is within 10° of the straight leg raising angle on tightest side—the validity criterion)*

Value to total range of lumbosacral motion is 75%.

Sacral (Hip) Flexion Angle	True Lumbar Flexion Angle	% Impairment of Whole Person
45°+	60°+	0
45°+	45°-60°	2
45°+	30°-45°	4
45°+	15°-30°	7
45°+	0°-15°	10
30°-45°	40°+	4
30°-45°	20°-40°	7
30°-45°	0°-20°	10
0°-30°	30°+	5
0°-30°	15°-30°	8
0°-30°	0°-15°	11

True lumbar extension from neutral position (0°) to:	Degrees of Lumbosacral Motion Lost	Retained	% Impairment of Whole Person
0°	25°	0°	7
10°	15°	10°	5
15°	10°	15°	3
20°	5°	20°	2
25°	0°	25°	0

*See text for discussion of Ankylosis.

Table 57. Impairment Due to Abnormal Motion and Ankylosis of the Lumbosacral Region—Lateral Flexion

Average range of *Lateral Flexion* is 50°.
Value of total range of lumosacral motion is 25%.

Abnormal Motion

Right lateral flexion from neutral position (0°) to:	Degrees of Lumbosacral Motion Lost	Retained	% Impairment of Whole Person
0°	25°	0°	5
10°	15°	10°	3
15°	10°	15°	2
20°	5°	20°	1
25°	0°	25°	0

Left lateral flexion from neutral position (0°) to:	Degrees of Lumbosacral Motion Lost	Retained	% Impairment of Whole Person
0°	25°	0°	5
10°	15°	10°	3
15°	10°	15°	2
20°	5°	20°	1
25°	0°	25°	0

Ankylosis

Region ankylosed at:	% Impairment of Whole Person
0° (neutral position)	10
30°	20
45°	30
60°	40
75° (full lumbosacral right/left lateral flexion)	50

process and the sacrum. Place the first inclinometer aligned in the coronal plane over the T12 spinous process while holding the second over the sacrum (Figure 94a). The trunk should be in the neutral position while the inclinometers are "zeroed out."

2. Instruct the subject to bend the trunk maximally to the right and record both angles. Subtract the sacral (hip) inclination from the T12 inclination for the *lumbar right lateral flexion angle* (Figure 94b). Return the trunk to the neutral position so that both inclinometers read "0" again.

3. Instruct the subject to bend the trunk maximally to the left as far as possible, again recording both inclinometer angles and subtracting the sacral (hip) angle from the T12 inclinometer angle to obtain the *lumbar left lateral flexion angle*. Again ask the subject to return to the neutral position.

4. Repeat the procedure three times. Only the *left and right lateral flexion angles* need be consistently measured to within +/-10% or 5°, whichever is greater. The final measurement for impairment evaluation is the greatest angle measured.

Figure 93. 2-inclinometer measurement technique for lumbosacral flexion/extension *(a) Neutral position and (b) flexion shown with the inclinometers at T12 and over the sacrum; (c) True lumbar extension = T12 inclination − sacral inclination (hip motion); (d) Straight leg raise on the tightest side should be within 10° of the total hip motion (hip flexion + hip extension).*

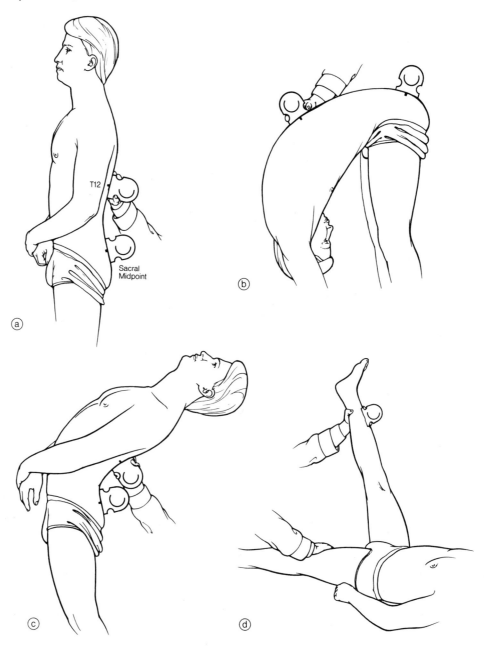

5. Consult the Abnormal Motion Section of Table 57 to determine the impairment of the whole person.

Measurement of lumbosacral spine lateral flexion using single inclinometer method
(for automated devices capable of calculating compound joint motions)

1. With the subject standing erect with knees straight, locate and place skin marks over the T12 spinous process and the sacrum. Place the inclinometer aligned in coronal plane over T12 skin mark and set first "0" reading. Move the inclinometer to the sacrum and set the second "0" reading.

2. Ask the subject to bend the trunk maximally to the right and record the sacral (hip) flexion angle. Move the inclinometer to the T12 skin mark duplicating original inclinometer position and record the angle. Then ask the subject to resume the neutral position, rerecord the "0" readings and calculate the *lumbar right lateral flexion angle*.

3. Record the "0" readings first at T12 then over the sacrum. Ask the subject to produce full lumbosacral left flexion and rerecord angles at the sacrum and T12 sequentially to obtain the calculated *lumbar left lateral flexion angle*.

4. Repeat the procedure three times. Only the *left and right lateral flexion angles* need be consistently measured to within +/-10% or 5°, whichever is greater. The final measurement for impairment evaluation is the greatest angle measured.

5. Consult the Abnormal Motion Section of Table 57 to determine the impairment of the whole person.

Example: T12 lateral flexion to the right measures 20°, 20°, 30°, and 25°, respectively. Sacral (hip) lateral flexion measures 15°, 5°, 10°, and 10°, respectively. The lumbosacral right lateral flexion angle measures 5°, 15°, 20°, and 15°, respectively. The first measurement was discarded as an invalid measure, necessitating a fourth measurement, but the succeeding three consecutive measures fulfilled validation criteria. The best right lateral flexion angle is 20°, and the impairment is 1%.

Ankylosis
Ankylosis in the lumbosacral lateral flexion generally represents a scoliosis, usually producing only limited impairment. Mark the T12 and sacral spinous processes and ask the subject to stand in the most erect position possible (correcting the deformity). Using the simple measurement mode in the coronal plane, subtract the sacral (hip) inclination from the T12 inclination and record the ankylosis angle. Obtain the impairment from Table 57.

Figure 94. 2-inclinometer Measurement Technique for Lumbosacral Lateral Bend *(a) Set the inclinometers at T12 and over the sacrum in the coronal plane with the inclinometers "zeroed out" in the erect position; (b) With the subject bending maximally to the right, subtract the sacral inclinometer reading from the T12 reading to obtain the true lumbar lateral bend angle to the right. Repeat the procedure to the left.*

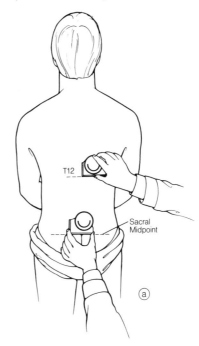

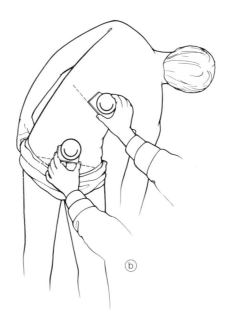

3.4 The Pelvis

The following shows impairment values associated with disorders of the pelvis:

Disorder	% Impairment of Whole Person
1. Healed fracture *without* displacement or residuals	0
2. Healed fracture *with* displacement and *without* residuals, involving:	
a. Single ramus	0
b. Rami, bilateral	0
c. Ilium	0
d. Ischium	0
e. Symphysis pubis, without separation	5
f. Sacrum	5
g. Coccyx	0
3. Healed fracture *with* displacement, deformity and residuals:	
a. Single ramus	0
b. Rami, bilateral	5
c. Ilium	2
d. Ischium, displaced 1 inch or more	10
e. Symphysis pubis, displaced or separated	15
f. Sacrum, into sacro-iliac joint	10
g. Coccyx, non-union or excision	5
h. Fracture into acetabulum	evaluate on basis of restricted motion of hip joint

The impairment value for hemipelvectomy is 50% of the whole person (Table 43).

Addendum to Chapter 3

A. Introduction

Sections 3.3a through 3.3e introduce the inclinometer technique in evaluating impairments due to loss of range of motion of the spine. Realizing that many users of the *Guides* may not be able to convert immediately to this newer technique, or that they may be consulting on cases that originated at a time prior to the adoption of this new technique as the preferred method for evaluating spinal impairment, we provide in this addendum a modification of the goniometer technique for evaluating range of motion of the spine. This addendum should be used only until the examiner develops the skills to use the inclinometer technique—we recommend that such skills should be in place by one year after the publication date of this third edition of the *Guides*. After that time only the inclinometer will be valid, and the goniometer should be used only for cases that pre-date the publication of the third edition, which, for consistency, must be evaluated using the goniometer.

Oftentimes, two or more physicians are asked to evaluate the impairment of one individual. If one physician uses the inclinometer technique and one the goniometer technique for evaluating range of motion of the spine, all other differences aside, the AMA considers the report of the physician who has used the inclinometer more valid than the report of the physician who has used the goniometer.

Principles for Calculating Impairment
The spine consists of three major regions: cervical, thoracic, and lumbar. Each region is considered only a portion of the whole spine (Figure 82, p. 71) as follows:

cervical = 80%; thoracic = 40%; lumbar = 90%. The spine as a whole is considered equivalent to the whole person for purposes of impairment evaluation. For the sake of simplicity, all impairments in this section have been adjusted for each regional percentage, permitting their expression as a percent impairment of the whole person.

In order to calculate total spine impairment:

A. Select the primarily impaired region (cervical, thoracic, lumbar).

1. If applicable, use Table 49 (p. 73) to obtain a diagnosis-based percentage of impairment.

2. When using the goniometer, skin marks *must* be placed over the end points (extremes) of the area of the spine being tested. Furthermore, the lower arc of the goniometer *must* move with the lower skin mark, thereby accounting for movement that may occur in other joints that may add to the perceived excursion of the area of the spine being evaluated.

3. Perform at least three measurements of each range of motion, and calculate the permitted variability (+/-10% or 5°) based on either the *maximum* or *median* motion values. That is, check whether all three measurements fall within reproducibility guidelines by varying less than those amounts from either the maximum or median value.

4. If consistency requirements are *not* met, perform additional tests up to a maximum of six until reproducibility criteria are satisified. If testing remains inconsistent after six measurements, consider the test invalid and re-examine at a later date.

Figure A1. Placement of Goniometer in Neutral Position of Cervical Spine: Flexion/Extension

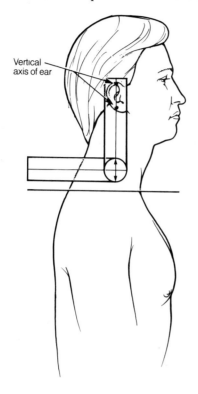

Vertical axis of ear

Figure A2. Flexion of Cervical Spine

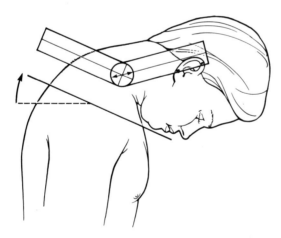

5. Use the *maximum* range of motion and find the percentage of impairment in the appropriate tables, most of which are found in Sections 3.3c to 3.3e of Chapter 3.

6. *Add* all range of motion impairment values for the one region; if the region is ankylosed, use the largest ankylosis impairment value.

7. To obtain the impairment of the whole person due to the impairment of the region of the spine, use the Combined Values Chart to combine the diagnosis-based impairment(s) with the impairment due to limited range of motion or ankylosis.

B. Repeat the above steps for secondarily impaired spinal regions, if applicable.

C. Combine all regional spine impairments into a single impairment of the whole person using the Combined Values Chart.

D. Identify impairments due to neurological deficits (Sections 3.1i and 3.2f) including radiculopathy and peripheral nerve injury, if applicable. Be sure to equate these to impairment of the whole person.

E. Combine all radicular and peripheral nerve injury impairments with the impairment of the whole person due to impairments of the spine.

Note: For the purpose of impairment evaluation, ankylosis is defined as either: (a) complete absence of motion, or (b) planar restriction of motion preventing the subject from reaching the neutral position of motion in that plane. The use of an impairment rating for ankylosis *excludes* the simultaneous use of abnormal motion measurements from the same table. Use Table 50 (p. 79) if radiographic methods are used to determine impairment due to ankylosis.

B. Impairments Due to Specific Disorders of the Spine

Consult Table 49 (p. 73) for the rating of impairments due to specific disorders of the spine.

C. Impairments Due to Range of Motion Abnormalities

Cervical Region—Flexion and Extension Abnormal Motion

1. Place the patient in the neutral position (Figure A1).

2. Center the goniometer (Figure A1), with its base in line with the superior border of the larynx (C5) and its arm extended vertically along skin marks on the ear. Record the goniometer reading.

3. Flexion: With the patient bending the head as far forward as possible (Figure A2), follow the range of motion with the goniometer arm. Keep the goniometer arm parallel to a line between skin marks. Note that shoulder motion moves the "stable" arm of the goniometer. Record the angle that subtends the arc of motion.

4. Extension: Starting from the neutral position with the patient bending the head as far backward as possible (Figure A3), follow the range of motion with the goniometer arm. Keep the goniometer arm parallel to a line between skin marks. Record the angle that subtends the arc of motion.

5. Consult the Abnormal Motion Section of Table 51 (p. 81) to determine the impairment of the whole person.

Example: 30° active flexion from neutral position (0°) is equivalent to 1% impairment of the whole person.

6. *Add* the impairment values contributed by flexion and extension. Their sum is the impairment of the whole person that is contributed by flexion and extension abnormalities of the cervical region.

Ankylosis

1. Place the goniometer base as if measuring the neutral position (Figure A1). Measure the deviation from the neutral position with the goniometer arm and record the reading.

2. Consult the Ankylosis Section of Table 51 (p. 81) to determine the impairment of the whole person.

Example: A cervical region with ankylosis at 30° flexion is equivalent to 23% impairment of the whole person.
    Consult Table 50 (p. 79) if radiographic methods are chosen to determine impairment due to ankylosis.

Cervical Region—Lateral Flexion
Abnormal Motion

1. Place the patient in the neutral position (Figure A4). Note the lateral extension or abduction of the arms to steady the shoulders. Place a skin mark over the T1 spinous process.

2. Center the goniometer over the back of the neck (Figure A4), with lower arm on the T1 skin mark and the goniometer axis along midline of the neck.

3. Right lateral flexion: Starting from the neutral position with the patient bending the neck to the right as far as possible (Figure A5), follow the range of motion with the goniometer arms. Note that shoulder motion moves the "stable" arm of the goniometer which is kept perpendicular to the T1 skin mark while the upper arm follows the occiput. Record the angle that subtends the arc of motion.

Figure A3. Extension of Cervical Spine

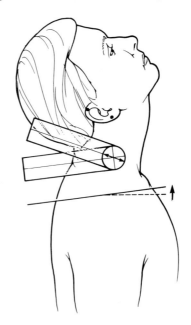

Figure A4. Placement of Goniometer in Neutral Position of Cervical Spine Lateral Flexion

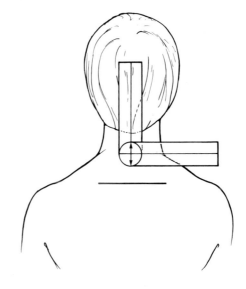

Figure A5. Right Lateral Flexion of Cervical Spine·

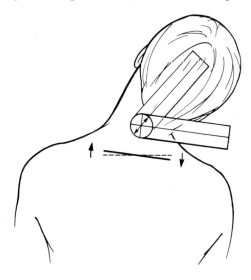

Figure A6. Placement of Goniometer in Neutral Position of Cervical Rotation

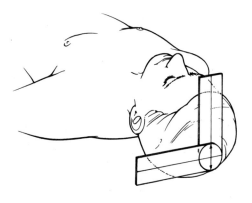

Figure A7. Left Rotation of Cervical Spine

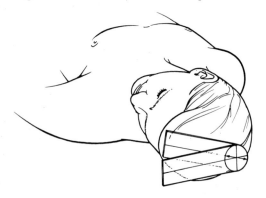

4. Left lateral flexion: Starting from the neutral position with the patient bending the neck to the left as far as possible, follow the range of motion with the goniometer arm. Note that shoulder motion moves the "stable" arm of the goniometer. Record the angle that subtends the arc of motion.

5. Consult the Abnormal Motion Section of Table 52 (p. 83) to determine the impairment of the whole person.

Example: 30° active left lateral flexion from neutral position (0°) is equivalent to 1% impairment of the whole person.

6. *Add* the impairment values contributed by left lateral flexion and right lateral flexion. Their sum represents the impairment of the whole person that is contributed by abnormal lateral flexion of the cervical region.

Ankylosis

1. Place the goniometer base as if measuring the neutral position (Figure A4). Measure the deviation from the neutral position with the goniometer arm and record the reading.

2. Consult the Ankylosis Section of Table 52 (p. 83) for the cervical region to determine the impairment of the whole person.

Example: A cervical region with ankylosis at 30° right lateral flexion is equivalent to 25% impairment of the whole person.

Consult Table 50 (p. 79) if radiographic methods are chosen to determine impairment due to ankylosis.

Cervical Region—Rotation
Abnormal Motion

1. Place the patient in the neutral position (Figure A6) while supine; place the goniometer in the coronal plane at the crown of the head.

2. With patient rotating the head to the right and left as far as possible (Figure A7), record the range of motion in each direction.

3. Consult the Abnormal Motion Section of Table 53 (p. 83) to determine the impairment of the whole person.

Example: 20° active left rotation from neutral position (0°) is equivalent to 3% impairment of the whole person.

4. *Add* the impairment values contributed by left rotation and right rotation. Their sum is the impairment of the whole person that is contributed by abnormal rotation of the cervical region.

Ankylosis

1. Estimate by the position of the chin the angle at which the cervical region is ankylosed.

2. Consult the Ankylosis Section of Table 53 (p. 83) to determine the impairment of the whole person.

Example: A cervical region with ankylosis at 20° right rotation is equivalent to 20% impairment of the whole person.

      Consult Table 50 (p. 79) if radiographic methods are chosen to determine impairment due to ankylosis.

Thoracolumbar Region—Flexion and Extension Abnormal Motion

1. Place the patient in the neutral position (Figure A8).

2. Center the goniometer axis at the midlumbar level (Figure A8). Record the goniometer reading with the upper arm parallel to T12 and the lower arm parallel to the skin mark over the sacral midpoint.

3. Flexion: With patient bending as far forward as possible (Figure A9), follow the range of motion. Note that the lower, "stable" arm of the goniometer moves as well as the upper. Record the angle that subtends the arc of motion keeping both arms parallel to the T12 and sacral skin marks.

4. Extension: Starting from the neutral position with the patient bending as far backward as possible, follow the range of motion with the goniometer arm. Record the angle that subtends the arc of motion.

5. Consult the Abnormal Motion Section of Table A1 to determine the impairment of the whole person.

Example: 20° active flexion from neutral position (0°) is equivalent to 7% impairment of the whole person.

6. *Add* the impairment values contributed by flexion and extension. Their sum represents the impairment of the whole person that is contributed by flexion and extension abnormalities of the thoracolumbar region.

Figure A8. Placement of Goniometer in Neutral Position of Thoracolumbar Flexion/Extension

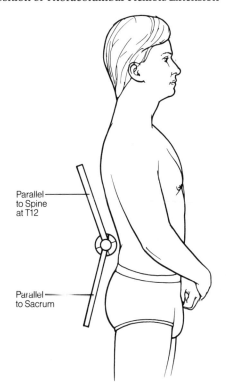

Parallel to Spine at T12

Parallel to Sacrum

Figure A9. Flexion of Thoracolumbar Spine

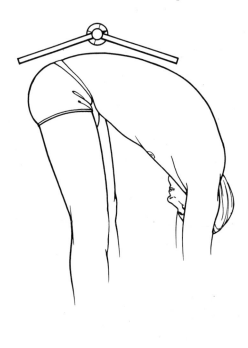

Figure A10. Placement of Goniometer in Neutral Position of Thoracolumbar Lateral Flexion

Figure A11. Left Lateral Flexion of Thoracolumbar Spine

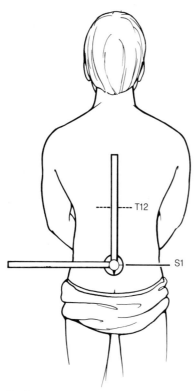

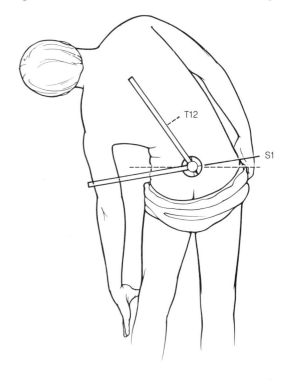

Ankylosis

1. Place the goniometer base as if measuring the neutral position (Figure A8). Measure the deviation from the neutral position with the goniometer arm and record the reading.

2. Consult the Ankylosis Section of Table A1 to determine the impairment of the whole person.

Example: A thoracolumbar region with ankylosis at 20° flexion is equivalent to 24% impairment of the whole person.

      Consult Table 50 (p. 79) if radiographic methods are chosen to determine impairment due to ankylosis.

Thoracolumbar Region—Lateral Flexion Abnormal Motion

1. Place the patient in the neutral position (Figure A10).

2. Center the goniometer with the lower arm over a skin mark over the sacrum and the goniometer axis along the midline of spine (Figure A10). The upper arm should cross a skin mark over the T12 spinous process.

3. Left lateral flexion: With the patient bending to the left as far as possible (Figure A11), follow the range of motion with the goniometer arms. Note that hip motion moves the "stable" arm of the goniometer. Record the angle that subtends the arc of motion keeping the arm perpendicular to the skin marks.

4. Right lateral flexion: Starting from the neutral position with the patient bending to the right as far as possible, follow the range of motion with the goniometer arms. Note that hip motion moves the "stable" arm of the goniometer. Record the angle that subtends the arc of motion.

5. Consult the Abnormal Motion Section of Table 57 (p. 91) to determine the impairment of the whole person.

Example: 10° active left lateral flexion from neutral position (0°) is equivalent to 3% impairment of the whole person.

6. *Add* the impairment values contributed by left lateral flexion and right lateral flexion. Their sum represents impairment of the whole person due to lateral flexion abnormalities of the thoracolumbar region.

Ankylosis

1. Place the goniometer base as if measuring the neutral position (Figure A10). Measure the deviation from the neutral position with the goniometer arm and record the reading.

2. Consult the Ankylosis Section of Table 57 (p. 91) to determine the impairment of the whole person.

Example: A thoracolumbar region with ankylosis at 10° right lateral flexion is equivalent to 10% impairment of the whole person.

Consult Table 50 (p. 79) if radiographic methods are chosen to determine impairment of the whole person.

Thoracolumbar Region—Rotation
Abnormal Motion

Since a goniometer cannot be used to measure thoracolumbar rotation, reproducibility that satisfies validity criteria is impossible. Therefore, rotation is not measured.

Table A1. Impairment Due to Abnormal Motion of the Thoracolumbar Region—Flexion/Extension

Abnormal Motion

Flexion from neutral (0°) position	% Impairment of Whole Person
60°+	0
45°-60°	2
30°-45°	4
15°-30°	7
0°-15°	10

Extension from neutral (0°) position	
25°	0
20°	2
10°	3
15°	5
0°	7

Ankylosis

Region ankylosed at:	% Impairment of Whole Person
0° (neutral position)	20
10°	22
20°	24
30°	27
40°	29
50°	31
60°	34
70°	36
80°	38
90° (full flexion)	40

Region ankylosed at:	
0° (neutral position)	20
10°	27
20°	34
25° (full extension)	40

Chapter 4

The Nervous System

4.0 Introduction

This chapter provides criteria for the evaluation of permanent impairment resulting from dysfunction of the brain, spinal cord, and cranial nerves, and those peripheral nerves not covered in Chapter 3.

Before using the information in this chapter, the reader is urged to review Chapters 1 and 2, which provide a general discussion of the purpose of the *Guides* and of the situations in which they are useful; and which discuss techniques for the evaluation of the subject and for preparation of reports. The report should include the information found in the following outline, which is developed more fully in Chapter 2.

A. Medical Evaluation
1. Narrative history of medical conditions
2. Results of the most recent clinical evaluation
3. Assessment of current clinical status and statement of future plans
4. Diagnoses and clinical impressions
5. Expected date of full or partial recovery

B. Analysis of Findings
1. Impact of medical condition(s) on life activities
2. Explanation for concluding that the medical condition(s) has or has not become static or well-stabilized
3. Explanation for concluding that the individual is or is not likely to suffer from sudden or subtle incapacitation
4. Explanation for concluding that the individual is or is not likely to suffer injury or further impairment by engaging in life activities or by attempting to meet personal, social, and occupational demands

5. Explanation for concluding that accommodations and/or restrictions are or are not warranted

C. Comparison of Results of Analysis with Impairment Criteria
1. Description of clinical findings, and how these findings relate to specific criteria in the chapter
2. Explanation of each percent of impairment rating
3. Summary list of all impairment ratings
4. Overall rating of impairment of the whole person

4.1 The Central Nervous System

Special Considerations: The emphasis in this chapter is upon organic deficits of the central nervous system (CNS) as demonstrated by loss of function. Categories for evaluating impairment are established in the chapter in terms of restrictions or limitations of the patient's ability to perform the activities of daily living and not in terms of specific diagnoses. However, before evaluating or classifying the impairment of any patient, the physician must establish, if possible, an accurate neurological diagnosis.

Evaluation of CNS impairment is difficult because of the complex relationships between the brain and the mind. It is impossible to avoid consideration of associated mental, emotional, and personality processes. When appropriate, Chapter 14 should be used in conjunction with this chapter.

When a patient has clinical findings indicative of both brain and spinal cord impairment, evaluation should be made of each, and the percentages of impairment should be combined by using the Combined Values Chart.

4.1a The Brain

The brain is a central regulatory organ and mediator of voluntary acts that includes areas in which consciousness, sensations, emotions, memory, and judgment are integrated. Permanent impairment can result from various disorders. The effects on the patient with the established disorder provide the criteria by which the permanent impairment is evaluated.

The more common categories of impairment resulting from brain disorders and the order in which they will be discussed are: 1) sensory and motor disturbances; 2) communication disturbances; 3) complex, integrated disturbances of cerebral function; 4) emotional disturbances; 5) disturbances of consciousness; 6) episodic neurological disorders; and 7) sleep and arousal disorders.

More than one category of impairment may result from brain disorders. In such cases the various degrees of impairment from the several categories are not added or combined, but the largest value, or greatest percentage of the seven categories of impairment, is used to represent the impairment for all of the types.

For example, a patient was determined to have a communication impairment of 35%, a complex integrated cerebral-function impairment of 15%, an emotional disturbance resulting in an impairment rating of 30%, and a disturbance of consciousness resulting in an impairment rating of 5%. The patient's impairment of brain function would be rated at 35% of the whole person and not at the sum of the values, 85%, or at "the combined value" of 64%.

Sensory and Motor Disturbances

A patient seldom has an isolated sensory or motor disturbance if the brain is involved. Evaluation of such disturbances is based on their ultimate effects on the activities of daily living. In evaluating the degree of impairment the physician should determine whether the disturbance is unilateral or bilateral and whether the preferred side is affected.

When *sensory* disturbances are evaluated, consideration should be given to: 1) pain and dysesthesias; 2) disorders in the recognition of the size, shape, and form of objects (astereognosis); 3) disturbances of two-point and position sense; 4) paresthesias of central origin; and 5) disturbances that might be identified by more elaborate testing, such as disorders of body image.

Organic lesions involving the optic nerve, optic chiasm, optic tracts, optic radiations, or the optic cortex may result in disturbances in the visual fields, such as homonymous hemianopsia, homonymous quadrantanopsia (superior and inferior), and bitemporal hemianopsia. Such lesions should be evaluated in terms of loss of the visual fields as described in Chapter 8. Lesions that cause central scotomata are, of course, manifested by disturbances in central vision and are evaluated as disturbances of central visual acuity.

It is recognized that certain isolated disturbances, such as thalamic pain, phantom limb sensations, or other subjective disturbances of the body image, may result in impairment. Evaluation of the effects of such disturbances calls for critical judgment on the part of examiners.

Motor disorders include hemiparesis and hemiplegias and variations thereof. The most common condition is hemiparesis, which may be of variable severity and responsible for different ratings of impairment, depending on how the patient's daily activities are affected. In addition, there is a large list of motor disorders that includes, but is not limited to: 1) involuntary movement, such as tremor, athetosis, chorea, or hemiballism; 2) disturbances of tone and posture; 3) various forms of akinesia and bradykinesia, such as Parkinsonism, in which voluntary and semiautomatic movement may be severely impaired; 4) impairment of associated and cooperative (synergistic) movements, as in certain diseases of the basal ganglia; 5) complex manual and gait disturbances, including the ataxias, especially those of frontal and cerebellar origin; and 6) motor seizure disorders, including generalized, focal, akinetic, and myoclonic seizures.

The *evaluation* of sensory and motor impairments due to brain disorders should be based on the patient's ability to perform various functions, for example, standing, walking, using the upper extremities, controlling bladder and bowel, breathing, and speaking. Methods of evaluating these functions are described in sections of this chapter dealing with the cranial nerves or spinal cord, or in other chapters of the *Guides*. When more than one function is involved, the percentage of impairment is derived by combining appropriate values by using the Combined Values Chart.

Language Disturbances

Impairment of speaking that involves the structures of the brain stem is discussed in detail in Chapter 9, and also briefly in the cranial nerves section of this chapter. Here the concern is with the central mechanism for language comprehension, storage, and production, which is mediated by the brain, and disturbance of which has to do with the clinical conditions known as aphasia and dysphasia.

Forms of disturbed communication, such as agraphia, alexia, or acalculia, are reflected in the following criteria for evaluating the impairment of communication due to brain damage. These criteria consider not only the comprehension and understanding of language by the patient, but also the patient's ability to produce discernible and appropriate language symbols.

Description	% Impairment of the Whole Person
1. Minimal disturbance in comprehension and production of language symbols of daily living	0-15
2. Moderate impairment in comprehension and production of language symbols for daily living	20-45
3. *Cannot* comprehend language symbols, therefore has an unintelligible or inappropriate production of language for daily living	50-90
4. *Cannot* comprehend *or* produce language symbols sufficient for daily living	95

Disturbances of Complex, Integrated Cerebral Functions

Disturbances of these functions constitute the well-known organic brain syndrome. The resulting deficits may include defects in orientation; ability to abstract or understand concepts; memory, both immediate and remote; judgment; ability to initiate decisions and perform planned action; and acceptable social behavior.

The restrictions placed on patients with established organic brain syndromes provide criteria by which the permanent impairment may be evaluated. These criteria are:

Description	% Impairment of the Whole Person
1. There is a degree of impairment of complex integrated cerebral functions, but there is ability to carry out most activities of daily living as well as before onset	5-15
2. There is a degree of impairment of complex integrated cerebral functions such that daily activities need some supervision and/or direction	20-45
3. There is a degree of impairment of complex integrated cerebral functions that limits daily activities to directed care under confinement at home or in other domicile	50-90
4. There is such a severe degree of impairment of complex integrated cerebral functions that the individual is unable to care for self in any situation or manner	95

Emotional Disturbances

Emotional disturbances may be one of the results of organic brain damage. These disturbances may range from irritability to outbursts of severe rage and aggression, or at the other extreme, to an absence of normal emotional response. The abnormalities include inappropriate euphoria, depression, degrees of fluctuation of emotional state, impairment of normal emotional interactions with others, involuntary laughing and crying, akinetic mutism, and other disturbances in the emotional sphere. The criteria for evaluating such disturbances are:

Description	% Impairment of the Whole Person
1. There is mild to moderate emotional disturbance under unusual stress	5-15
2. There is mild to moderate emotional disturbance under ordinary stress	20-45
3. There is moderate to severe emotional disturbance under ordinary to minimal stress, which requires sheltering	50-90
4. There is severe emotional disturbance that continually endangers self or others	95

Consciousness Disturbances

Disturbances of consciousness that are not covered in the episodic disorders or in the sleep and arousal disorders, which are described below, include organic confusional state (hyper- or hypoactive), stupor (poorly organized responses to noxious stimuli), and coma (no response).

Determination of grades of impairment of consciousness may be made by judging the patient's reaction to noxious stimuli; this may vary from a well-organized reaction to none at all.

Description	% Impairment of the Whole Person
1. Neurological disorder results in mild alteration in the state of consciousness	5-35
2. Neurological disorder results in moderate alteration in the state of consciousness	40-70
3. Neurological disorder results in a state of stupor	75-90
4. Neurological disorder results in a state of coma	95

Episodic Neurological Disorders

Episodic neurological disorders include, but are not limited to, syncope, epilepsy, and the convulsive disorders. Criteria for evaluating such impairments are based on the frequency, severity, and duration of attacks as they affect the patient's performance of the activities of daily living. These criteria are:

Description	% Impairment of the Whole Person
1. An episodic neurological disorder is of slight severity and under such control that most of the activities of daily living can be performed	5-15
2. An episodic neurological disorder is of such severity as to interfere moderately with the activities of daily living	20-45
3. An episodic neurological disorder is of such severity and constancy as to limit activities to supervised or protected care or confinement	50-90
4. An episodic neurological disorder is of such severity and constancy as to totally incapacitate the individual in terms of daily living	95

Sleep and Arousal Disorders

The disorders of sleep and arousal include such syndromes as the disorders of initiating and maintaining sleep, or insomnia; disorders of excessive somnolence, including those associated with sleep-induced respiratory impairment; disorders of the sleep-wake schedule; and dysfunctions associated with sleep, sleep stages, or parasomnias.

The categories of impairment that may arise from sleep disorders relate to: 1) the nervous system, with reduced daytime attention, concentration, and other cognitive capacities; 2) mental and behavioral factors, including depression, irritability, interpersonal difficulties, and social problems; and 3) the cardiovascular system, with systemic and pulmonary hypertension, cardiac enlargement and congestive heart failure, cardiac arrhythmias, and polycythemia.

In assessing permanent impairment due to sleep and arousal disorders, the physician must complete a thorough diagnostic evaluation and allow time for appropriate treatment to take effect. The physician should then evaluate the permanent impairment of each affected organ system and combine the impairment ratings using the Combined Values Chart. The criteria for the cardiovascular and for the mental and behavioral impairments are found in Chapters 6 and 14, respectively. The criteria for the central nervous system impairment due to excessive daytime sleepiness are:

Description	% Impairment of the Whole Person
1. There is reduced daytime alertness due to sleepiness or sleep episodes, or disturbed nocturnal sleep affecting complex integrated cerebral functions, but ability remains to carry out most activities of daily living	5-15
2. There is reduced daytime alertness due to sleepiness or sleep episodes, or disturbed nocturnal sleep affecting complex integrated cerebral functions that requires some supervision to carry out activities of daily living	20-45
3. There is reduced daytime alertness due to sleepiness or sleep episodes, or disturbed nocturnal sleep that significantly limits activities of daily living and requires supervision by caretakers	50-90
4. There is such a severe reduction of daytime alertness due to sleepiness or sleep episodes or disturbed nocturnal sleep, that activities of daily living are severely limited so as to cause the patient to be unable to care for self in any situation or manner	95

4.1b The Spinal Cord

The spinal cord is concerned with sensory, motor, and visceral functions. Permanent impairment can result from various disorders affecting these functions. The restrictions placed upon the patient who has an established spinal cord disorder provide criteria by which the permanent impairment may be evaluated.

The more common impairments resulting from spinal cord disorders and the order in which they will be discussed, involve: 1) station and gait; 2) use of upper extremities; 3) respiration; 4) urinary bladder function; 5) anorectal function; and 6) sexual function.

Sensory disturbances, including the loss of touch, pain, temperature, vibration, or position senses, and paresthesias and phantoms, may be a part of spinal cord disorders. Autonomic (vegetative) disorders, such as disturbance of sweating, circulation, and temperature regulation, may also occur in the course of spinal cord disorders. The rating of impairment due to such sensory disturbances or autonomic disorders should be determined by the amount of functional impairment according to the criteria given below.

Accompanying disorders, such as trophic lesions, urinary calculi, osteoporosis, nutritional disturbances, infections, and reactive psychological states may occur. The degree to which any of these augment impairment from a dysfunction of the spinal cord should be based on the criteria given in the chapters of the *Guides* that deal with those disorders.

Station and Gait

The ability to stand and walk provides criteria for evaluating spinal cord disorders affecting the lower extremities. These criteria are:

Description	% Impairment of the Whole Person
1. Patient can rise to a standing position and can walk *but* has difficulty with elevations, grades, steps, and distances	5-20
2. Patient can rise to a standing position and can walk with difficulty *but* is limited to level surfaces. There is variability as to the distance the patient can walk	25-35
3. Patient can rise to a standing position and can maintain it with difficulty *but* cannot walk	40-60
4. Patient cannot stand without a prosthesis or the help of others	65

Use of Upper Extremities

Because the basic tasks of everyday living are more dependent upon the preferred upper extremity, dysfunction or loss of the preferred extremity results in greater impairment than impairment of the nonpreferred extremity.

Evaluation of impairment of the preferred extremity should be subject to periodic review, because the originally nonpreferred extremity sometimes becomes as accomplished as the originally preferred extremity. The criteria for the evaluation of spinal cord impairment affecting *ONLY* one upper extremity are:

Description	% Impairment of the Whole Person	
	Preferred Extremity	Nonpreferred Extremity
1. Can use the involved extremity for self care, grasping, and holding *but* has difficulty with digital dexterity	5-10	0-5
2. Can use the involved extremity for self care, can grasp and hold objects with difficulty, *but* has no digital dexterity	15-25	10-15
3. Can use the involved extremity *but* has difficulty with self care activities	30-35	20-25
4. *Cannot* use the involved extremity for self care	40-60	30-40

When the spinal cord disorder affects both upper extremities, the resulting impairment to the whole person is greater than a simple combination of the values of "preferred" and "nonpreferred." The criteria for evaluating spinal cord disorders affecting both upper extremities are:

Description	% Impairment of the Whole Person
1. Can use both upper extremities for self care, grasping, and holding *but* has difficulty with digital dexterity	5-15
2. Can use both upper extremities for self care, can grasp and hold objects with difficulty *but* has no digital dexterity	20-40
3. Can use both upper extremities *but* has difficulty with self care activities	45-80
4. *Cannot* use upper extremities	85

Respiration

Respiration in this guide is limited to the individual's ability to perform the act of breathing. Criteria for evaluating the limitations placed on the patient with respiratory difficulty due to spinal cord disorders are:

Description	% Impairment of the Whole Person
1. Capable of spontaneous respiration *but* has difficulty in activities of daily living that require extra exertion	5-20

2. Capable of spontaneous respiration *but* of a degree that restricts patient to sitting, standing, or limited ambulation   25-50

3. Capable of spontaneous respiration *but* of a degree that limits patient to bed existence   75-90

4. No capacity for spontaneous respiration   95

Urinary Bladder Function

The ability to control bladder emptying provides the criteria for evaluating permanent bladder impairment resulting from spinal cord disorders. These criteria are:

Description	% Impairment of the Whole Person
1. Patient has varying degree of voluntary bladder control *but* is impaired by urgency	5-10
2. Patient has good bladder reflex activity *but* no voluntary control (limited capacity with intermittent emptying times)	15-20
3. Patient's bladder has poor reflex activity (intermittent dribbling) and no voluntary control	25-35
4. Patient has no reflex or voluntary control of the bladder (continuous dribbling)	40-60

Anorectal Function

The ability to control anorectal emptying provides criteria for evaluating the permanent impairment resulting from spinal cord disorders. These criteria are:

Description	% Impairment of the Whole Person
1. Anorectum has reflex regulation *but* only limited voluntary control	0-5
2. Anorectum has reflex regulation *but* no voluntary control	10-15
3. Anorectum has no reflex regulation and no voluntary control	20-25

Sexual Function

Sexual capability and awareness of sexual function provide the criteria for evaluating permanent impairment resulting from spinal cord disorders. These criteria are:

Description	% Impairment of the Whole Person (Ages 40-65 Years)
1. Sexual function is possible *but* with varying degree of difficulty of erection or ejaculation in males, or awareness in both sexes	5-10
2. Reflex sexual function is possible *but* there is no awareness	10-15
3. There is no sexual function	20

These values may be increased by 50% of the given value for those below the age of 40 years, and decreased by 50% for those over the age of 65 years. For instance, in a 25-year-old man, a 50% increase of a 20% impairment would yield a 30% impairment of function.

Table 1 summarizes the percentage values for the impairment of the spinal cord and brain.

4.1c The Cranial Nerves

The cranial nerves are discussed in this chapter by their respective names. Reference also is made to them in other chapters dealing with specific organs, such as the eye and the ear.

Twelve pairs of cranial nerves emerge from the base of the brain. These are identified by Roman numerals I through XII, and by their names. Some of the nerves are mixed, having sensory, autonomic, and motor fibers, while others have only one or two types of fibers.

Ratings of impairments that involve these nerves are made as follows:

I-Olfactory: The olfactory nerve is concerned with the sense of smell. In cases of complete bilateral involvement with total inability to detect any odors (anosmia), the impairment is placed at 3% of the whole person. Parosmia, or perversion of the sense of smell, may be sufficiently disturbing to constitute an impairment, and the physician should consider that fact when evaluating olfactory nerve function. The value of 3% for anosmia would be combined with the value of any other permanent impairment of the patient.

II-Optic: The optic nerve is concerned with the sense of vision. Impairment resulting from the complete destruction of an optic nerve, which causes total loss of vision in one eye, is rated at 24% of the whole person. Impairment of the whole person from complete loss of both optic nerves, which causes total blindness, would be 85%. Evaluation of partial impairments of the optic nerve is considered in Chapter 8.

Table 1. Spinal Cord and Brain Impairment Values

A. Spinal Cord and/or Brain	% Impairment of the Whole Person			B. Brain	% Impairment of the Whole Person
Station and gait				**Language disturbances**	
Can stand but walks with difficulty	5-20			Mild difficulties	0-15
Can stand but walks only on the level	25-35			Comprehends but cannot produce	
Can stand but cannot walk	40-60			sufficient or appropriate language	20-45
Can neither stand nor walk	65			Cannot comprehend or produce	
Use of upper extremities	(Preferred Extremity)	(Nonpreferred Extremity)	(Both)	intelligible or appropriate language	50-90
				Cannot comprehend or produce language	95
Some difficulty with digital dexterity	5-10	0- 5	5-15	**Complex integrated cerebral function disturbances**	
Has no digital dexterity	15-25	10-15	20-40	Can carry out daily living tasks	5-15
Has difficulty with self care	30-35	20-25	45-80	Needs some supervision	20-45
Cannot carry out self care	40-60	30-40	85	Needs confinement	50-90
Respiration				Cannot care for self	95
Difficulty only where extra exertion required	5-20			**Emotional disturbances**	
Restricted to limited ambulation	25-50			Only present under unusual stress	5-15
Restricted to bed	75-90			Present in mild to moderate	
Has no spontaneous respiration	95			degree under ordinary stress	20-45
Urinary bladder function				Present in moderate to severe	
Impairment in form of urgency	5-10			degree under ordinary stress	50-90
Good reflex activity without voluntary control	15-20			Severe degree; continually endangers self or others	95
Poor reflex activity and no voluntary control	25-35			**Consciousness disturbances**	
No reflex or voluntary control	40-60			Mild alterations	5-35
Anorectal function				Moderate alterations	40-70
Limited voluntary control	0- 5			Stupor	75-90
Has reflex regulation but no voluntary control	10-15			Coma	95
No reflex regulation or voluntary control	20-25			**Episodic neurological disorders**	
Sexual function	age— (below 40)	(40-65)	(over 65)	Slight interference with daily living	5-15
				Moderate interference with daily living	20-45
				Requires constant supervision or confinement	50-90
Mild difficulties	8-15	5-10	3- 5	Totally incapacitated for daily living	95
Reflex function possible but no awareness	15-23	10-15	5- 8	**Sleep and arousal disorders**	
No sexual function	30	20	10	Slight interference with daily activities	5-15
				Requires some supervision to carry out daily activities	20-45
				Requires supervision of care by caretakers	50-90
				Patient unable to care for self	95

III-Oculomotor; IV-Trochlear; and VI-Abducens: These nerves are responsible for the motility of the eyeballs and for regulating the size of the pupil.

If there is loss of any one of these nerves or of combinations of them, with resulting inability to perceive a single image (permanent diplopia), the condition is equivalent to the loss of vision in one eye and the impairment is set at 24% of the whole person. This is true as well in patients who can correct the affected eye by covering the other eye.

In instances where loss of function of the eyeball musculature secondary to nerve involvement requires special positioning of the head for effective vision, consideration should be given to combining appropriate values for impairment to locomotion, station, and so forth. If partial visual impairment must be evaluated, Chapter 8 should be consulted.

V-Trigeminal: This is a mixed nerve with sensory fibers to the face, cornea, anterior scalp, nasal and oral cavities, tongue, and the supratentorial dura mater; and with motor fibers to the muscles of mastication.

Sensation in the area served by the trigeminal nerve, including the cornea, is tested with the usual techniques of evaluating tactile appreciation and pain. Loss of sensation on one side results in some dysfunction, and this should be rated at 3% to 10% impairment of the whole person. Bilateral trigeminal sensory loss, which is rare, is more disturbing, and the impairment of the whole person in that instance would be 20% to 35%. The impairment rating for loss of sensation of the trigeminal nerve is to be combined with any impairment rating for pain and for motor loss.

Intractable unilateral or bilateral trigeminal neuralgia, "tic douloureux," may entail impairment ranging from 10% to 50% of the whole person, depending on the frequency and severity of the attacks.

Impairment from the pain of "atypical trigeminal neuralgia" is to be made on the basis of how much the neuralgia interferes with daily activities of the patient and would be in the range of 0% to 20% impairment of the whole person.

Motor involvement of the trigeminal nerve not only affects chewing, but also causes difficulty in speaking and swallowing. This is particularly true when there is bilateral damage. Complete loss of the motor function of one trigeminal nerve would be rated at 3% to 5% impairment of the whole person. Complete bilateral motor loss would result in 30% to 45% impairment of the whole person, depending on the difficulty with speech and swallowing that the patient experiences.

Methods of evaluating speech impairment and ability to swallow are set forth in greater detail in Chapter 9.

VII-Facial: This is a mixed nerve with a sensory component carrying tactile sensory supply to a part of the external ear, the external auditory canal, tympanic membrane, soft palate and adjacent pharynx, and taste fibers to the anterior two-thirds of the tongue; motor fibers to the muscles of expression and to the accessory muscles of mastication and deglutition; and special fibers to the lacrimal and salivary glands.

Sensory loss from damage to one or even both facial nerves would not interfere with the patient's performance of daily activities, and in that instance no impairment rating would be given. Since taste also is mediated by the IX nerve, it is unlikely that even loss of both facial nerves would result in a complete loss of taste. If total loss of taste were to occur, the rating would be 3% impairment of the whole person.

Unilateral motor loss of the facial nerve causes the individual to have some difficulty with facial expression, blinking, chewing, and the control of salivation. Also the face is distorted. The permanent impairment in complete unilateral motor loss is 10% to 15% impairment of the whole person.

Bilateral motor loss of the facial nerve constitutes a more severe handicap, and the impairment of the whole person would be 30% to 45%. These values are established on the basis of the difficulties in food-taking and speech, and are correlated with impairment values for the IX, X, XI, and XII cranial nerves and with evaluations made in Chapter 9.

VIII-Auditory: This so-called single nerve actually consists of two separate components, a cochlear nerve that is concerned with hearing, and a vestibular nerve that affects equilibrium.

Unilateral loss of hearing is much less of an impairment than is bilateral, or total loss. Complete loss of one cochlear nerve carries a rating of impairment of 6% of the whole person, and complete bilateral loss of hearing has a rating of 35%. Tinnitus alone does not result in permanent impairment. However, tinnitus in the presence of a unilateral hearing loss may impair speech discrimination, and 3% to 5% should be added to the rating for the hearing loss. The procedure for evaluating hearing loss is given in Chapter 9.

The total loss of one vestibular nerve rarely results in permanent disturbance of equilibrium, and therefore, no percentage of permanent impairment is given. Total bilateral loss of the vestibular nerves is usually compensated to some degree by other neural mechanisms. The permanent impairment of the whole person may range from 0% to 25%, depending on the extent of such compensation. The full classification for vestibular impairment is given in Chapter 9.

IX-Glossopharyngeal; X-Vagus; and XI-Cranial Accessory: The glossopharyngeal and the vagus are mixed nerves that supply sensory fibers chiefly to the posterior part of the tongue, pharynx, larynx, and trachea. Motor fibers innervate the pharynx and the larynx. Autonomic fibers supply the thoracic and upper abdominal viscera.

The cranial accessory nerves assist the vagus in supplying some of the muscles of the larynx.

Sensory impairment of the glossopharyngeal and vagus nerves is difficult to evaluate and should be judged by how it contributes to the impairment of swallowing, breathing, speaking, and visceral function.

The glossopharyngeal nerves may be the source of severe neuralgia. This, however, is usually curable. In those rare cases where residual impairment results, the physician should assign a value that is consistent with other established values and that is based on the severity of the neuralgia and the degree to which it interferes with the daily activities of the patient.

The impairment of swallowing due to disorders of one or of a combination of these nerves may be evaluated as follows:

Description	% Impairment of the Whole Person
1. The diet is restricted to semi-solid foods or to soft foods	5-10
2. The diet is limited to liquid foods	20-30
3. The taking of food is by tube or by gastrostomy	40-60

The impairment of speech due to disorders of one or of combinations of these nerves is discussed in detail in Chapter 9.

XII-Hypoglossal: This is the motor nerve to the tongue. Unilateral loss of the function of this nerve does not ordinarily result in significant impairment.

Bilateral loss results in impairment of the functions of swallowing and speech. Evaluation of these impairments is based on the same criteria as for the glossopharyngeal, vagus, and cranial accessory nerves.

Table 2 is a summary of the percentage values for the impairments of the cranial nerves.

4.2 The Peripheral Spinal Nerves of the Head and Neck, Trunk, Inguinal Region, and Perineum

The peripheral spinal nerves constitute an intricate conduction system that serves as the conductor of neural impulses traveling in both directions between the spinal cord and other tissues of the body and through which many important bodily functions are regulated. Impairments due to disorders of the peripheral spinal nerves that innervate the head and neck, trunk, inguinal region, and perineum are described in this section. The peripheral nerves innervating the extremities are discussed in Chapter 3.

Functionally, the peripheral spinal nerves can be divided into three main groups of fibers: 1) sensory (afferent) fibers that carry impulses arising from various receptors in the skin, muscles, tendons, ligaments, bones, and joints to the central nervous system; 2) motor (efferent) fibers, the large alpha motor neuron fibers conducting impulses from the spinal cord to skeletal muscle fibers, and the small gamma motor neuron fibers carrying impulses to muscle spindles for feedback control; and 3) autonomic fibers, which are efferent and are concerned with the control of smooth muscles and glandular activities.

In evaluating peripheral nerve function, it is important to recognize two important concepts: 1) the metabolism of peripheral nerves occurs primarily in the cell body (neuron), either in the spinal cord, brainstem, or ganglions, and the peripheral parts of the nerves are dependent on neuronal function and on the process of axoplasmic transport of essential factors between the cell body and the nerve terminals; and 2) there are "trophic" effects of interactions between nerve fibers and other cells, which are illustrated by skeletal muscle atrophy following immobilization in spite of intact peripheral nerves, or "disuse atrophy."

Disorders of autonomic nerve function may impair an organ or body system. The chapter that is concerned with the body system affected should be consulted when determining the degree of impairment due to these disorders.

Permanent impairment related to a peripheral spinal nerve may be described as an alteration of sensory or motor function that has become static or well stabilized after an appropriate course of medical management and rehabilitation therapy for a period of time sufficient to permit regeneration and other physiologic recovery.

Method of Evaluation

In order to evaluate impairment resulting from the effects of peripheral spinal nerve lesions, it is necessary to determine the extent of loss of function due to: 1) sensory deficit, pain, or discomfort; and 2) loss of muscle strength and motor control of muscles. Although atrophy, vasomotor and trophic changes, reflex changes, and certain characteristic deformities are also effects of peripheral nerve lesions, it is not necessary to evaluate all of these separately, because they would be reflected in the sensory disturbance, and loss of muscle strength or control.

Table 2. Values for Impairment of Cranial Nerves

	% Impairment of the Whole Person
I. Olfactory	
Complete unilateral loss	0
Complete bilateral loss	3
II. Optic	
Complete unilateral loss	24
Complete bilateral loss	85
III,IV, VI. Oculomotor, Trochlear, Abducens (Alone or in Combinations)	
Complete loss of ability to perceive single image, but with a condition which can be corrected by covering one eye and then having clear vision	24
V. Trigeminal	
Complete unilateral sensory loss	3-10
Complete bilateral sensory loss	20-35
Intractable typical trigeminal neuralgia, or tic douloureux	10-50
Atypical facial neuralgia	0-20
Complete unilateral motor loss	3- 5
Complete bilateral motor loss	30-45
VII. Facial	
Complete loss of taste (unlikely)	3
Complete unilateral paralysis	10-15
Complete bilateral paralysis	30-45
VIII. Auditory refer to chapter 9	
IX, X, XI. Glossopharyngeal, Vagus, Cranial Accessory	
Swallowing impairment due to any one or two combinations of these nerves	
diet restricted to semi-solids	5-10
diet restricted to liquids	20-30
diet by tube feeding or gastrostomy	40-60
Speech refer to chapter 9	
XII. Hypoglossal	
Unilateral paralysis	0
Bilateral paralysis	
Swallowing impairment	
diet restricted to semi-solids	5-10
diet restricted to liquids	20-30
diet by tube feeding or gastrostomy	40-60
Speech impairment refer to chapter 9	

Table 3. Grading Scheme and Procedure for Determining Impairment of Affected Body Part Due to Pain, Discomfort, or Loss of Sensation

Description	Grade
a. Grading Scheme	
1. No loss of sensation or no spontaneous abnormal sensations	0%
2. Decreased sensation with or without pain, which is forgotten during activity	5-25%
3. Decreased sensation with or without pain, which interferes with activity	30-60%
4. Decreased sensation with or without pain, which may prevent activity (minor or causalgia)	65-80%
5. Decreased sensation with severe pain, which may cause outcries as well as prevent activity (major causalgia)	85-95%
6. Decreased sensation with pain, which may prevent all activity	100%
b. Procedure	
1. Identify the area of involvement, using the dermatome chart.	
2. Identify the nerve(s) that innervate the area(s).	
3. Find the value for maximum loss of function of the nerve(s) due to pain or loss of sensation or pain, using the appropriate table.*	
4. Grade the degree of decreased sensation or pain according to the grading scheme above.	
5. Multiply the value of the nerve (from the appropriate table) by the degree of decreased sensation or pain.	

*Table 5 for nerves to the head and neck; Table 6 for thoracic nerves; Table 7 for nerves to the inguinal region and the perineum.

Restrictions of motion and ankyloses may result from peripheral spinal nerve impairments. Consideration was given to such impairments when the percentage values set forth in this section were derived. Therefore, if an impairment results strictly from a peripheral nerve lesion, the evaluator *should not* apply the impairment values from both Chapter 3 and from this chapter, because this would result in a duplication of the impairment rating. However, when restricted motion or ankylosis exists but cannot be attributed to sensory involvement or muscle weakness, then values from Chapter 3 may be combined with values of this chapter using the Combined Values Chart.

It is necessary for the physician to establish as accurately as possible the anatomic distribution of sensory and/or motor loss and verify that the distribution relates to a specific peripheral nerve or nerves before determining the percentage of permanent impairment. The diagnosis is based firmly on the patient's signs and symptoms. With a carefully obtained history, a thorough medical and neurological examination, and appropriate laboratory aids, the physician should characterize the pain, discomfort, and loss of sensation occurring in the areas innervated by the affected nerve, and also the degree of muscle strength and fine motor control that has been lost.

Pain: In evaluating pain that is associated with peripheral spinal nerve disorders, the physician should consider: 1) how the pain interferes with the individual's performance of the activities of daily living; 2) to what extent the pain follows the defined anatomical pathways of the root, plexus, or peripheral nerve; 3) to what extent the description of the pain indicates that it is caused by the peripheral spinal nerve abnormality; that is, the pain should correspond to other kinds of disturbances of the involved nerve or nerve root.

Complaints of pain that cannot be characterized as above are not considered within the scope of this chapter (for a discussion of categories of pain and their characterization, see Appendix B). The examiner must determine whether the sensory or motor deficit is due to involvement of one or more peripheral nerves in order to use the appropriate table (Table 5 for nerves to the head and neck, Table 6 for thoracic nerves, Table 7 for nerves to the inguinal region and perineum).

A grading scheme and procedure for determining impairment of a body part that is affected by pain, discomfort, or loss of sensation are found in Table 3.

Strength: Involvement of peripheral spinal nerves or nerve roots may lead to paralysis or to weakness of the muscles supplied by them. In the case of weakness, the patient often will attempt to substitute stronger muscles to accomplish the desired motion. Thus, the physician should have an understanding of the muscles that are involved in the performance of the various movements of the body and its parts.

Muscle testing, including tests for strength, duration, repetition of contraction, and function, aids evaluation of the functions of specific nerves. Muscle testing is based on the principle of gravity and resistance, that is, the ability to raise a segment of the body through its range of motion against gravity and to hold the segment at the end of its range of motion against resistance.

A grading scheme and procedure for determining impairment of a body part that is affected by loss of strength are found in Table 4.

After the individual values for loss of function due to sensory deficit, pain, or discomfort, and loss of function due to loss of strength have been determined, the impairment to the part of the body or to the whole person is calculated by combining the values using the Combined Values Chart.

Determination of Impairment

The order in which permanent impairment of the peripheral spinal nerves will be discussed is: 1) the spinal nerve roots; 2) the spinal nerve plexuses; and 3) the named spinal nerves.

The Spinal Nerve Roots

The roots of the spinal nerves can be impaired by various diseases or by injuries that produce partial or complete, and unilateral or bilateral, effects. The degree of permanent impairment resulting from a spinal nerve root dysfunction would be reflected in the loss of function of the named spinal nerves having fibers from the specific nerve root. Since the named spinal nerves have fibers from more than one root, a dysfunction affecting two or more roots that supply fibers to the same nerves usually will be more impairing than a combination of the individual root impairment values.

Impairment ratings for the spinal nerve roots can be determined by combining appropriate values for impairment of named spinal nerves that are derived from those roots (see below, "The Named Spinal Nerves"). When there is bilateral involvement, the two unilateral ratings should be determined separately and combined using the Combined Values Chart.

The Lumbosacral Plexus

Impairments due to dysfunction of the lumbosacral plexus are found in Chapter 3. The loss of those functions of the trunk and perineum associated with the lumbosacral plexus (bowel, bladder, and reproductive functions, and trunk stabilization) should be taken into account when using the appropriate section of Chapter 3.

Table 4. Grading Scheme and Procedure for Determining Impairment of Affected Body Part Due to Loss of Strength

Description	Grade
a. Grading Scheme	
1. Complete range of motion against gravity and full resistance	0%
2. Complete range of motion against gravity and some resistance, or reduced fine movements and motor control	5-20%
3. Complete range of motion against gravity and only without resistance	25-50%
4. Complete range of motion with gravity eliminated	55-75%
5. Slight contractibility, but no joint motion	80-90%
6. No contractibility	100%
b. Procedure	
1. Identify the motion involved, such as flexion, extension, etc.	
2. Identify the muscle(s) performing the motion.	
3. Determine the nerve(s) that innervate the muscle(s), and find the value for maximum percent loss, due to loss of strength, according to the appropriate table.*	
4. Grade degree of loss of strength according to the grading scheme above.	
5. Multiply the value of the nerve (from the appropriate table) by the degree of loss of strength.	

*Table 5 for nerves to the head and neck; Table 6 for thoracic nerves; Table 7 for nerves to the inguinal region and perineum.

Table 5. Specific Unilateral Spinal Nerve Impairment Affecting the Head and Neck

Nerve	Maximum % Loss of Function Due to Sensory Deficit, Pain or Discomfort	Maximum % Loss of Function Due to Loss of Strength	% Impairment of The Whole Person*
Greater occipital	5	0	0- 5
Lesser occipital	3	0	0- 3
Great auricular	3	0	0- 3
Accessory (spinal accessory)	0	10	0-10

*See Tables 3 and 4 for grading schemes for determining impairment of the whole person due to sensory deficit or loss of strength.

The Named Spinal Nerves

The named spinal nerves most frequently associated with impairments are grouped below according to the involved parts of the body, that is, the head, neck, and diaphragm; and the trunk, inguinal region, and perineum. By consulting the sections below, the physician can determine how the clinical findings can be translated into percentages of loss of function of the whole person. The absence from the sections of some of the named spinal nerves and the absence of certain impairment values indicate that impairment associated with the particular nerve seldom occurs or is considered to be of little significance.

The percentages are expressed in terms of unilateral involvement. When there is bilateral involvement, the unilateral impairments should be determined separately and each converted to whole person impairment. Finally, the unilateral values are combined by using the Combined Values Chart.

Head, Neck, and Diaphragm

A unilateral phrenic nerve disorder would result in minimal to no functional impairment, inasmuch as the patient would compensate and continue to carry on the activities of daily living. The impairment to the whole person for unilateral phrenic involvement would be 0% to 5%. On the other hand, bilateral phrenic involvement would result in a demonstrable reduction in ventilatory function, and would be evaluated in terms of the criteria set forth in the section on the central nervous system.

Table 5 presents impairments due to loss of function of specific nerves to the head and neck.

Trunk, Inguinal Region, and Perineum

Evaluation of impairment of intercostal and abdominal nerves, which derive from T2-L1, is based on the number of nerves involved. The percentages in Table 6 are in terms of complete loss of function in the involved nerves. The percentages for bilateral impairment are derived by combining the figures for unilateral impairment by means of the Combined Values Chart. Where intercostal neuralgia persists, the impairment of the whole person is 0% to 3%.

Table 7 provides ratings for unilateral impairment of the iliohypogastric, ilioinguinal, and coccygeal nerves, and for unilateral and bilateral impairment of the pudendal nerves (including branches to the inferior hemorrhoidal nerve, perineal nerve, and dorsal nerve of the penis or clitoris).

References

1. Baker AB, Joynt RJ (eds): *Clinical Neurology,* vol 1-4. Philadelphia, JB Lippincott (updated annually).

2. Rowland LP (ed): *Merritts' Textbook of Neurology,* ed 7. Philadelphia, Lea and Febiger, 1984.

3. Sunderland S: *Nerves and Nerve Injuries,* ed 2. Edinburgh, Churchill Livingstone, 1978.

4. Strub RL, Black FW: *The Mental Status Examination in Neurology,* ed 2. Philadelphia, FA Davis, 1985.

Table 6. Impairment of Thoracic Nerve

	% Impairment of the Whole Person	
	Unilateral Involvement	Bilateral Involvement
Any 2 thoracic nerves	0- 5	0-10
Any 2 to 5 thoracic nerves	5-15	10-28
Any 5 or more thoracic nerves	15-35	28-58

Table 7. Unilateral Spinal Nerve Impairment Affecting Inguinal Region and Perineum

Nerve	Maximum % Loss of Function Due to Sensory Deficit, Pain or Discomfort	Maximum % Loss of Function Due to Loss of Strength	% Impairment of the Whole Person*
Iliohypogastric	3	0	0- 3
Ilioinguinal	5	0	0- 5
Pudendal (unilateral)	5	5	0-10
Pudendal (bilateral)	20	20	0-36
Coccygeal	5	0	0- 5

*See Tables 3 and 4 for grading scheme for determining impairment of the whole person due to sensory deficit or loss of strength.

Chapter 5

The Respiratory System

5.0 Introduction

The major topic of this chapter is the evaluation of respiratory impairment by the use of physiologic tests such as spirometry and diffusing capacity. Guidelines for determining impairment not related to these tests are also provided.

Before using the information in this chapter, the reader is urged to review Chapters 1 and 2, which provide a general discussion of the purpose of the *Guides* and of the situations in which they are useful; and which discuss techniques for the evaluation of the subject and for preparation of a report. The report should include the information found in the following outline, which is developed more fully in Chapter 2.

A. Medical Evaluation
1. Narrative history of medical conditions
2. Results of the most recent clinical evaluation
3. Assessment of current clinical status and statement of future plans
4. Diagnoses and clinical impressions
5. Expected date of full or partial recovery

B. Analysis of Findings
1. Impact of medical condition(s) on life activities
2. Explanation for concluding that the medical condition(s) has or has not become static or well-stabilized
3. Explanation for concluding that the individual is or is not likely to suffer from sudden or subtle incapacitation
4. Explanation for concluding that the individual is or is not likely to suffer injury or further impairment by engaging in life activities or by attempting to meet personal, social, and occupational demands
5. Explanation for concluding that accommodations and/or restrictions are or are not warranted

C. Comparison of Results of Analysis with Impairment Criteria
1. Description of clinical findings, and how these findings relate to specific criteria in the chapter
2. Explanation of each percent of impairment rating
3. Summary list of all impairment ratings
4. Overall rating of impairment of the whole person

5.1 Evaluation of Impairment Due to Respiratory Disease

General Considerations

There are several classification schemes used to define the degree of respiratory impairment. Some of these are based on actual values of pulmonary function tests, while others use predicted values. One scheme is based on severity of dyspnea. This chapter represents an attempt to develop criteria that would help standardize assessment of respiratory impairment.

The criteria presented in this chapter are based upon those developed by the Ad Hoc Committee on Impairment/Disability Criteria of the American Thoracic Society (ATS). The criteria are intended to apply to occupational as well as to nonoccupational respiratory diseases. The latter may include conditions such as hypoventilation states, vascular occlusive disease, and chest wall weakness.

Personal and Medical History

Identification:

The physician should record basic information about the patient, including name, address, age, sex, social security number, telephone number, and date and place of birth. Information about ethnicity, marital status, highest grade completed in school, and regularity and extent of exercise may be helpful in selected situations.

Dyspnea:

The physician should ask specific questions about whether or not dyspnea is present and whether it is increasing in severity. This could be related to reduced lung function and thus might be an indication of impairment. Table 1 provides a scale for determining the severity of dyspnea.

The causes of dyspnea are multiple and complex. Individual responses to a given degree of dyspnea vary and are influenced by factors unrelated to lung disease, such as cardiac disease, difficulty in verbal communication, and preoccupation with health. Therefore, the presence of dyspnea may provide clues to the evaluating physician that respiratory or other problems may be present. However, the severity of dyspnea itself does not constitute a criterion upon which impairment of lung function is based.

Table 1. Classification of Dyspnea

Mild	Dyspnea is present with fast walking on level ground or walking up a slight hill; the person can keep pace with other persons of same age and body build on level ground, but not on hills or stairs.
Moderate	Dyspnea is present while walking on level ground with persons of the same age and body build or walking up one flight of stairs.
Severe	Dyspnea is present after the person walks more than 4 to 5 minutes at own pace on level ground; the person may be short of breath with less exertion, or even at rest.

Cough and sputum production:

Although cough occurs frequently in patients with chronic obstructive pulmonary disease (COPD), only some patients will meet the accepted criterion of chronic bronchitis: cough that is productive of sputum each day for at least three months out of the year for at least two consecutive years, without other apparent causes. Thus, a detailed description of sputum volume, color, odor, and consistency, and how often it is expectorated, is important.

Wheezing:

The hallmark of airway obstruction is the wheeze. In addition to reversible airway obstruction (asthma) and emphysema, foreign bodies or tumors in airways can cause wheezing, but in the latter instances the wheezing is usually confined to one area of the chest. Wheezing may also occur in persons with congestive heart failure. Wheezing should be described in terms of frequency, the time of day or time of year it occurs, what are the possible etiologic factors involved, whether it occurs as paroxysms along with shortness of breath, and whether the shortness of breath limits the person's capacity to function.

Environmental exposure, tobacco usage, and chronological occupational data:

A detailed history of the individual's employment in chronological order should be obtained. It is easiest to begin with the most recent job and work back to the earliest job. The examiner should ask about the specific activities in each job, rather than about only the job title. An employee should be questioned about exposures to dusts, gases, vapors and fumes. The specific information required should include (1) the year he or she was first exposed to an agent; (2) the extent of the exposure; (3) the total number of years of exposure; (4) his or her estimate of the hazard that the agent posed; and (5) the number of years since exposure ceased. The physician should be aware that hobbies that generate dust, such as woodworking, may cause lung disease as well.

Individuals should be classified as nonsmokers, present smokers, and ex-smokers; the latter are those who have stopped for at least one year. The smoking history should list type(s) of tobacco smoked (cigarette, pipe, or cigar) and should emphasize cigarette smoking history. The history should include information about the age at which the person started to smoke and if and when the use of cigarettes was discontinued. The cumulative dose of exposure should be estimated in terms of "pack-years," which is the product of the usual number of packs of cigarettes the patient smoked per day multiplied by the total number of years the individual was a smoker. The maximum level of tobacco used should be described.

Data on environmental exposures and use of tobacco are especially important when the examining physician is asked to give an opinion on apportionment between causes of a lung disorder. The reader should consult Appendix A for a definition of *apportionment*.

Physical Examination

The physician should take the person's blood pressure and heart and respiratory rates after the person has rested at least five minutes, and should note the person's position when these measurements are taken. The physician should check for the following: *en bloc* movement of the chest, use of the sternocleidomastoid and

Figure 1: Lung Capacities and Volumes in the Normal State and in Three Abnormal Conditions**

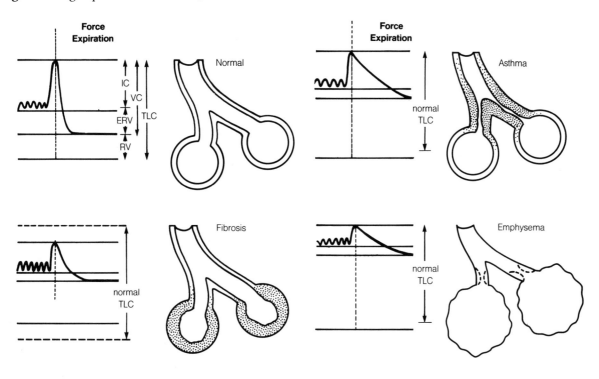

IC: Inspiratory capacity, **VC:** Vital capacity, **TLC:** Total lung capacity, **RV:** Residual volume, **ERV:** Expiratory reserve volume
**Residual volume, and therefore total lung capacity, cannot be measured by spirometry alone.

other accessory muscles of respiration, paradoxical movement of the intercostal spaces posterolaterally, and an attempt to elevate the chest cage by fixing the shoulders and leaning forward. The physician should record the degree of thoracic muscle wasting, the position and extent of diaphragmatic motion, and the presence of paradoxical movement between the rib cage and the abdomen.

Description of breathing:
The physician should record the presence of tachypnea, hyperpnea, labored breathing at rest, inability to complete sentences because of dyspnea, as well as exhalation through pursed lips. Duration of forced expiratory flow following a maximal inspiration can be measured while listening over the trachea with a stethoscope. Normally the duration is less than four seconds, but it may be several times longer in a patient with airflow obstruction.

Cyanosis and clubbing:
The physician should note the presence of cyanosis of the buccal mucosa or lips; if there is a normal hemoglobin concentration, cyanosis may not be seen until the arterial blood oxygen saturation is less than 75%. Club-

bing, almost invariably absent in persons with COPD alone, may occur when lung abscess, empyema, bronchiectasis, lung cancer, mesothelioma, or asbestosis is present as well.

Adventitious lung sounds:
The physician should note the character of the lung sounds during quiet, deep breathing. Noting the relative duration of expiration and inspiration and listening to the quality and intensity of breath sounds can provide valuable information concerning obstruction to airflow.

Intensity and location of wheezing, rhonchi, and rales should be described, as well as whether they are heard during inspiration, expiration, or both. Crackles may be present in two-thirds of persons with chronic interstitial disease such as asbestosis and desquamative interstitial pneumonia. These crackles usually occur during late inspiration. Early inspiratory crackles may be heard in diseases of airflow obstruction and particularly in bronchiolitis obliterans.

Cor pulmonale:
The physician should look for evidence of cor pulmonale, which may be associated with conditions such as chronic bronchitis and emphysema and with chronic diffuse interstitial disease. If right heart failure

Table 2. Predicted Normal FVC Values (Liters) For Men (BTPS)

Age	Height (cm) 146	148	150	152	154	156	158	160	162	164	166	168	170	172	174	176	178	180	182	184	186	188	190	192	194
18	3.72	3.84	3.96	4.08	4.20	4.32	4.44	4.56	4.68	4.80	4.92	5.04	5.16	5.28	5.40	5.52	5.64	5.76	5.88	6.00	6.12	6.24	6.36	6.48	6.60
20	3.68	3.80	3.92	4.04	4.16	4.28	4.40	4.52	4.64	4.76	4.88	5.00	5.12	5.24	5.36	5.48	5.60	5.72	5.84	5.96	6.08	6.20	6.32	6.44	6.56
22	3.64	3.76	3.88	4.00	4.12	4.24	4.36	4.48	4.60	4.72	4.84	4.96	5.08	5.20	5.32	5.44	5.56	5.68	5.80	5.92	6.04	6.16	6.28	6.40	6.52
24	3.60	3.72	3.84	3.95	4.08	4.20	4.32	4.44	4.56	4.68	4.80	4.92	5.04	5.16	5.28	5.40	5.52	5.64	5.76	5.88	6.00	6.12	6.24	6.36	6.48
26	3.55	3.67	3.79	3.91	4.03	4.15	4.27	4.39	4.51	4.63	4.75	4.87	4.99	5.11	5.23	5.35	5.47	5.59	5.71	5.83	5.95	6.07	6.19	6.31	6.43
28	3.51	3.63	3.75	3.87	3.99	4.11	4.23	4.35	4.47	4.59	4.71	4.83	4.95	5.07	5.19	5.31	5.43	5.55	5.67	5.79	5.91	6.03	6.15	6.27	6.39
30	3.47	3.59	3.71	3.83	3.95	4.07	4.19	4.31	4.43	4.55	4.67	4.79	4.91	5.03	5.15	5.27	5.39	5.51	5.63	5.75	5.87	5.99	6.11	6.23	6.35
32	3.43	3.55	3.67	3.79	3.91	4.03	4.15	4.27	4.39	4.51	4.63	4.75	4.87	4.99	5.11	5.23	5.35	5.47	5.59	5.71	5.83	5.95	6.07	6.19	6.31
34	3.38	3.50	3.62	3.74	3.86	3.98	4.10	4.22	4.34	4.46	4.58	4.70	4.82	4.94	5.06	5.18	5.30	5.42	5.54	5.66	5.78	5.90	6.02	6.14	6.26
36	3.34	3.46	3.58	3.70	3.82	3.94	4.06	4.18	4.30	4.42	4.54	4.66	4.78	4.90	5.02	5.14	5.26	5.38	5.50	5.62	5.74	5.86	5.98	6.10	6.22
38	3.30	3.42	3.54	3.66	3.78	3.90	4.02	4.14	4.26	4.38	4.50	4.62	4.74	4.86	4.98	5.10	5.22	5.34	5.46	5.58	5.70	5.82	5.94	6.06	6.18
40	3.25	3.37	3.49	3.61	3.73	3.85	3.97	4.09	4.21	4.33	4.45	4.57	4.69	4.81	4.93	5.05	5.17	5.29	5.41	5.53	5.65	5.77	5.89	6.01	6.13
42	3.21	3.33	3.45	3.57	3.69	3.81	3.93	4.05	4.17	4.29	4.41	4.53	4.65	4.77	4.89	5.01	5.13	5.25	5.37	5.49	5.61	5.73	5.85	5.97	6.09
44	3.17	3.29	3.41	3.53	3.65	3.77	3.89	4.01	4.13	4.25	4.37	4.49	4.61	4.73	4.85	4.97	5.09	5.21	5.33	5.45	5.57	5.69	5.81	5.93	6.05
46	3.13	3.25	3.37	3.49	3.61	3.73	3.85	3.97	4.09	4.21	4.33	4.45	4.57	4.69	4.81	4.93	5.05	5.17	5.29	5.41	5.53	5.65	5.77	5.89	6.01
48	3.08	3.20	3.32	3.44	3.56	3.68	3.80	3.92	4.04	4.16	4.28	4.40	4.52	4.64	4.76	4.88	5.00	5.12	5.24	5.36	5.48	5.60	5.72	5.84	5.96
50	3.04	3.16	3.28	3.40	3.52	3.64	3.76	3.88	4.00	4.12	4.24	4.36	4.48	4.60	4.72	4.84	4.96	5.08	5.20	5.32	5.44	5.56	5.68	5.80	5.92
52	3.00	3.12	3.24	3.36	3.48	3.60	3.72	3.84	3.96	4.08	4.20	4.32	4.44	4.56	4.68	4.80	4.92	5.04	5.16	5.28	5.40	5.52	5.64	5.76	5.88
54	2.95	3.07	3.19	3.31	3.43	3.55	3.67	3.79	3.91	4.03	4.15	4.27	4.39	4.51	4.63	4.75	4.87	4.99	5.11	5.23	5.35	5.47	5.59	5.71	5.83
56	2.91	3.03	3.15	3.27	3.39	3.51	3.63	3.75	3.87	3.99	4.11	4.23	4.35	4.47	4.59	4.71	4.83	4.95	5.07	5.19	5.31	5.43	5.55	5.67	5.79
58	2.87	2.99	3.11	3.23	3.35	3.47	3.59	3.71	3.83	3.95	4.07	4.19	4.31	4.43	4.55	4.67	4.79	4.91	5.03	5.15	5.27	5.39	5.51	5.63	5.75
60	2.83	2.95	3.07	3.19	3.31	3.43	3.55	3.67	3.79	3.91	4.03	4.15	4.27	4.39	4.51	4.63	4.75	4.87	4.99	5.11	5.23	5.35	5.47	5.59	5.71
62	2.78	2.90	3.02	3.14	3.26	3.38	3.50	3.62	3.74	3.86	3.98	4.10	4.22	4.34	4.46	4.58	4.70	4.82	4.94	5.06	5.18	5.30	5.42	5.54	5.66
64	2.74	2.86	2.98	3.10	3.22	3.34	3.46	3.58	3.70	3.82	3.94	4.06	4.18	4.30	4.42	4.54	4.66	4.78	4.90	5.02	5.14	5.26	5.38	5.50	5.62
66	2.70	2.82	2.94	3.06	3.18	3.30	3.42	3.54	3.66	3.78	3.90	4.02	4.14	4.26	4.38	4.50	4.62	4.74	4.86	4.98	5.10	5.22	5.34	5.46	5.58
68	2.65	2.77	2.89	3.01	3.13	3.25	3.37	3.49	3.61	3.73	3.85	3.97	4.09	4.21	4.33	4.45	4.57	4.69	4.81	4.93	5.05	5.17	5.29	5.41	5.53
70	2.61	2.73	2.85	2.97	3.09	3.21	3.33	3.45	3.57	3.69	3.81	3.93	4.05	4.17	4.29	4.41	4.53	4.65	4.77	4.89	5.01	5.13	5.25	5.37	5.49
72	2.57	2.69	2.81	2.93	3.05	3.17	3.29	3.41	3.53	3.65	3.77	3.89	4.01	4.13	4.25	4.37	4.49	4.61	4.73	4.85	4.97	5.09	5.21	5.33	5.45
74	2.53	2.65	2.77	2.89	3.01	3.13	3.25	3.37	3.49	3.61	3.73	3.85	3.97	4.09	4.21	4.33	4.45	4.57	4.69	4.81	4.93	5.05	5.17	5.29	5.41

FVC in liters = 0.0600 H − 0.0214 A − 4.650. R^2 = 0.54, SEE = 0.644, 95% Confidence Interval = 1.115.

Definitions of abbreviations: R^2 = coefficient of determination, SEE = standard error of estimate, H = height in cm, and A = age in years. BTPS = body temperature, ambient pressure and saturated with water vapor at these conditions.

The axes of the table are age (in years) at the side, and height (in cm) at the top. The predicted normal FVC in liters for the male patient is found at the intersection of the row for his age, and the column for his height.

Adapted from Crapo RO, Morris AH, Gardner RM: Reference spirometric values using techniques and equipment that meet ATS recommendations. *Am Rev Respir Dis* 1981; 123:659-664.

accompanies cor pulmonale, neck vein distention occurs above the manubrium sterni when the patient lies supine: the veins fill from below, and their volume does not decrease when the thorax is elevated 45 degrees from the horizontal. If there is such a sign, the physician should determine impairment of the cardiovascular system (see Chapter 6), which should be combined with the impairment rating for pulmonary disease using the Combined Values Chart.

Chest roentgenograms:
Minimal radiographic examination should consist of posterior-anterior (PA) and lateral views taken on deep inspiration. Chest radiographic findings often correlate poorly with physiologic findings in diseases of airflow limitation such as asthma and emphysema. No correlation between ability to work and roentgenographic findings has been noted.

If there is obstructive disease, the chest radiograph should be described in terms of hyperinflation, loss of vascular markings, presence of bullae, flattened diaphragms, and an increase in the retrosternal air space, sternophrenic angle, and PA diameter. Cardiac abnormalities or evidence of cor pulmonale with enlargement of the central pulmonary arteries with small distal pulmonary arterial branches should be noted.

In interstitial diseases with small rounded or irregular opacities, such as coal workers' pneumoconiosis or asbestosis, respectively, the correlation between physiologic and radiographic abnormalities is poor. The only exception is when there is radiographic evidence of progressive massive fibrosis (PMF). As the PMF intensifies, there is frequently a significant reduction in the ventilatory capacity.

The physician should be familiar with the 1980 International Labor Organization (ILO) Classification of Pneumoconioses, and use that Classification in describing radiographic findings.

Table 3. Predicted Normal FVC Values For Women (BTPS)

Age	Height (cm) 146	148	150	152	154	156	158	160	162	164	166	168	170	172	174	176	178	180	182	184	186	188	190	192	194
18	3.19	3.29	3.39	3.48	3.58	3.68	3.78	3.88	3.98	4.07	4.17	4.27	4.37	4.47	4.56	4.66	4.76	4.86	4.96	5.06	5.15	5.25	5.35	5.45	5.55
20	3.15	3.24	3.34	3.44	3.54	3.64	3.74	3.83	3.93	4.03	4.13	4.23	4.32	4.42	4.52	4.62	4.72	4.82	4.91	5.01	5.11	5.21	5.31	5.41	5.50
22	3.10	3.20	3.30	3.40	3.50	3.59	3.69	3.79	3.89	3.99	4.09	4.18	4.28	4.38	4.48	4.58	4.67	4.77	4.87	4.97	5.07	5.17	5.26	5.36	5.46
24	3.06	3.16	3.26	3.35	3.45	3.55	3.65	3.75	3.85	3.94	4.04	4.14	4.24	4.34	4.43	4.53	4.63	4.73	4.83	4.93	5.02	5.12	5.22	5.32	5.42
26	3.02	3.12	3.21	3.31	3.41	3.51	3.61	3.70	3.80	3.90	4.00	4.10	4.20	4.29	4.39	4.49	4.59	4.69	4.78	4.88	4.98	5.08	5.18	5.28	5.37
28	2.97	3.07	3.17	3.27	3.37	3.46	3.56	3.66	3.76	3.86	3.96	4.05	4.15	4.25	4.35	4.45	4.54	4.64	4.74	4.84	4.94	5.04	5.13	5.23	5.33
30	2.93	3.03	3.13	3.23	3.32	3.42	3.52	3.62	3.72	3.81	3.91	4.01	4.11	4.21	4.31	4.40	4.50	4.60	4.70	4.80	4.89	4.99	5.09	5.19	5.29
32	2.89	2.99	3.08	3.18	3.28	3.38	3.48	3.57	3.67	3.77	3.87	3.97	4.07	4.16	4.26	4.36	4.46	4.56	4.65	4.75	4.85	4.95	5.05	5.15	5.24
34	2.84	2.94	3.04	3.14	3.24	3.34	3.43	3.53	3.63	3.73	3.83	3.92	4.02	4.12	4.22	4.32	4.42	4.51	4.61	4.71	4.81	4.91	5.00	5.10	5.20
36	2.80	2.90	3.00	3.10	3.19	3.29	3.39	3.49	3.59	3.68	3.78	3.88	3.98	4.08	4.18	4.27	4.37	4.47	4.57	4.67	4.76	4.86	4.96	5.06	5.16
38	2.76	2.86	2.95	3.05	3.15	3.25	3.35	3.45	3.54	3.64	3.74	3.84	3.94	4.03	4.13	4.23	4.33	4.43	4.53	4.62	4.72	4.82	4.92	5.02	5.11
40	2.71	2.81	2.91	3.01	3.11	3.21	3.30	3.40	3.50	3.60	3.70	3.79	3.89	3.99	4.09	4.19	4.29	4.38	4.48	4.58	4.68	4.78	4.87	4.97	5.07
42	2.67	2.77	2.87	2.97	3.06	3.16	3.26	3.36	3.46	3.56	3.65	3.75	3.85	3.95	4.05	4.14	4.24	4.34	4.44	4.54	4.64	4.73	4.83	4.93	5.03
44	2.63	2.73	2.82	2.92	3.02	3.12	3.22	3.32	3.41	3.51	3.61	3.71	3.81	3.90	4.00	4.10	4.20	4.30	4.40	4.49	4.59	4.69	4.79	4.89	4.98
46	2.58	2.68	2.78	2.88	2.98	3.08	3.17	3.27	3.37	3.47	3.57	3.67	3.76	3.86	3.96	4.06	4.16	4.25	4.35	4.45	4.55	4.65	4.75	4.84	4.94
48	2.54	2.64	2.74	2.84	2.93	3.03	3.13	3.23	3.33	3.43	3.52	3.62	3.72	3.82	3.92	4.01	4.11	4.21	4.31	4.41	4.51	4.60	4.70	4.80	4.90
50	2.50	2.60	2.69	2.79	2.89	2.99	3.09	3.19	3.28	3.38	3.48	3.58	3.68	3.78	3.87	3.97	4.07	4.17	4.27	4.36	4.46	4.56	4.66	4.76	4.86
52	2.46	2.55	2.65	2.75	2.85	2.95	3.04	3.14	3.24	3.34	3.44	3.54	3.63	3.73	3.83	3.93	4.03	4.12	4.22	4.32	4.42	4.52	4.62	4.71	4.81
54	2.41	2.51	2.61	2.71	2.80	2.90	3.00	3.10	3.20	3.30	3.39	3.49	3.59	3.69	3.79	3.89	3.98	4.08	4.18	4.28	4.38	4.47	4.57	4.67	4.77
56	2.37	2.47	2.57	2.66	2.76	2.86	2.96	3.06	3.15	3.25	3.35	3.45	3.55	3.65	3.74	3.84	3.94	4.04	4.14	4.23	4.33	4.43	4.53	4.63	4.73
58	2.33	2.42	2.52	2.62	2.72	2.82	2.91	3.01	3.11	3.21	3.31	3.41	3.50	3.60	3.70	3.80	3.90	4.00	4.09	4.19	4.29	4.39	4.49	4.58	4.68
60	2.28	2.38	2.48	2.58	2.68	2.77	2.87	2.97	3.07	3.17	3.26	3.36	3.46	3.56	3.66	2.76	3.85	3.95	4.05	4.15	4.25	4.34	4.44	4.54	4.64
62	2.24	2.34	2.44	2.53	2.63	2.73	2.83	2.93	3.02	3.12	3.22	3.32	3.42	3.52	3.61	3.71	3.81	3.91	4.01	4.11	4.20	4.30	4.40	4.50	4.60
64	2.20	2.29	2.39	2.49	2.59	2.69	2.79	2.88	2.98	3.08	3.18	3.28	3.37	3.47	3.57	3.67	3.77	3.87	3.96	4.06	4.16	4.26	4.36	4.45	4.55
66	2.15	2.25	2.35	2.45	2.55	2.64	2.74	2.84	2.94	3.04	3.14	3.23	3.33	3.43	3.53	3.63	3.72	3.82	3.92	4.02	4.12	4.22	4.31	4.41	4.51
68	2.11	2.21	2.31	2.40	2.50	2.60	2.70	2.80	2.90	2.99	3.09	3.19	3.29	3.39	3.48	3.58	3.68	3.78	3.88	3.98	4.07	4.17	4.27	4.37	4.47
70	2.07	2.16	2.26	2.36	2.46	2.56	2.66	2.75	2.85	2.95	3.05	3.15	3.24	3.34	3.44	3.54	3.64	3.74	3.83	3.93	4.03	4.13	4.23	4.33	4.42
72	2.02	2.12	2.22	2.32	2.42	2.51	2.61	2.71	2.81	2.91	3.01	3.10	3.20	3.30	3.40	3.50	3.59	3.69	3.79	3.89	3.99	4.09	4.18	4.28	4.38
74	1.98	2.08	2.18	2.27	2.37	2.47	2.57	2.67	2.77	2.86	2.96	3.06	3.16	3.26	3.36	3.45	3.55	3.65	3.75	3.85	3.94	4.04	4.14	4.24	4.34

FVC in liters = 0.0491H − 0.0216 A − 3.590. R^2 = 0.74, SEE = 0.393, 95% Confidence Interval = 0.676.

Definitions of abbreviations: R^2 = coefficient of determination, SEE = standard error of estimate, H = height in cm, and A = age in years. BTPS = body temperature, ambient pressure and saturated with water vapor at these conditions.

The axes of the table are age (in years) at the side, and height (in cm) at the top. The predicted normal FVC in liters for the female patient is found at the intersection of the row for her age, and the column for her height.

Adapted from Crapo RO, Morris AH, Gardner RM: Reference spirometric values using techniques and equipment that meet ATS recommendations. *Am Rev Respir Dis* 1981; 123:659-664.

5.2 Physiologic Tests of Pulmonary Function: Techniques, Use, and Interpretation

Forced expiratory maneuvers (simple spirometry):
A forced expiratory maneuver, illustrated diagramatically in Figure 1, is performed in all examinations of permanent impairment. The maneuver measures the mechanical ventilatory capacity of the lungs. There are three component parts: forced vital capacity, or FVC; forced expiratory volume in the first second, or FEV_1; and the ratio of these measurements expressed as a percentage, or the FEV_1/FVC ratio. Correlation between work status and FEV_1 values is usually good, and most patients with an FEV_1 of less than one liter are not working. Gener-

ally, individuals with an FEV_1/FVC ratio of less than 40% have a shortened life span. For interstitial lung disease, the FVC has proved to be a reliable and valid index of significant impairment.

The spirometric tests should be performed as described in the 1987 ATS Statement on Standardization of Spirometry. The equipment, methods of calibration, and techniques should meet the ATS criteria. The spirogram that is technically acceptable and demonstrates the best efforts by the patient should be used to calculate the FEV_1 and FVC. The examiner should include copies of all spirometric tracings in his or her report.

Height should be measured in centimeters with the individual standing in his or her stocking feet. If the individual cannot stand or suffers from spinal deformities, his or her height should be considered as equal to

Table 4. Predicted Normal FEV$_1$ Values For Men

Age	146	148	150	152	154	156	158	160	162	164	166	168	170	172	174	176	178	180	182	184	186	188	190	192	194
18	3.42	3.50	3.58	3.66	3.75	3.83	3.91	3.99	4.08	4.16	4.24	4.33	4.41	4.49	4.57	4.66	4.74	4.82	4.91	4.99	5.07	5.15	5.24	5.32	5.40
20	3.37	3.45	3.53	3.61	3.70	3.78	3.86	3.95	4.03	4.11	4.19	4.28	4.36	4.44	4.53	4.61	4.69	4.77	4.86	4.94	5.02	5.11	5.19	5.27	5.35
22	3.32	3.40	3.48	3.57	3.65	3.73	3.81	3.90	3.98	4.06	4.15	4.23	4.31	4.39	4.48	4.56	4.64	4.73	4.81	4.89	4.97	5.05	5.14	5.22	5.30
24	3.27	3.35	3.43	3.52	3.60	3.68	3.77	3.85	3.93	4.01	4.10	4.18	4.26	4.35	4.43	4.51	4.59	4.68	4.76	4.84	4.92	5.01	5.09	5.17	5.26
26	3.22	3.30	3.39	3.47	3.55	3.63	3.72	3.80	3.88	3.97	4.05	4.13	4.21	4.30	4.38	4.46	4.54	4.63	4.71	4.79	4.88	4.90	5.04	5.12	5.21
28	3.17	3.25	3.34	3.42	3.50	3.59	3.67	3.75	3.83	3.92	4.00	4.08	4.16	4.25	4.33	4.41	4.50	4.58	4.66	4.74	4.83	4.91	4.99	5.08	5.16
30	3.12	3.21	3.29	3.37	3.45	3.54	3.62	3.70	3.78	3.87	3.95	4.03	4.12	4.20	4.28	4.36	4.45	4.53	4.61	4.70	4.78	4.86	4.94	5.03	5.11
32	3.07	3.16	3.24	3.32	3.40	3.49	3.57	3.65	3.74	3.82	3.90	3.98	4.07	4.15	4.23	4.32	4.40	4.48	4.56	4.65	4.73	4.81	4.90	4.98	5.06
34	3.02	3.11	3.19	3.27	3.36	3.44	3.52	3.60	3.69	3.77	3.85	3.94	4.02	4.10	4.18	4.27	4.35	4.43	4.52	4.60	4.68	4.76	4.85	4.93	5.01
36	2.98	3.06	3.14	3.22	3.31	3.39	3.47	3.56	3.64	3.72	3.80	3.89	3.97	4.05	4.14	4.22	4.30	4.38	4.47	4.55	4.63	4.71	4.80	4.88	4.96
38	2.93	3.01	3.09	3.18	3.26	3.34	3.42	3.51	3.59	3.67	3.76	3.84	3.92	4.00	4.09	4.17	4.25	4.33	4.42	4.50	4.58	4.67	4.75	4.83	4.91
40	2.88	2.96	3.04	3.13	3.21	3.29	3.38	3.46	3.54	3.62	3.71	3.79	3.87	3.95	4.04	4.12	4.20	4.29	4.37	4.45	4.53	4.62	4.70	4.78	4.87
42	2.83	2.91	3.00	3.08	3.16	3.24	3.33	3.41	3.49	3.57	3.66	3.74	3.82	3.91	3.99	4.07	4.15	4.24	4.32	4.40	4.49	4.57	4.65	4.73	4.82
44	2.78	2.86	2.95	3.03	3.11	3.19	3.28	3.36	3.44	3.53	3.61	3.69	3.77	3.86	3.94	4.02	4.11	4.19	4.27	4.35	4.44	4.52	4.60	4.69	4.77
46	2.73	2.81	2.90	2.98	3.06	3.15	3.23	3.31	3.39	3.48	3.56	3.64	3.73	3.81	3.89	3.97	4.06	4.14	4.22	4.31	4.39	4.47	4.55	4.64	4.72
48	2.68	2.77	2.85	2.93	3.01	3.10	3.18	3.26	3.35	3.43	3.51	3.59	3.68	3.76	3.84	3.93	4.01	4.09	4.17	4.25	4.34	4.42	4.50	4.59	4.67
50	2.63	2.72	2.80	2.88	2.97	3.05	3.13	3.21	3.30	3.38	3.46	3.55	3.63	3.71	3.79	3.88	3.96	4.04	4.12	4.21	4.29	4.37	4.46	4.54	4.62
52	2.59	2.67	2.75	2.83	2.92	3.00	3.08	3.17	3.25	3.33	3.41	3.50	3.58	3.66	3.74	3.83	3.91	3.99	4.08	4.16	4.24	4.32	4.41	4.49	4.57
54	2.54	2.62	2.70	2.79	2.87	2.95	3.03	3.12	3.20	3.28	3.36	3.45	3.53	3.61	3.70	3.78	3.86	3.94	4.03	4.11	4.19	4.28	4.36	4.44	4.52
56	2.49	2.57	2.65	2.74	2.82	2.90	2.98	3.07	3.15	3.23	3.32	3.40	3.48	3.56	3.65	3.73	3.81	3.90	3.98	4.06	4.14	4.23	4.31	4.39	4.48
58	2.44	2.52	2.60	2.69	2.77	2.85	2.94	3.02	3.10	3.18	3.27	3.35	3.43	3.52	3.60	3.68	3.76	3.85	3.93	4.01	4.10	4.18	4.26	4.34	4.43
60	2.39	2.47	2.55	2.64	2.72	2.80	2.89	2.97	3.05	3.14	3.22	3.30	3.38	3.47	3.55	3.63	3.72	3.80	3.88	3.96	4.05	4.13	4.21	4.29	4.38
62	2.34	2.42	2.51	2.59	2.67	2.76	2.84	2.92	3.00	3.09	3.17	3.25	3.34	3.42	3.50	3.58	3.67	3.75	3.83	3.91	4.00	4.08	4.16	4.25	4.33
64	2.29	2.38	2.46	2.54	2.62	2.71	2.79	2.87	2.96	3.04	3.12	3.20	3.29	3.37	3.45	3.53	3.62	3.70	3.78	3.87	3.95	4.03	4.11	4.20	4.28
66	2.24	2.33	2.41	2.49	2.58	2.66	2.74	2.82	2.91	2.99	3.07	3.15	3.24	3.32	3.40	3.49	3.57	3.65	3.73	3.82	3.90	3.98	4.07	4.15	4.23
68	2.20	2.28	2.36	2.44	2.53	2.61	2.69	2.77	2.86	2.94	3.02	3.11	3.19	3.27	3.35	3.44	3.52	3.60	3.69	3.77	3.85	3.93	4.02	4.10	4.18
70	2.15	2.23	2.31	2.39	2.48	2.56	2.64	2.73	2.81	2.89	2.97	3.06	3.14	3.22	3.31	3.39	3.47	3.55	3.64	3.72	3.80	3.89	3.97	4.05	4.13
72	2.10	2.18	2.26	2.35	2.43	2.51	2.59	2.68	2.76	2.84	2.93	3.01	3.09	3.17	3.26	3.34	3.42	3.51	3.59	3.67	3.75	3.84	3.92	4.00	4.08
74	2.05	2.13	2.21	2.30	2.38	2.46	2.55	2.63	2.71	2.79	2.88	2.96	3.04	3.13	3.21	3.29	3.37	3.46	3.54	3.62	3.70	3.79	3.87	3.95	4.04

FEV$_1$ in liters = 0.0414 H − 0.0244 A − 2.190. R^2 = 0.64, SEE = 0.486, 95% Confidence Interval = 0.842.

Definitions of abbreviations: R^2 = coefficient of determination, SEE = standard error of estimate, H = height in cm, and A = age in years. BTPS = body temperature, ambient pressure and saturated with water vapor at these conditions.

The axes of the table are age (in years) at the side, and height (in cm) at the top. The predicted normal FEV$_1$ in liters for the male patient is found at the intersection of the row for his age, and the column for his height.

Adapted from Crapo RO, Morris AH, Gardner RM: Reference spirometric values using techniques and equipment that meet ATS recommendations. *Am Rev Respir Dis* 1981; 123:659-664.

the arm span, which is the distance between the tips of the middle fingers when the arms are stretched horizontally against the wall.

An individual should be evaluated after he or she has received optimum therapy or is in optimum health. If wheezing or other evidence of bronchospasm is evident at the time of examination, the ventilatory studies should be done before and after the administration of a bronchodilator. The post-bronchodilator test should be done after an appropriate waiting period (10 to 20 minutes). The spirogram indicating the best effort, either before or after administration of the bronchodilator, should be used to calculate the FVC and FEV$_1$.

The person's FVC and FEV$_1$ results should be compared to predicted "normal" values. Such values for both adult males and females are presented in Tables 2 through 5. To find the "normal" value, find the person's age in the left-hand column and the height along the top row, and locate the predicted value at the intersection of the respective row and column. The spirometry measurements for black persons and persons of

Asian descent tend to be smaller than for whites of the same age, height, and sex. Therefore, the evaluating physician should multiply the predicted value by 0.9 before comparing a black or Asian individual's values to the appropriate tables. To date no other ethnic groups have been studied sufficiently to determine if there are differences from the predicted values, which are based upon a white population.

The person's actual FEV$_1$/FVC ratio, expressed as a percentage figure, should be used for determining impairment based on this parameter.

Diffusing capacity of carbon monoxide (D$_{CO}$): The single breath D$_{CO}$ should be used for the evaluation of all levels of impairment. The methodology for performing single breath D$_{CO}$ described by the ATS should be followed.

The D$_{CO}$ measures the amount of CO which diffuses across the alveolar-capillary membrane in a specified amount of time. It is especially useful in detecting

Table 5. Predicted Normal FEV$_1$ Values For Women

Age	Height (cm) 146	148	150	152	154	156	158	160	162	164	166	168	170	172	174	176	178	180	182	184	186	188	190	192	194
18	2.96	3.02	3.09	3.16	3.23	3.30	3.37	3.43	3.50	3.57	3.64	3.71	3.78	3.85	3.91	3.98	4.05	4.12	4.19	4.26	4.32	4.39	4.46	4.53	4.60
20	2.91	2.97	3.04	3.11	3.18	3.25	3.32	3.38	3.45	3.52	3.59	3.66	3.73	3.79	3.86	3.93	4.00	4.07	4.14	4.20	4.27	4.34	4.41	4.48	4.55
22	2.85	2.92	2.99	3.06	3.13	3.20	3.26	3.33	3.40	3.47	3.54	3.61	3.67	3.74	3.81	3.88	3.95	4.02	4.09	4.15	4.22	4.29	4.36	4.43	4.50
24	2.80	2.87	2.94	3.01	3.08	3.15	3.21	3.28	3.35	3.42	3.49	3.56	3.62	3.69	3.76	3.83	3.90	3.97	4.03	4.10	4.17	4.24	4.31	4.38	4.44
26	2.75	2.82	2.89	2.96	3.03	3.09	3.16	3.23	3.30	3.37	3.44	3.50	3.57	3.64	3.71	3.78	3.85	3.91	3.98	4.05	4.12	4.19	4.26	4.33	4.39
28	2.70	2.77	2.84	2.91	2.97	3.04	3.11	3.18	3.25	3.32	3.39	3.45	3.52	3.59	3.66	3.73	3.80	3.86	3.93	4.00	4.07	4.14	4.21	4.27	4.34
30	2.65	2.72	2.79	2.86	2.92	2.99	3.06	3.13	3.20	3.27	3.33	3.40	3.47	3.54	3.61	3.68	3.74	3.81	3.88	3.95	4.02	4.09	4.15	4.22	4.29
32	2.60	2.67	2.74	2.80	2.87	2.94	3.01	3.08	3.15	3.21	3.28	3.35	3.42	3.49	3.56	3.63	3.69	3.76	3.83	3.90	3.97	4.04	4.10	4.17	4.24
34	2.55	2.62	2.68	2.75	2.82	2.89	2.96	3.03	3.10	3.16	3.23	3.30	3.37	3.44	3.51	3.57	3.64	3.71	3.78	3.85	3.92	3.98	4.05	4.12	4.19
36	2.50	2.57	2.63	2.70	2.77	2.84	2.91	2.98	3.04	3.11	3.18	3.25	3.32	3.39	3.45	3.52	3.59	3.66	3.73	3.80	3.87	3.93	4.00	4.07	4.14
38	2.45	2.51	2.58	2.65	2.72	2.79	2.86	2.92	2.99	3.06	3.13	3.20	3.27	3.34	3.40	3.47	3.54	3.61	3.68	3.75	3.81	3.88	3.95	4.02	4.09
40	2.40	2.46	2.53	2.60	2.67	2.74	2.81	2.87	2.94	3.01	3.08	3.15	3.22	3.28	3.35	3.42	3.49	3.56	3.63	3.69	3.76	3.83	3.90	3.97	4.04
42	2.34	2.41	2.48	2.55	2.62	2.69	2.75	2.82	2.89	2.96	3.03	3.10	3.17	3.23	3.30	3.37	3.44	3.51	3.58	3.64	3.71	3.78	3.85	3.92	3.99
44	2.29	2.36	2.43	2.50	2.57	2.64	2.70	2.77	2.84	2.91	2.98	3.05	3.11	3.18	3.25	3.32	3.39	3.46	3.52	3.59	3.66	3.73	3.80	3.87	3.93
46	2.24	2.31	2.38	2.45	2.52	2.58	2.65	2.72	2.79	2.86	2.93	2.99	3.06	3.13	3.20	3.27	3.34	3.41	3.47	3.54	3.61	3.68	3.75	3.82	3.88
48	2.19	2.26	2.33	2.40	2.46	2.53	2.60	2.67	2.74	2.81	2.88	2.94	3.01	3.08	3.15	3.22	3.29	3.35	3.42	3.49	3.56	3.63	3.70	3.76	3.83
50	2.14	2.21	2.28	2.35	2.41	2.48	2.55	2.62	2.69	2.76	2.82	2.89	2.96	3.03	3.10	3.17	3.23	3.30	3.37	3.44	3.51	3.58	3.65	3.71	3.78
52	2.09	2.16	2.23	2.29	2.36	2.43	2.50	2.57	2.64	2.70	2.77	2.84	2.91	2.98	3.05	3.12	3.18	3.25	3.32	3.39	3.46	3.53	3.59	3.66	3.73
54	2.04	2.11	2.18	2.24	2.31	2.38	2.45	2.52	2.59	2.65	2.72	2.79	3.86	3.93	3.00	3.06	3.13	3.20	3.27	3.34	3.41	3.47	3.54	3.61	3.68
56	1.99	2.06	2.12	2.19	2.26	2.33	2.40	2.47	2.53	2.60	2.67	2.74	2.81	2.88	2.94	3.01	3.08	3.15	3.22	3.29	3.36	3.42	3.49	3.56	3.63
58	1.94	2.00	2.07	2.14	2.21	2.28	2.35	2.42	2.48	2.55	2.62	2.69	2.76	2.83	2.89	2.96	3.03	3.10	3.17	3.24	3.30	3.37	3.44	3.51	3.58
60	1.89	1.95	2.02	2.09	2.16	2.23	2.30	2.36	2.43	2.50	2.57	2.64	2.71	2.77	2.84	2.91	2.98	3.05	3.12	3.18	3.25	3.32	3.39	3.46	3.53
62	1.83	1.90	1.97	2.04	2.11	2.18	2.24	2.31	2.38	2.45	2.52	2.59	2.66	2.72	2.79	2.86	2.93	3.00	3.07	3.13	3.20	3.27	3.34	3.41	3.48
64	1.78	1.85	1.92	1.99	2.06	2.13	2.19	2.26	2.33	2.40	2.47	2.54	2.60	2.67	2.74	2.81	2.88	2.95	3.01	3.08	3.15	3.22	3.29	3.36	3.42
66	1.73	1.80	1.87	1.94	2.01	2.07	2.14	2.21	2.28	2.35	2.42	2.48	2.55	2.62	2.69	2.76	2.83	2.90	2.96	3.03	3.10	3.17	3.24	3.31	3.37
68	1.68	1.75	1.82	1.89	1.95	2.02	2.09	2.16	2.23	2.30	2.37	2.43	2.50	2.57	2.64	2.71	2.78	2.84	2.91	2.98	3.05	3.12	3.19	3.25	3.32
70	1.63	1.70	1.77	1.84	1.90	1.97	2.04	2.11	2.18	2.25	2.31	2.38	2.45	2.52	2.59	2.66	2.72	2.79	2.86	2.93	3.00	3.07	3.14	3.20	3.27
72	1.58	1.65	1.72	1.78	1.85	1.92	1.99	2.06	2.13	2.19	2.26	2.33	2.40	2.47	2.54	2.61	2.67	2.74	2.81	2.88	2.95	3.02	3.08	3.15	3.22
74	1.53	1.60	1.67	1.73	1.80	1.87	1.94	2.01	2.08	2.14	2.21	2.28	2.35	2.42	2.49	2.55	2.62	2.69	2.76	2.83	2.90	2.96	3.03	3.10	3.17

FEV$_1$ in liters = $0.0342\,H - 0.0255\,A - 1.578$. $R^2 = 0.80$, SEE = 0.326, 95% Confidence Interval = 0.561.

Definitions of abbreviations: R^2 = coefficient of determination, SEE = standard error of estimate, H = height in cm, and A = age in years. BTPS = body temperature, ambient pressure and saturated with water vapor at these conditions.

The axes of the table are age (in years) at the side, and height (in cm) at the top. The predicted normal FEV$_1$ in liters for the female patient is found at the intersection of the row for her age, and the column for her height.

Adapted from Crapo RO, Morris AH, Gardner RM: Reference spirometric values using techniques and equipment that meet ATS recommendations. *Am Rev Respir Dis* 1981; 123:659-664.

abnormalities that limit gas transference, such as emphysema or interstitial fibrosis of the lung parenchyma. However, measurement of diffusing capacity is affected by many factors. A decrease in hemoglobin concentration of 2.5 to 3.0 gm/100 ml will reduce the value of the diffusing capacity by approximately 10%; corrections can be made for severe anemia or polycythemia. The change in alveolar oxygen tension that occurs at moderate altitudes, such as 5,000 feet above sea level affects D_{CO} measurement by as much as 7%. However, these effects are usually of little significance, and in fact are smaller than the variability of the test itself, which is quite large.

Predicted "normal" values are presented in Tables 6 and 7. These tables are to be used in a manner similar to the tables on spirometry. A laboratory that performs the D_{CO} under conditions or with procedures that are different from the ATS recommendations should either develop and verify its own prediction equations or use an accepted and verified equation that is appropriate to its needs.

The interpretations of the FVC, FEV$_1$, FEV$_1$/FVC ratio and D_{CO} are given in Table 8. Results for all four measures of lung function must be in the normal range for a person to be considered not impaired according to physiologic parameters. At least one of these measures should be abnormal to the degree described in a given class definition if an impairment is to be rated in that class.

Measured exercise capacity:
Testing to measure exercise capacity should not be done when an individual's spirometry and D_{CO} measurements indicate severe impairment. Measured exercise capacity testing may be done when (1) the individual's complaint of dyspnea is more severe than spirometry or D_{CO} would indicate; OR (2) the individual

Table 6. Predicted Normal Single Breath D_{CO} Values For Men (STPD)

Age	Height (cm) 146	148	150	152	154	156	158	160	162	164	166	168	170	172	174	176	178	180	182	184	186	188	190	192	194
18	29.8	30.6	31.4	32.2	33.1	33.9	34.7	35.5	36.3	37.1	38.0	38.8	39.6	40.4	41.2	42.1	42.9	43.7	44.5	45.4	46.2	47.0	47.8	48.6	49.4
20	29.3	30.2	31.0	31.8	32.6	33.4	34.3	35.1	35.9	36.7	37.5	38.4	39.2	40.0	40.8	41.6	42.5	43.3	44.1	44.9	45.7	46.6	47.4	48.2	49.0
22	28.9	29.7	30.6	31.4	32.2	33.0	33.8	34.7	35.5	36.3	37.1	37.9	38.8	39.6	40.4	41.2	42.0	42.9	43.7	44.5	45.3	46.1	47.0	47.8	48.6
24	28.5	29.3	30.1	31.0	31.8	32.6	33.4	34.2	35.1	35.9	36.7	37.5	38.3	39.2	40.0	40.8	41.6	42.4	43.3	44.1	44.9	45.7	46.5	47.4	48.2
26	28.1	28.9	29.7	30.5	31.4	32.2	33.0	33.8	34.6	35.5	36.3	37.1	37.9	38.7	39.6	40.4	41.2	42.0	42.8	43.7	44.5	45.3	46.1	46.9	47.8
28	27.7	28.5	29.3	30.1	30.9	31.8	32.6	33.4	34.2	35.0	35.9	36.7	37.5	38.3	39.1	40.0	40.8	41.6	42.4	43.2	44.1	44.9	45.7	46.5	47.3
30	27.2	28.1	28.9	29.7	30.5	31.3	32.2	33.0	33.8	34.6	35.4	36.3	37.1	37.9	38.7	39.6	40.4	41.2	42.0	42.8	43.6	44.5	45.3	46.1	46.9
32	26.8	27.6	28.5	29.3	30.1	30.9	31.7	32.6	33.4	34.2	35.0	35.8	36.7	37.5	38.3	39.1	39.9	40.8	41.6	42.4	43.2	44.1	44.9	45.7	46.5
34	26.4	27.2	28.1	28.9	29.7	30.5	31.3	32.1	33.0	33.8	34.6	35.4	36.2	37.1	37.9	38.7	39.5	40.4	41.2	42.0	42.8	43.6	44.4	45.3	46.1
36	26.0	26.8	27.6	28.4	29.3	30.1	30.9	31.7	32.5	33.4	34.2	35.0	35.8	36.6	37.5	38.3	39.1	39.9	40.7	41.6	42.4	43.2	44.0	44.8	45.7
38	25.6	26.4	27.2	28.0	28.8	29.7	30.5	31.3	32.1	32.9	33.8	34.6	35.4	36.2	37.0	37.9	38.7	39.5	40.3	41.1	42.0	42.8	43.6	44.4	45.2
40	25.1	26.0	26.8	27.6	28.4	29.2	30.1	30.9	31.7	32.5	33.3	34.2	35.0	35.8	36.6	37.4	38.3	39.1	39.9	40.7	41.5	42.4	43.2	44.0	44.8
42	24.7	25.5	26.4	27.2	28.0	28.8	29.6	30.5	31.3	32.1	32.9	33.7	34.6	35.4	36.2	37.0	37.8	38.7	39.5	40.3	41.1	41.9	42.8	43.6	44.4
44	24.3	25.1	25.9	26.8	27.6	28.4	29.2	30.0	30.9	31.7	32.5	33.3	34.1	35.0	35.8	36.6	37.4	38.2	39.1	39.9	40.7	41.5	42.3	43.2	44.0
46	23.9	24.7	25.5	26.3	27.2	28.0	28.8	29.6	30.4	31.3	32.1	32.9	33.7	34.6	35.4	36.2	37.0	37.8	38.6	39.5	40.3	41.1	41.9	42.7	43.6
48	23.5	24.3	25.1	25.9	26.7	27.6	28.4	29.2	30.0	30.8	31.7	32.5	33.3	34.1	34.9	35.8	36.6	37.4	38.2	39.1	39.9	40.7	41.5	42.3	43.1
50	23.1	23.9	24.7	25.5	26.3	27.1	28.0	28.8	29.6	30.4	31.2	32.1	32.9	33.7	34.5	35.4	36.2	37.0	37.8	38.6	39.4	40.3	41.1	41.9	42.7
52	22.6	23.4	24.3	25.1	25.9	26.7	27.6	28.4	29.2	30.0	30.8	31.6	32.5	33.3	34.1	34.9	35.7	36.6	37.4	38.2	39.0	39.9	40.7	41.6	42.3
54	22.2	23.0	23.8	24.7	25.5	26.3	27.1	27.9	28.8	29.6	30.4	31.2	32.0	32.9	33.7	34.5	35.3	36.1	37.0	37.8	38.6	39.4	40.2	41.1	41.9
56	21.8	22.6	23.4	24.2	25.1	25.9	26.7	27.5	28.3	29.2	30.0	30.8	31.6	32.4	33.3	34.1	34.9	35.7	36.5	37.4	38.2	39.0	39.8	40.6	41.5
58	21.4	22.2	23.0	23.8	24.6	25.5	26.3	27.1	27.9	28.7	29.6	30.4	31.2	32.0	32.8	33.7	34.5	35.3	36.1	36.9	37.8	38.6	39.4	40.2	41.0
60	20.9	21.8	22.6	23.4	24.2	25.0	25.9	26.7	27.5	28.3	29.1	30.0	30.8	31.6	32.4	33.2	34.1	34.9	35.7	36.5	37.3	38.2	39.0	39.8	40.6
62	20.5	21.3	22.2	23.0	23.8	24.6	25.4	26.3	27.1	27.9	28.7	29.5	30.4	31.2	32.0	32.8	33.6	34.5	35.3	36.1	36.9	37.7	38.6	39.4	40.2
64	20.1	20.9	21.7	22.6	23.4	24.2	25.0	25.8	26.7	27.5	28.3	29.1	29.9	30.8	31.6	32.4	33.2	34.1	34.9	35.7	36.5	37.3	38.1	39.0	39.8
66	19.7	20.5	21.3	22.1	23.0	23.8	24.6	25.4	26.2	27.1	27.9	28.7	29.5	30.4	31.2	32.0	32.8	33.6	34.4	35.3	36.1	36.9	37.7	38.6	39.4
68	19.3	20.1	20.9	21.7	22.6	23.4	24.2	25.0	25.8	26.6	27.5	28.3	29.1	29.9	30.7	31.6	32.4	33.2	34.0	34.9	35.7	36.5	37.3	38.1	38.9
70	18.8	19.7	20.5	21.3	22.1	22.9	23.8	24.6	25.4	26.2	27.0	27.9	28.7	29.5	30.3	31.1	32.0	32.8	33.6	34.4	35.2	36.1	36.9	37.7	38.5
72	18.4	19.2	20.1	20.9	21.7	22.5	23.3	24.2	25.0	25.8	26.6	27.4	28.3	29.1	29.9	30.7	31.5	32.4	33.2	34.0	34.8	35.6	36.5	37.3	38.1
74	18.0	18.8	19.6	20.5	21.3	22.1	22.9	23.7	24.6	25.4	26.2	27.0	27.8	28.7	29.5	30.3	31.1	31.9	32.8	33.6	34.4	35.2	36.0	36.9	37.7

D_{CO} in ml/min/mm Hg = $0.410\,H - 0.210\,A - 26.31$. R^2 = 0.60, SEE = 4.82, 95% Confidence Interval = 8.2.

Definitions of abbreviations: R^2 = coefficient of determination, SEE = standard error of estimate, H = height in cm, and A = age in years. STPD = temperature 0°C, pressure 760 mm Hg and dry (0 water vapor).

The regression analysis has been normalized to a standard hemoglobin of 14.6 g/dl using Cotes' modification of the relationship described by Roughton and Forster.

The axes of the table are age (in years) at the side, and height (in cm) at the top. The predicted normal D_{CO} in ml/min/mm Hg for the male patient is found at the intersection of the row for his age, and the column for his height.

Adapted from Crapo RO, Morris AH: Standardized single breath normal values of carbon monoxide diffusing capacity. *Am Rev Respir Dis* 1981; 123:185-190.

states that he or she is physically unable to meet the demands of a specific job because of breathlessness; OR (3) the individual has not performed maximally or correctly in the spirometry or D_{CO} tests.

Exercise testing is not recommended for an individual who, in the opinion of the examining physician, has medical contraindications to such tests. A person's overall physical conditioning and cardiac status not only may significantly affect results of an exercise test, but also may determine whether such a test should be done at all.

Exercise capacity is measured by the $\dot{V}O_2$ in ml/(kg·min), or in METS, a unit equal to 3.5 ml/(kg·min) (see Chapter 6). Tables are available that equate specific work tasks with either $\dot{V}O_2$ or METS. Generally, working at his or her own pace, a person can sustain work output for an eight-hour period if the person does not exceed 40% of his or her maximum $\dot{V}O_2$ ($\dot{V}O_2$ max) as determined by exercise tests.

Arterial blood gases:
Blood gas determinations are considered invasive, and the results are difficult to standardize due to the effects of factors such as hyperventilation, breathholding, altitude, and obesity. Thus, this examination should be reserved for selected cases and performed under rigidly controlled laboratory conditions. Hypoxemia must be documented on two occasions at least four weeks apart. If hypoxemia is suspected, blood gas determinations can be done during an exercise capacity test. In general, for most persons with obstructive lung disease, the FEV_1 correlates better with exercise capacity than does the partial pressure of arterial oxygen.

Table 7. Predicted Normal Single Breath D_{CO} Values For Women (STPD)

Age	Height (cm) 146	148	150	152	154	156	158	160	162	164	166	168	170	172	174	176	178	180	182	184	186	188	190	192	194
18	26.0	26.5	27.0	27.6	28.1	28.6	29.2	29.7	30.2	30.8	31.3	31.9	32.4	32.9	33.5	34.0	34.5	35.1	35.6	36.1	36.7	37.2	37.7	38.3	38.8
20	25.7	26.2	26.7	27.3	27.8	28.4	28.9	29.4	30.0	30.5	31.0	31.6	32.1	32.6	33.2	33.7	34.2	34.8	35.3	35.8	36.4	36.9	37.4	38.0	38.5
22	25.4	25.9	26.5	27.0	27.5	28.1	28.6	29.1	29.7	30.2	30.7	31.3	31.8	32.3	32.9	33.4	33.9	34.5	35.0	35.5	36.1	36.6	37.1	37.7	38.2
24	25.1	25.6	26.2	26.7	27.2	27.8	28.3	28.8	29.4	29.9	30.4	31.0	31.5	32.0	32.6	33.1	33.6	34.2	34.7	35.2	35.8	36.3	36.8	37.4	37.9
26	24.8	25.3	25.9	26.4	26.9	27.5	28.0	28.5	29.1	29.6	30.1	30.7	31.2	31.7	32.3	32.8	33.3	33.9	34.4	34.9	35.5	36.0	36.5	37.1	37.6
28	24.5	25.0	25.6	26.1	26.6	27.2	27.7	28.2	28.8	29.3	29.8	30.4	30.9	31.4	32.0	32.5	33.0	33.6	34.1	34.6	35.2	35.7	36.2	36.8	37.3
30	24.2	24.7	25.3	25.8	26.3	26.9	27.4	27.9	28.5	29.0	29.5	30.1	30.6	31.1	31.7	32.2	32.7	33.3	33.8	34.3	34.9	35.4	35.9	36.5	37.0
32	23.9	24.4	25.0	25.5	26.0	26.6	27.1	27.6	28.2	28.7	29.2	29.8	30.3	30.8	31.4	31.9	32.4	33.0	33.5	34.1	34.6	35.1	35.7	36.2	36.7
34	23.6	24.1	24.7	25.2	25.7	26.3	26.8	27.3	27.9	28.4	28.9	29.5	30.0	30.6	31.1	31.6	32.2	32.7	33.2	33.8	34.3	34.8	35.4	35.9	36.4
36	23.3	23.8	24.4	24.9	25.4	26.0	26.5	27.1	27.6	28.1	28.7	29.2	29.7	30.3	30.8	31.3	31.9	32.4	32.9	33.5	34.0	34.5	35.1	35.6	36.1
38	23.0	23.6	24.1	24.6	25.2	25.7	26.2	26.8	27.3	27.8	28.4	28.9	29.4	30.0	30.5	31.0	31.6	32.1	32.6	33.2	33.7	34.2	34.8	35.3	35.8
40	22.7	23.3	23.8	24.3	24.9	25.4	25.9	26.5	27.0	27.5	28.1	28.6	29.1	29.7	30.2	30.7	31.3	31.8	32.3	32.9	33.4	33.9	34.5	35.0	35.5
42	22.4	23.0	23.5	24.0	24.6	25.1	25.6	26.2	26.7	27.2	27.8	28.3	28.8	29.4	29.9	30.4	31.0	31.5	32.0	32.6	33.1	33.6	34.2	34.7	35.2
44	22.1	22.7	23.2	23.7	24.3	24.3	25.3	25.9	26.4	26.9	27.5	28.0	28.5	29.1	29.6	30.1	30.7	31.2	31.7	32.3	32.8	33.3	33.9	34.4	34.9
46	21.8	22.4	22.9	23.4	24.0	24.5	25.0	25.6	26.1	26.6	27.2	27.7	28.2	28.8	29.3	29.8	30.4	30.9	31.4	32.0	32.5	33.0	33.6	34.1	34.6
48	21.5	22.1	22.6	23.1	23.7	24.2	24.7	25.3	25.8	26.3	26.9	27.4	27.9	28.5	29.0	29.5	30.1	30.6	31.1	31.7	32.2	32.8	33.3	33.8	34.4
50	21.2	21.8	22.3	22.8	23.4	23.9	24.4	25.0	25.5	26.0	26.6	27.1	27.6	28.2	28.7	29.3	29.8	30.3	30.9	31.4	31.9	32.5	33.0	33.5	34.1
52	20.9	21.5	22.0	22.5	23.1	23.5	24.1	24.7	25.2	25.8	26.3	26.8	27.4	27.9	28.4	29.0	29.5	30.0	30.6	31.1	31.6	32.2	32.7	33.2	33.8
54	20.6	21.2	21.7	22.3	22.8	23.3	23.9	24.4	24.9	25.5	26.0	26.5	27.1	27.6	28.1	28.7	29.2	29.7	30.3	30.8	31.3	31.9	32.4	32.9	33.5
56	20.4	20.9	21.4	22.0	22.5	23.0	23.6	24.1	24.6	25.2	25.7	26.2	26.8	27.3	27.8	28.4	28.9	29.4	30.0	30.5	31.0	31.6	32.1	32.6	33.2
58	20.1	20.6	21.1	21.7	22.2	22.7	23.3	23.8	24.3	24.9	25.4	25.9	26.5	27.0	27.5	28.1	28.6	29.1	29.7	30.2	30.7	31.3	31.8	32.3	32.9
60	19.8	20.3	20.8	21.4	21.9	22.4	23.0	23.5	24.0	24.6	25.1	25.6	26.2	26.7	27.2	27.8	28.3	28.8	29.4	29.9	30.4	31.0	31.5	32.0	32.6
62	19.5	20.0	20.5	21.1	21.6	22.1	22.7	23.2	23.7	24.3	24.8	25.3	25.9	26.4	26.9	27.5	28.0	28.5	29.1	29.6	30.1	30.7	31.2	31.7	32.3
64	19.2	19.7	20.2	20.8	21.3	21.8	22.4	22.9	23.4	24.0	24.5	25.0	25.6	26.1	26.6	27.2	27.7	28.2	28.8	29.3	29.8	30.4	30.9	31.5	32.0
66	18.9	19.4	19.9	20.5	21.0	21.5	22.1	22.6	23.1	23.7	24.2	24.1	25.3	25.8	26.3	26.9	27.4	28.0	28.5	29.0	29.6	30.1	30.6	31.2	31.7
68	18.6	19.1	19.6	20.2	20.7	21.2	21.8	22.3	22.8	23.4	23.9	24.5	25.0	25.5	26.1	26.6	27.1	27.7	28.2	28.7	29.3	29.8	30.3	30.9	31.4
70	18.3	18.8	19.3	19.9	20.4	21.0	21.5	22.0	22.6	23.1	23.5	24.2	24.7	25.2	25.8	26.3	26.8	27.4	27.9	28.4	29.0	29.5	30.0	30.6	31.1
72	18.0	18.5	19.1	19.6	20.1	20.7	21.2	21.1	22.3	22.8	23.3	23.9	24.4	24.9	25.5	26.0	26.5	27.1	27.6	28.1	28.7	29.2	29.7	30.3	30.8
74	17.7	18.2	18.8	19.3	19.8	20.4	20.9	21.4	22.0	22.5	23.0	23.6	24.1	24.6	25.2	25.7	26.2	26.8	27.3	27.8	28.4	28.9	29.4	30.0	30.5

D_{CO} in ml/min/mm Hg = 0.267 H − 0.148 A − 10.34. R^2 = 0.60, SEE = 3.40, 95% Confidence Interval = 5.74.

Definitions of abbreviations: R^2 = coefficient of determination, SEE = standard error of estimate, H = height in cm, and A = age in years. STPD = temperature 0°C, pressure 760 mm Hg and dry (0 water vapor).

The regression analysis has been normalized to a standard hemoglobin of 12.8 g/dl (the original equation was normalized to a standard hemoglobin of 14.6 g/dl) using Cotes' modification of the relationship described by Roughton and Forster.

The axes of the table are age (in years) at the side, and height (in cm) at the top. The predicted normal D_{CO} in ml/min/mm Hg for the female patient is found at the intersection of the row for her age, and the column for her height.

Adapted from Crapo RO, Morris AH: Standardized single breath normal values of carbon monoxide diffusing capacity. *Am Rev Respir Dis* 1981; 123:185-190.

5.3 Criteria for Evaluating Permanent Impairment

Table 8 presents the criteria for rating permanent impairment. The value of $\dot{V}O_2$ max less than 15 ml/(kg·min) is not a hard and fast criterion for severe impairment; a person may be considered severely impaired if 30% to 40% of his or her $\dot{V}O_2$ max is not sufficient to meet the $\dot{V}O_2$ costs of his or her occupational activity over an eight-hour period.

Arterial blood gas determination may itself indicate severe impairment when an individual is stable and receiving optimal therapy. A person with a resting PaO_2 of less than 60 mm Hg in room air may be deemed severely impaired if he or she has evidence of one or more of the secondary conditions related to arterial hypoxemia, such as pulmonary hypertension, cor pulmonale, increasingly severe hypoxemia during exercise testing, and erythrocytosis. A resting PaO_2 of less than 50 mm Hg in room air is by itself a criterion for severe impairment.

5.4 Examples of Permanent Respiratory Impairment

Example 1 of Class 1
Impairment of the Whole Person:
A 38-year-old nonsmoking male coal miner had worked in underground mining as a cutting machine operator for 20 years. On his most recent mandatory chest radiograph examination he was found to have Category 1, simple pneumoconiosis. He requested further evaluation of his pulmonary status because of complaints of

shortness of breath. He was 176 cm tall and had no positive physical flndings. Pulmonary function testing gave the following results:

	Observed Values	Percent of Predicted
FVC	5.0 liters	98
FEV_1	4.13 liters	99
FEV_1/FVC%	83	
D_{CO}	38 ml/min/mm Hg	100

The $\dot{V}O_2$ max was 32 ml/(kg·min).

Diagnosis: Uncomplicated coal workers' pneumoconiosis.

Impairment: 0% impairment of the whole person.

Comment: This individual has no demonstrable impairment even though he has an occupational disease that is recognized by radiography (see Table 9) and subjective complaints of dyspnea.

Example 2 of Class 1
Impairment of the Whole Person:
A 50-year-old male, driver of a beer delivery truck for the past 25 years, was referred for evaluation with the complaint that he had become too short of breath to carry three cases of beer up a flight of stairs. Approximately three months before referral, he had an anteroseptal myocardial infarction, and had been in the hospital for three weeks. Thereafter, he was allowed to return to work after beginning a progressive exercise program. He smoked one pack per day of unfiltered cigarettes.

Physical examination showed that the man was 190 cm tall and had no positive physical findings. By chest radiograph the lung fields were normal, but there was an unusual prominence of the left ventricular segment of the heart. Pulmonary function results were as follows:

	Observed Values	Percent of Predicted
FVC	5.39 liters	95
FEV_1	4.0 liters	90
FEV_1/FVC%	74	
D_{CO}	37 ml/min/mm Hg	90

The $\dot{V}O_2$ max was 18 ml/(kg·min).

The patient was considered to be in Class 1 insofar as the respiratory system was concerned. But because of the cardiac abnormality, he was to receive further evaluation for impairment of the cardiovascular system.

Diagnosis: Inadequate cardiac output as a result of myocardial infarction.

Impairment: 0% impairment due to respiratory disease.

Example of Class 2
Impairment of the Whole Person:
A 57-year-old man had a history of cough for six years' duration with slowly progressing dyspnea on exertion. Four months before examination he noticed an increase in the cough and noted also that he was becoming more dyspneic while walking one block on level ground at his own pace.

For a five-year period ending approximately 15 years ago, the man worked for a manufacturing company, spraying asbestos insulation on the interior walls of metal buildings. For the past three years his annual chest radiographs showed diminished lung volumes, interstitial fibrosis at both lung bases, and pleural plaques suggestive of asbestosis.

At examination the man weighed 87.5 kg (193 pounds) and was 172 cm tall. Auscultation of the lungs disclosed end-respiratory crackles at both lung bases.

	Observed Values	Percent of Predicted
FVC	3.30 liters	83
FEV_1	1.99 liters	62
FEV_1/FVC%	60	
D_{CO}	17.8 ml/min/mm Hg	77

The $\dot{V}O_2$ max was 22 ml/(kg·min).

Diagnosis: Asbestosis.

Impairment: 25% impairment of the whole person.

Comment: While at the time of this evaluation the man was in Class 2, the symptoms and signs of asbestosis could progress with time, impairing him further.

Example of Class 3
Impairment of the Whole Person:
A 56-year-old male, a foundry worker for 22 years, complains of progressing dyspnea of five years duration. He now has difficulty keeping up with other men his age. He usually has to stop on the second flight going up stairs, and he can walk only ½ mile on level ground at his own pace. He has had a productive cough for eight years that has produced more than two tablespoons of whitish, nonsmelling sputum per day. He has smoked a pack per day of nonfilter cigarettes since age 14 years.

In the foundry during the first 15 years of his employment, little effort was made to control dust, and

Table 8. Classes of Respiratory Impairment

	Class 1 0% No Impairment of the Whole Person	Class 2 10-25% Mild Impairment of the Whole Person	Class 3 30-45% Moderate Impairment of the Whole Person	Class 4 50-100% Severe Impairment of the Whole Person
FVC FEV_1 FEV_1/FVC (as percent) D_{CO}	FVC ≥ 80% of predicted, *and* FEV_1 ≥ 80% of predicted, *and* FEV_1/FVC ≥ 70% and D_{CO} ≥ 80% of predicted.	FVC between 60% and 79% of predicted, *or* FEV_1 between 60% and 79% of predicted, *or* FEV_1/FVC between 60% and 69%, *or* D_{CO} between 60% and 79% of predicted.	FVC between 51% and 59% of predicted, *or* FEV_1 between 41% and 59% of predicted, *or* FEV_1/FVC between 41% and 59%, *or* D_{CO} between 41% and 59% of predicted.	FVC ≤ 50% of predicted *or* FEV_1 ≤ 40% of predicted, *or* FEV_1/FVC ≤ 40%, *or* D_{CO} ≤ 40% of predicted.
	or	**or**	**or**	**or**
$\dot{V}O_2$ Max	> 25 ml/(kg · min)	Between 20 and 25 ml/(kg · min)	Between 15 and 20 ml/(kg · min)	< 15 ml/(kg · min)

FVC is Forced Vital Capacity, FEV_1 is Forced Expiratory Volume in the first second, D_{CO} is diffusing capacity of carbon monoxide. The D_{CO} is primarily of value for persons with restrictive lung disease. In Classes 2 and 3, if the FVC, FEV_1 and FEV_1/FVC ratio are normal and the D_{CO} is between 41% and 79%, then an exercise test is required.

$\dot{V}O_2$ Max, or measured exercise capacity, is useful in assessing whether a person's complaint of dyspnea (see Table 1) is a result of respiratory or other conditions. A person's cardiac and conditioning status must be considered in performing the test and in interpreting the results.

there was considerable sand dust from the molds. Recently, dust control measures have been better.

Examination shows that the man is 170 cm tall and he has bilateral, basilar, end-inspiratory, fine-pitched crackles. The examination otherwise is unremarkable and chest radiograph is normal. Pulmonary function studies show the following:

	Observed Values	Percent of Predicted
FVC	3.48 liters	80
FEV_1	1.60 liters	45
FEV_1/FVC%	46	
D_{CO}	16 ml/min/mm Hg	51

The $\dot{V}O_2$ max was 16 ml/(kg·min).

Diagnosis: Chronic bronchitis and pulmonary emphysema.

Impairment: 35% impairment of the whole person.

Comment: This man has an obvious obstructive ventilatory defect with impairment of his diffusion capacity. His oxygen intake is limited, probably because of his decreased ventilatory ability.

Example of Class 4
Impairment of the Whole Person:
A 60-year-old male worked as an insulator for 40 years. He had particularly heavy exposure to asbestos over a five-year period during the construction of a steam generating plant. He had no known asbestos exposure during the past eight years, during which time he worked with fiberglass. He smoked two packs of ciga-

rettes per day from the age of 15 years to that of 50 years, at which time he cut down to one pack per day. During the past 10 years he noted gradually increasing fatigue and shortness of breath. While at first he was unable to keep up with others when walking up hills, during the past three years he became unable to walk as rapidly as others on level ground. Therefore he stopped working about two months before he was examined. He denied having a productive cough.

Examination disclosed that the man was 186 cm tall. He had digital clubbing and cyanosis of the nail beds, ear lobes, and tip of the nose. He had fine respiratory crackles over the lower half of both lung bases posteriorly. No other abnormalities were noted.

Chest radiograph disclosed bilateral pleural thickening, a small linear calcification near the left side of the heart, a linear calcification in the dome of the right hemidiaphragm, and linear densities in the lower half of each lung field. Pulmonary function testing revealed:

	Observed Values	Percent of Predicted
FVC	3.13 liters	60
FEV_1	1.0 liters	25
FEV_1/FVC%	31	
D_{CO}	7.46 ml/min/mm Hg	20

The $\dot{V}O_2$ max was 11 ml/(kg·min).

Diagnosis: Asbestosis and pulmonary emphysema.

Impairment: 70% impairment of the whole person.

Comment: This person had a severe combined restrictive and obstructive ventilatory impairment with marked reduction of his diffusing capacity and a decreased $\dot{V}O_2$ max.

Table 9. Impairment Not Directly Related to Lung Function

Condition	Comment
Asthma	An asthmatic person, who despite optimum medical therapy, including daily administration of a bronchodilator under regular physician care, and whose physiologic tests of impairment fall under Class 4 (Table 2) after administration of an inhaled bronchodilator in a laboratory, is considered to be severely impaired. This level of impairment should be found on three successive tests, performed at least one week apart.
	(It is recognized that persons whose asthma causes less-than-severe impairment, or whose asthma is related directly to a job-related exposure (such as toluene diisocyanate) may occasionally be evaluated for the purposes of determining employability or employment-related disability. The final determination, which is a nonmedical decision, relies in part on medical evidence. The physician's thorough documentation of the nature of the asthmatic condition, as well as nonmedical evidence, such as exposure data and reports of supervisors or fellow employees, are crucial to this determination.)
Hypersensitivity pneumonitis	A person with this condition may need to be removed from exposure to the causative agent or other agents with similar sensitizing properties, in order to avoid future attacks and chronic sequelae.
Pneumoconiosis	Although pneumoconiosis may cause no physiologic impairment, its presence usually requires removal from exposure to the dust that caused the condition.
Sleep disorders	Obstructive sleep apnea, central sleep apnea and Cheyne-Stokes respiration may prevent progression through normal stages of sleep, and may lead to hypersomnolence, hypoxia, hemodynamic changes and personality disorders. Impairment due to sleep disorders should be evaluated according to criteria in Chapters 4, 6, and 14, and combined using the Combined Values Chart.
Lung cancers	All persons with lung cancers are to be considered severely impaired at the time of diagnosis. At a re-evaluation at one year after the diagnosis is established, if the person is found to be free of all evidence of tumor recurrence, then he or she should be rated according to the physiologic parameters in Table 8. If there is evidence of tumor, the person remains severely impaired. If the tumor recurs at a later date, the person immediately is considered to be severely impaired.

Impairment Not Directly Related to Lung Function

Certain respiratory conditions may cause impairment that is not readily quantifiable by spirometry, diffusing capacity, or measured exercise testing. Table 9 highlights these conditions, with some general comments. The evaluation of impairment of persons with these conditions should be done by physicians with expertise in lung disease, and the final impairment rating should be left to the physician's judgment.

References

1. American Thoracic Society Ad Hoc Committee on Impairment/Disability Criteria: Evaluation of impairment/disability secondary to respiratory disorders. *Am Rev Respir Dis* 1986;134:1205-1209.

2. American Thoracic Society Committee on Proficiency Standards for Pulmonary Function Laboratories: Standardization of spirometry-1987 update. *Am Rev Respir Dis* 1987;136:1285-1298.

3. American Thoracic Society D_{LCO} Standardization Conference: Single breath carbon monoxide diffusing capacity (transfer factor): Recommendations for a standard technique. *Am Rev Respir Dis* 1987;136:1299-1307.

4. Crapo RO, Morris AH, Gardner RM: Reference spirometric values using techniques and equipment that meet ATS recommendations. *Am Rev Respir Dis* 1981;123:659-664.

5. Crapo RO, Morris AH: Standardized single breath normal values for carbon monoxide diffusing capacity. *Am Rev Respir Dis* 1981;123: 185-190.

6. American College of Sports Medicine: Guidelines for Graded Testing and Exercise Prescription, ed 2. Philadelphia, Lea and Febiger, 1980, pp 29-32.

7. Oren A, Sue KD, Hansen JE, et al: The role of exercise testing in impairment evaluation. *Am Rev Respir Dis* 1987; 135:230-235.

Chapter 6

The Cardiovascular System

6.0 Introduction

The purpose of this chapter is to assist the physician by providing criteria for the evaluation of permanent impairment of the cardiovascular system according to the person's ability to perform the activities of daily living. The cardiovascular system consists of the heart, the aorta, the systemic arteries, and the pulmonary arteries; impairment of the system includes abnormal elevation of pressure in either the aorta, or systemic hypertension, or in the pulmonary artery, or pulmonary hypertension. The coronary and peripheral circulations are considered to be part of the cardiovascular system; however, impairment from disorders of the cerebral circulation is considered in Chapter 4.

Before using the information in this chapter, the reader is urged to review Chapters 1 and 2, which provide a general discussion of the purpose of the *Guides* and of the situations in which they are useful; and which discuss techniques for the evaluation of the subject and for preparation of a report. The report should include the information found in the following outline, which is developed more fully in Chapter 2.

A. *Medical Evaluation.*
1. Narrative history of medical conditions
2. Results of the most recent clinical evaluation
3. Assessment of current clinical status and statement of future plans
4. Diagnoses and clinical impressions
5. Expected date of full or partial recovery

B. *Analysis of Findings*
1. Impact of medical condition(s) on life activities
2. Explanation for concluding that the medical condition(s) has or has not become static or well-stabilized
3. Explanation for concluding that the individual is or is not likely to suffer from sudden or subtle incapacitation
4. Explanation for concluding that the individual is or is not likely to suffer injury or further impairment by engaging in life activities or by attempting to meet personal, social, and occupational demands
5. Explanation for concluding that accommodations and/or restrictions are or are not warranted

C. *Comparison of Results of Analysis with Impairment Criteria*
1. Description of clinical findings, and how these findings relate to specific criteria in the chapter
2. Explanation of each percent of impairment rating
3. Summary list of all impairment ratings
4. Overall rating of impairment of the whole person

Symptomatic Limitation

In this chapter reference is made to limitation of activities of daily living because of symptoms. Information about such limitation is subjective, and it is open to interpretation on the part of both patient and examiner. Therefore, when it is possible, the examiner should obtain objective data about the extent of the limitation before attempting to estimate the degree of permanent impairment. When estimating the extent of a limitation due to symptoms, the physician should use the functional classification in Table 1.

Exercise Testing

In most circumstances the physician should attempt to quantitate limitations due to symptoms by observing the patient during exercise. The most widely used and standardized exercise protocols involve the use of a motor-driven treadmill with varying grades and speeds. The protocols vary slightly, but they all attempt to relate the exercise to excess energy expended and to functional class. The excess energy expended usually is expressed with the "MET," a term that represents the multiples of resting metabolic energy utilized for any given activity. One MET is considered to be 3.5 ml/(kg·min). The 70 kg man who burns 1.2 kilocalories per minute sitting at rest uses approximately three METS when walking 4 kilometers per hour.

Table 2 displays the relationship of excess energy expenditures in METS to functional class according to the protocols of several investigators. With all protocols, the exercise periods last for three minutes; the periods are represented in the table by boxes with numbers giving the estimated METS involved.

If a treadmill is not available, steps may be used to attempt to quantitate the exercise capacity of a patient. Table 3 shows the relationships of exercise with steps of various heights, excess energy expenditure, and

---

Table 1. Functional Classifications*

Class 1:
The patient has cardiac disease but no resulting limitation of physical activity. Ordinary physical activity does not cause undue fatigue, palpitation, dyspnea, or anginal pain.

Class 2:
The patient has cardiac disease resulting in slight limitation of physical activity. The patient is comfortable at rest and in the performance of ordinary, light, daily activities. Greater than ordinary physical activity, such as heavy physical exertion, results in fatigue, palpitation, dyspnea, or anginal pain.

Class 3:
The patient has cardiac disease resulting in marked limitation of physical activity. The patient is comfortable at rest. Ordinary physical activity results in fatigue, palpitation, dyspnea, or anginal pain.

Class 4:
The patient has cardiac disease resulting in inability to carry on any physical activity without discomfort. Symptoms of inadequate cardiac output, pulmonary congestion, systemic congestion, or of the anginal syndrome may be present, even at rest. If any physical activity is undertaken, discomfort is increased.

---

*Adapted from: Criteria Committee of the New York Heart Association: *Diseases of the Heart and Blood Vessels: Nomenclature and Criteria for Diagnosis*, ed 6, Boston, Little Brown and Company, 1964, pp 112-113. Copyright © 1964, Little Brown and Company. For the purposes of assessing impairment this well established classification is to be preferred over the newer classification introduced in the 7th edition in 1973.

---

functional class. Estimations of excess energy expenditure also can be made with a bicycle ergometer (Table 4).

Some laboratories are equipped to measure oxygen consumption and carbon dioxide production during exercise. Data on a patient acquired by these techniques may become the most accurate method of estimating a patient's exercise capacity.

A major problem with using any exercise testing technique to attempt to quantitate an individual's functional capacity is the marked variability in patients' abilities and willingness to cooperate. Therefore, the physician also must estimate the individual's cooperation and effort during the test; some patients will continue far beyond where they should, while others will stop after minimal effort because they feel fatigued.

6.1 Valvular Heart Disease

Valvular heart disease may be caused by congenital, rheumatic, infectious, or traumatic factors, or a combination. Valvular disease may result in (1) an increased work load on either the left or right ventricle, leading to hypertrophy and/or dilation of the ventricle, and eventually to ventricular failure with congestion of the lungs or other organs; (2) obstruction to inflow of the ventricle as in mitral or tricuspid stenosis, causing congestion of organs even in the absence of ventricular failure; and (3) decreased cardiac output.

Valvular heart disease can be detected and its severity assessed by a thorough history and physical examination. The precision of the estimate of impairment often can be improved by obtaining appropriate laboratory studies, which may include electrocardiogram (ECG), chest radiograph, echocardiogram, exercise testing, radioisotope studies, hemodynamic measurements, or angiography.

The severity of valvular heart disease can be reduced, but not fully reversed, by operative procedures on the valves or by replacement of the valve with a prosthetic device. After such a procedure, sufficient time from the date of operation must elapse to allow maximum recovery of the heart, lungs, and other organs before estimating permanent impairment due to the valvular disease.

In addition, medications may affect the severity of valvular heart disease, especially limitations due to symptoms. Therefore, sufficient time must be allowed for these medications to be introduced and adjusted, and for them to exert their effects, before an estimate of permanent impairment is made.

Table 2. Relationship of METS and Functional Class According to 5 Treadmill Protocols

METS Treadmill Tests	1.6	2	3	4	5	6	7	8	9	10	11	12	13	14	15	16
Ellestad					1.7	3.0			4.0						5.0	
				←———————————————— 10 per cent grade ————————————————→												
Bruce					1.7		2.5		3.4				4.2			
					10		12		14				16			
Balke			←———————————————— 3.4 miles per hour ————————————————→													
				2	4	6	8	10	12	14	16	18	20	22	24	26
Balke			←——————————— 3.0 miles per hour ———————————→													
				0	2.5	5	7.5	10	12.5	15	17.5	20	22.5			
Naughton	1.0	←—— 2.0 miles per hour ——→														
		0	0	3.5	7	10.5	14	17.5								
METS	1.6	2	3	4	5	6	7	8	9	10	11	12	13	14	15	16
Clinical Status	Symptomatic Patients															
		Diseased, Recovered														
				Sedentary Healthy												
					Physically Active Subjects											
Functional Class	IV	III				II		I and Normal								

In the Ellestad protocol, the numbers in the boxes are miles per hour (mph); in the Bruce protocol the top numbers are mph and the bottom numbers are the percent grade. In the Balke and Naughton protocols the numbers are the percent grade.

Adapted from: Fox SM III, Naughton JP, Haskell WL: Physical activity and the prevention of coronary heart disease. *Annals of Clinical Research* 1971; 3:404-432. Copyright © 1971 The Finnish Medical Society Duodecim

Criteria for Evaluating Impairment Due to Valvular Disease

Class 1—Impairment of the Whole Person, 0-10%:
A patient belongs in Class 1 when (a) the patient has evidence by physical examination or laboratory test of valvular heart disease, but no symptoms in the performance of ordinary daily activities or even upon moderately heavy exertion (functional Class 1); *and* (b) the patient does not require continuous treatment, although prophylactic antibiotics may be recommended at the time of a surgical procedure to reduce the risk of bacterial endocarditis; *and* (c) the patient remains free of signs of congestive heart failure; *and* (d) there are no signs of ventricular hypertrophy or dilation, and the severity of the stenosis or regurgitation is estimated to be mild; *or* (e) in the patient who has recovered from valvular heart surgery, all of the above criteria are met.

Example 1: A 22-year-old woman has a midsystolic click and a late systolic murmur. She has no symptoms, and there are no signs of cardiac enlargement, or congestive heart failure, or cardiac rhythm disturbance. Physical examination reveals slight pectus excavatum. Chest radiograph and electrocardiogram (ECG) are normal. An echocardiogram shows prolapse of the mitral valve and normal left atrial and left ventricular size and function.

Diagnosis: Mitral valve prolapse syndrome.

Impairment: 0% impairment of the whole person.

Comment: If the ECG showed definite T wave abnormalities, or the echocardiogram showed slight enlargement of the left atrium or left ventricle, then the valve disorder would be estimated at 1% to 10% impairment, depending on the severity of the abnormality as shown by the laboratory studies.

A patient who has the murmur of aortic regurgitation or the signs of a bicuspid aortic valve, but who has no symptoms, no signs of cardiac enlargement, and no signs of congestive heart failure, might be estimated to have an impairment of 1% to 10%, depending on the estimated severity of the aortic valve disease.

The echocardiogram is not necessary to establish the diagnosis or degree of impairment.

Table 3. Relationship of METS and Functional Class According to Two Step Protocol

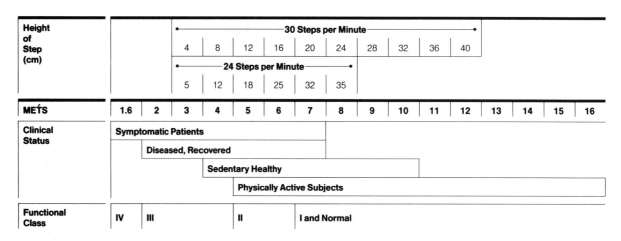

Source: Fox SM III, Naughton JP, Haskell WL: Physical activity and the prevention of coronary heart disease. *Annals of Clinical Research* 1971; 3:404-432. Copyright © 1971 The Finnish Medical Society Duodecim

Table 4. Energy Expenditure in METS During Bicycle Ergometry

Body Weight		Work Rate on Bicycle Ergometer (kg m⁻¹ min⁻¹ and Watts)												
(kg)	(lb)	75 12	150 25	300 50	450 75	600 100	750 125	900 150	1050 175	1200 200	1350 225	1500 250	1650 275	1800 300 (kg m⁻¹ min⁻¹) (Watts)
20	44	4.0	6.0	10.0	14.0	18.0	22.0							
30	66	3.4	4.7	7.3	10.0	12.7	15.3	17.9	20.7	23.3				
40	88	3.0	4.0	6.0	8.0	10.0	12.0	14.0	16.0	18.0	20.0	22.0		
50	110	2.8	3.6	5.2	6.8	8.4	10.0	11.5	13.2	14.8	16.3	18.0	19.6	21.1
60	132	2.7	3.3	4.7	6.0	7.3	8.7	10.0	11.3	12.7	14.0	15.3	16.7	18.0
70	154	2.6	3.1	4.3	5.4	6.6	7.7	8.8	10.0	11.1	12.2	13.4	14.0	15.7
80	176	2.5	3.0	4.0	5.0	6.0	7.0	8.0	9.0	10.0	11.0	12.0	13.0	14.0
90	198	2.4	2.9	3.8	4.7	5.6	6.4	7.3	8.2	9.1	10.0	10.9	11.8	12.6
100	220	2.4	2.8	3.6	4.4	5.2	6.0	6.8	7.6	8.4	9.2	10.0	10.8	11.6
110	242	2.4	2.7	3.4	4.2	4.9	5.6	6.3	7.1	7.8	8.5	9.3	10.0	10.7
120	264	2.3	2.7	3.3	4.0	4.7	5.3	6.0	6.7	7.3	8.0	8.7	9.3	10.0

Source: American College of Sports Medicine. *Guidelines for Graded Exercise Testing and Exercise Prescription.* Philadelphia, Lea and Febiger, 1975, p. 17. Copyright © 1975, American College of Sports Medicine.

Example 2: A 30-year-old woman has recovered from mitral commissurotomy, is asymptomatic, and has returned to an active life. She had rheumatic fever at age 8 and has had no recurrences.

Physical examination reveals a well healed surgical wound without tenderness. There are no abnormal precordial pulsations or signs of congestive heart failure. The first heart sound is loud; an opening snap is heard approximately 100 milliseconds after the second heart sound and there is a short rumble in mid-diastole. A grade 1/6 to 2/6 holosystolic murmur is heard at the apex.

Chest radiograph shows a heart of normal size and no signs of pulmonary congestion. An ECG has minimal P wave abnormalities. Echocardiogram shows slight enlargement of the left atrium and no enlargement or dysfunction of the ventricles.

Diagnosis: Mitral stenosis and postmitral commissurotomy.

Impairment: 5% to 10% impairment of the whole person.

Comment: The estimated degree of impairment will depend on the estimated severity of mitral regurgitation, residual stenosis, etc. Echocardiogram, cardiac catheterization, and angiography are not necessary and should not be obtained solely to help estimate the impairment.

Class 2—Impairment of the Whole Person, 15-25%:
A patient belongs in Class 2 when (a) the patient has evidence by physical examination or laboratory studies

of valvular heart disease, and there are no symptoms in the performance of ordinary daily activities, but symptoms develop on moderately heavy physical exertion (functional Class 2); *or* (b) the patient requires moderate dietary adjustment or drugs to prevent symptoms or to remain free of the signs of congestive heart failure or other consequences of valvular heart disease, such as syncope, chest pain, and emboli; *or* (c) the patient has signs or laboratory evidence of cardiac chamber hypertrophy and/or dilation, and the severity of the stenosis or regurgitation is estimated to be moderate, and surgical correction is not feasible or advisable; *or* (d) the patient has recovered from valvular heart surgery and meets the above criteria.

Example 1: A 63-year-old man was noted during a routine examination five years ago to have the murmur of aortic regurgitation and mild heart failure. He is an office worker, and he plays 18 holes of golf regularly, using an electric cart. The patient has been advised to restrict his salt intake and to take digoxin 0.25 mg daily.

At present, the patient's blood pressure is 160/50 mm Hg, the pulse is 70 beats per minute and regular, and the peripheral pulses are bounding. There are no signs of congestive heart failure. The apical impulse is just outside the midclavicular line, is slightly larger than normal, and is slightly prolonged. There is a grade 3/6 harsh, short, systolic ejection murmur in the aortic area, and a grade 3/6 long decrescendo diastolic murmur along the left lower sternal border. A faint mid-diastolic rumble is heard at the apex. The first and second heart sounds are normal.

An ECG shows tall R waves in V5 and V6 with low but upright T waves. Chest radiograph shows prominence of the apical portion of the cardiac silhouette and no cardiomegaly or pulmonary congestion. Echocardiogram shows a normal-sized aortic root, delicate aortic valve leaflets, fluttering of the anterior leaflet of the mitral valve, and ventricular volumes and volume indices at the upper limits of normal.

Cardiac catheterization and angiography show the following pressures: aorta 160/40 mm Hg, left ventricle 160/12 mm Hg, left atrium "a" 12 mm Hg and "v" 10 mm Hg. Aortography reveals moderate aortic regurgitation.

Diagnosis: Moderately severe aortic regurgitation of uncertain etiology.

Impairment: 20% to 25% impairment of the whole person.

Comment: Even though the patient is asymptomatic, impairment would be estimated to be greater if there were cardiomegaly, deeply inverted T waves in

leads 1, L, V5 and V6, or a dilated left ventricle on the echocardiogram. The cardiac catheterization and angiography were not necessary in this case to estimate the degree of impairment.

Example 2: A 66-year-old woman had several syncopal episodes three years ago, was found to have severe calcific stenosis of the aortic valve, and underwent aortic valve replacement with a large Bjork-Shiley prosthesis. She has returned to an active life, which includes walking two miles each morning. She takes oral anticoagulants to maintain the prothrombin time in the therapeutic range, the level being tested every three weeks. She takes antibiotics before dental or operative procedures but no other medication.

Physical examination discloses normal blood pressure and pulse and no signs of heart failure. The apical impulse has a slightly sustained quality. On auscultation a grade 1/6 early systolic murmur is heard in the first right intercostal space. The first heart sound is normal and the second heart sound is very sharp.

ECG reveals a normal rhythm and QRS pattern, and low T waves in leads 1, L, V5, and V6. Chest radiograph shows slight prominence of the apex of the heart, a properly positioned prosthesis, and no evidence of pulmonary congestion. Echocardiogram discloses a properly positioned prosthesis and ventricles of normal size with thickening of the left ventricular wall.

Cardiac catheterization and angiography show normal pressure in the left ventricle and a 15 mm Hg pressure gradient between the left ventricle and aorta. Aortography shows minimal aortic regurgitation.

Diagnosis: Calcific aortic stenosis, probably related to congenital bicuspid aortic valve, valve replacement with a Bjork-Shiley prosthesis.

Impairment: 20% impairment of the whole person.

Comment: The degree of impairment in this person might be greater if a faint decrescendo diastolic murmur were heard along the left sternal border, or if the gradient across the valve were slightly higher.

Class 3—Impairment of the Whole Person, 30-50%: A patient belongs in Class 3 when (a) the patient has signs of valvular heart disease and has slight to moderate symptomatic discomfort during the performance of ordinary daily activities (functional Class 3); *and* (b) dietary therapy or drugs do not completely control symptoms or prevent congestive heart failure; *and* (c) the patient has signs or laboratory evidence of cardiac chamber hypertrophy or dilation, the severity of the stenosis or regurgitation is estimated to be moderate or severe, and surgical correction is not feasible; *or* (d) the patient has recovered from heart valve surgery but continues to have symptoms and signs of congestive heart failure including cardiomegaly.

Example 1: A 71-year-old man with idiopathic thrombocytopenia that does not respond to medications has had moderate exertional dyspnea for the past two years despite the continued use of diuretics and digoxin. Presently, he is comfortable at rest, but he becomes short of breath when climbing to the second floor. He sleeps on two pillows and has not awakened short of breath since the dose of diuretics was increased one year ago.

Physical examination reveals a patient able to lie flat comfortably. Blood pressure is 110/80 mm Hg, and pulse rate is 84 beats per minute and irregular. The venous pressure is normal and there is no edema. Breath sounds are harsh at each base, but there are no rales. The apical impulse is large, hyperdynamic and displaced to the anterior axillary line. There is a slight parasternal heave. The first and second heart sounds are loud, and a grade 4/6 holosystolic murmur is heard at the lower sternal border, apex, and axilla. A third heart sound is audible.

The ECG shows atrial fibrillation with an irregular ventricular response of about 80 per minute. There are low T waves, but the QRS pattern is normal. The chest radiograph shows cardiomegaly with a large left atrium. There is prominence of the vasculature of the upper lobes. Echocardiogram shows slight enlargement of the left and right ventricles and definite enlargement of the left atrium with "hammocking" that suggests mitral valve prolapse.

Diagnosis: Severe mitral regurgitation due to mitral valve prolapse.

Impairment: 50% impairment of the whole person.

Comment: Greater exercise tolerance and less cardiomegaly would suggest a lower degree of impairment.

Example 2: A 60-year-old woman had surgery to replace the aortic and mitral valves one year ago. Despite taking oral anticoagulants, digoxin, and diuretics and restricting salt in her diet, she does not have much stamina. She tires easily and must rest each afternoon. Ankle edema sometimes develops, but it clears promptly after she takes an extra diuretic tablet. She sleeps on one pillow and has no nocturnal dyspnea. While able to do light house work, the patient has not felt so well

that she wishes to return to her work as a seamstress. Her weight remains about 15 pounds below preoperative weight.

Physical examination reveals the patient to be comfortable when lying flat. Blood pressure is 110/70 mm Hg; pulse is 80 beats per minute and irregular. Venous pressure is normal and there is no edema. The lungs are clear. The apical impulse is enlarged, is located at the anterior axillary line, and is sustained through all of systole; there is no parasternal heave. The prosthetic valve sounds are normal. A grade 1/6 early systolic murmur is heard in the first right interspace and along the left sternal border.

The ECG shows atrial fibrillation with an irregular ventricular response of about 80 per minute. Chest radiograph shows cardiomegaly with left ventricular and left atrial enlargement. There is prominence of the vasculature in the upper lobes. Echocardiogram shows no evidence of prosthetic valve malfunction or displacement. There is slight enlargement of the ventricles and left atrium. Ventricular function is good.

Diagnosis: Aortic and mitral valve disease, probably rheumatic in origin; surgical replacement of valves.

Impairment: 40% impairment of the whole person.

Class 4—Impairment of the Whole Person, 55-100%: A patient belongs in Class 4 when (a) the patient has signs by physical examination of valvular heart disease, and symptoms at rest or in the performance of less than ordinary daily activities (functional Class 4); *and* (b) dietary therapy and drugs cannot control symptoms or prevent signs of congestive heart failure; *and* (c) the patient has signs or laboratory evidence of cardiac chamber hypertrophy and/or dilation; and the severity of the stenosis or regurgitation is estimated to be moderate or severe, and surgical correction is not feasible; *or* (d) the patient has recovered from valvular heart surgery but continues to have symptoms or signs of congestive heart failure.

Example 1: A 45-year-old woman has had treatment for congestive heart failure over a 10-year period. In spite of properly using diuretics and digoxin and, for the past year, a peripheral vasodilator, the patient continues to become breathless on minimal exertion. Even going to the bathroom causes breathlessness and fatigue. She sleeps on three pillows. For years, her ankles have been swollen, and over the last year her abdomen has become protuberant.

Physical examination shows a woman who is pale and weak. Her face is thin, showing temporal depression, and jaundice is present. She is breathing 22

Table 5. Impairment Classification for Valvular Heart Disease

Class 1 0-10% Impairment of Whole Person	Class 2 15-25% Impairment of Whole Person	Class 3 30-50% Impairment of Whole Person	Class 4 55-100% Impairment of Whole Person
The patient has evidence by physical examination or laboratory studies of valvular heart disease, but no symptoms in the performance of ordinary daily activities or even upon moderately heavy exertion (functional class 1); **and** The patient does not require continuous treatment, although prophylactic antibiotics may be recommended at the time of a surgical procedure to reduce the risk of bacterial endocarditis; **and** The patient remains free of signs of congestive heart failure; **and** There are no signs of ventricular hypertrophy or dilation, and the severity of the stenosis or regurgitation is estimated to be mild; **or** In the patient who has recovered from valvular heart surgery, all of the above criteria are met.	The patient has evidence by physical examination or laboratory studies of valvular heart disease, and there are no symptoms in the performance of ordinary daily activities, but symptoms develop on moderately heavy physical exertion (functional class 2); **or** The patient requires moderate dietary adjustment or drugs to prevent symptoms or to remain free of the signs of congestive heart failure or other consequences of valvular heart disease, such as syncope, chest pain and emboli; **or** The patient has signs or laboratory evidence of cardiac chamber hypertrophy and/or dilation, and the severity of the stenosis or regurgitation is estimated to be moderate, and surgical correction is not feasible or advisable; **or** The patient has recovered from valvular heart surgery and meets the above criteria.	The patient has signs of valvular heart disease and has slight to moderate symptomatic discomfort during the performance of ordinary daily activities (functional class 3); **and** Dietary therapy or drugs do not completely control symptoms or prevent congestive heart failure; **and** The patient has signs or laboratory evidence of cardiac chamber hypertrophy or dilation, the severity of the stenosis or regurgitation is estimated to be moderate or severe, and surgical correction is not feasible; **or** The patient has recovered from heart valve surgery but continues to have symptoms and signs of congestive heart failure including cardiomegaly.	The patient has signs by physical examination of valvular heart disease, and symptoms at rest or in the performance of less than ordinary daily activities (functional class 4); **and** Dietary therapy and drugs cannot control symptoms or prevent signs of congestive heart failure; **and** The patient has signs or laboratory evidence of cardiac chamber hypertrophy and/or dilation; and the severity of the stenosis or regurgitation is estimated to be moderate or severe, and surgical correction is not feasible; **or** The patient has recovered from valvular heart surgery but continues to have symptoms or signs of congestive heart failure.

times per minute, and blood pressure is 110/70 mm Hg; the pulse rate is about 80 beats per minute and irregular. The patient prefers the sitting position, and in that position, the neck veins are distended to the midneck and show prominent V waves.

There are rales at both lung bases. There is a parasternal heave. On auscultation there is a grade 3/6 harsh systolic murmur in the second right interspace; this murmur is long but stops in late systole. After a time gap, a long, loud decrescendo diastolic murmur is heard. At the lower sternal border and at the apex, respectively, are a blowing holosystolic murmur and a mid-diastolic rumble. The first heart sound is diminished and the second heart sound is loud in the second left interspace. The liver is large and pulsatile, and it has a span of approximately 12 cm. Ascites and 3-plus pitting edema of the thighs, sacral area, and legs are present.

The ECG shows atrial fibrillation and an irregular ventricular response of about 80 per minute. There is low voltage of the QRS and T waves. The chest radiograph shows massive cardiomegaly suggesting enlargement of all chambers. There is prominence of the vasculature in the upper lobes, and Kerley B lines are seen on both sides. The echocardiogram shows enlargement of all chambers. The left ventricular ejection fraction is 20%.

Diagnosis: Aortic and mitral stenosis and regurgitation, and tricuspid regurgitation, of rheumatic etiology.

Impairment: 100% impairment of the whole person.

Example 2: A 50-year-old male with mitral valve disease had advanced symptoms and signs of heart failure resulting in congestion of the pulmonary and systemic circulations. He underwent mitral valve replacement two years ago. Since then, despite restriction of activities and salt and the use of digoxin and diuretics, the patient's activities remained limited by dyspnea upon minimal exertion. Vigorous use of diuretics eliminated peripheral edema but resulted in chemical evidence of pre-renal azotemia. The patient was able to walk a city block at a normal pace, drive an automobile, and sleep comfortably, but he became breathless after climbing one flight of stairs.

Physical examination reveals a comfortable patient with a blood pressure of 110/70 mm Hg; pulse is 80 beats per minute and irregular. The venous pressure is normal and there is no peripheral edema. There are rales at the left base. The apical impulse is normal, but there is a parasternal heave. The prosthetic valve sounds are normal but there is a grade 1/6 holosystolic murmur at the apex.

ECG shows atrial fibrillation with irregular ventricular response at about 80 per minute and low T waves. Chest radiograph shows cardiomegaly with enlargement of the left and right ventricles and left atrium. There is prominence of the pulmonary vasculature in all lung fields. No Kerley B lines are seen. The prosthetic valve is properly positioned. Echocardiogram shows enlargement of the ventricles and the left atrium. The prosthetic valve is properly positioned and functioning.

Cardiac catheterization and angiography reveal a left ventricular pressure of 110/18 mm Hg and a mean left atrial pressure of 20 mm Hg. The pulmonary artery pressure is 45/18 mm Hg. Left ventricular angiogram shows mild mitral regurgitation and reduction of ventricular contraction.

Diagnosis: Mitral valve replacement with a prosthesis; left ventricular dysfunction. The etiology probably is rheumatic.

Impairment: 80% impairment of the whole person.

The criteria for impairment due to valvular heart disease are shown in Table 5.

6.2 Coronary Heart Disease

Coronary heart disease is most commonly due to arteriosclerosis of the coronary arteries, a process that results in reduced coronary blood flow. Other causes of limited or reduced coronary blood flow include coronary artery spasm, emboli, congenital abnormality, and trauma. Also, inflammatory processes and arteritis can obstruct the coronary arteries, especially the coronary ostia.

Reduced coronary flow may result in injury to the myocardium, leading to infarction or diffuse fibrosis. The degree of impairment of the individual is determined by the consequences of both the reduced coronary blood flow and the reduced ventricular function. Reduced coronary blood flow also can cause angina pectoris, which itself may impair a person's ability to perform his or her usual activities. In addition, reduced coronary blood flow and myocardial damage may cause cardiac arrhythmias, which are discussed in a separate section.

The physician must obtain a detailed history in order to estimate the degree of impairment due to coronary heart disease. The physical examination may contribute to estimating the severity of the disorder and especially to estimating the degree of impairment

of ventricular function. In most patients laboratory studies also will be necessary. Studies obtained at rest, during exercise, and after exercise are especially useful in evaluating patients suspected of having coronary heart disease. Coronary angiography may be necessary in some patients.

Impairment due to coronary heart disease can be reduced but not eliminated by diet, exercise training programs, cessation of cigarette smoking, use of medications, and surgical procedures. Sufficient time must be allowed for these measures to have an effect before an estimate of permanent impairment is made.

Criteria for Evaluating Permanent Impairment Due to Coronary Heart Disease

Class 1—Impairment of the Whole Person, 0-10%:
Because of the serious implications of reduced coronary blood flow, it is not reasonable to classify the degree of impairment as 0% to 10% in any patient who has symptoms of coronary heart disease corroborated by physical examination or laboratory tests. This class of impairment should be reserved for the patient with an equivocal history of angina pectoris on whom coronary angiography is performed, or for a patient on whom coronary angiography is performed for other reasons, and in whom is found less than 50% reduction in the cross-sectional area of a coronary artery.

Class 2—Impairment of the Whole Person, 15-25%:
A patient belongs in Class 2 when (a) the patient has history of a myocardial infarction or angina pectoris that is documented by appropriate laboratory studies, but at the time of evaluation the patient has no symptoms while performing ordinary daily activities or even moderately heavy physical exertion (functional Class 1); *and* (b) the patient may require moderate dietary adjustment and/or medication to prevent angina or to remain free of signs and symptoms of congestive heart failure; *and* (c) the patient is able to walk on the treadmill or bicycle ergometer and obtain a heart rate of 90% of his or her predicted maximum heart rate without developing significant ST segment shift, ventricular tachycardia, or hypotension; if the patient is uncooperative or unable to exercise because of disease affecting another organ system, this requirement may be omitted; *or* (d) the patient has recovered from coronary artery surgery or angioplasty, remains asymptomatic during ordinary daily activities, and is able to

Table 6. Maximal and 90% of Maximal Achievable Heart Rate, by Age and Sex

Heart Rate		Age							
		30	35	40	45	50	55	60	65
Men	Maximal	193	191	189	187	184	182	180	178
	90% Maximal	173	172	170	168	166	164	162	160
Women	Maximal	190	185	181	177	172	168	163	159
	90% Maximal	171	167	163	159	155	151	147	143

Source: Sheffield LH: Exercise stress testing, in Braunwald E (ed): *Heart Disease—A Textbook of Cardiovascular Medicine,* ed 3, Philadelphia, WB Saunders Company, 1988, p. 227. Copyright © 1988, WB Saunders Company.

exercise as outlined above. If the patient is taking a beta adrenergic blocking agent, he or she should be able to exercise on the treadmill or bicycle ergometer to a level estimated to cause an energy expenditure of at least 10 METS as a substitute for the heart rate target.

Any of the exercise protocols in Table 2 may be used. The maximum and 90% of maximum predicted heart rates by age and sex group are presented in Table 6.

Example 1: A 50-year-old man had an acute myocardial infarction six months ago. He was hospitalized for 10 days, at which time serial ECGs showed classical changes of an inferior wall infarction. After recovering, the patient returned to his work as an attendant in a service station. At present, the man is following a diet to maintain a weight of 160 lb, which is 25 lb less than his weight one year ago. He has no symptoms and is receiving no medication.

Physical examination and chest radiographs are normal. The ECG shows Q waves in leads 2, 3, and F and flat T waves in the same leads. When he exercises, his heart rate is 152 beats per minute, and he has an adequate rise in blood pressure; there are no ECG pattern changes indicating ischemia or arrhythmias.

Diagnosis: Recent inferior wall myocardial infarction.

Impairment: 20% impairment of the whole person.

Comment: An uncomplicated recovery from an anterior wall infarction would equal 25% impairment.

Example 2: A 52-year-old woman underwent coronary artery bypass surgery six months ago for relief of angina. A vein graft was placed into the left anterior descending coronary artery and another into the right coronary artery. Preoperative coronary angiography had shown no significant obstruction in the circumflex coronary artery. Since surgery the patient has done well and has returned to work as a client service specialist for an insurance firm. She has had no symptoms but has

avoided heavy physical exertion. She is taking 0.3 gm aspirin daily but no other medications. An exercise test 10 days ago showed a heart rate of 144 beats per minute after 10 minutes of exercise, and no ST segment shifts or arrhythmias.

Physical examination reveals a well healed scar and a normal heart. The resting ECG shows low T waves in leads 1, L, V4, V5 and V6 and no Q waves. The chest radiograph shows normal heart and lungs.

Diagnosis: Coronary heart disease with coronary artery bypass surgery.

Impairment: 15% impairment of the whole person.

Class 3—Impairment of the Whole Person, 30-50%: A patient belongs in Class 3 when (a) the patient has a history of myocardial infarction that is documented by appropriate laboratory studies, or angina pectoris that is documented by changes on a resting or exercise ECG or radioisotope study that are suggestive of ischemia; *or* (b) the patient has either a fixed or dynamic focal obstruction of at least 50% of a coronary artery, demonstrated by angiography; *and* (c) the patient requires moderate dietary adjustment or drugs to prevent frequent angina or to remain free of symptoms and signs of congestive heart failure, but may develop angina pectoris or symptoms of congestive heart failure after moderately heavy physical exertion (functional Class 2); *or* (d) the patient has recovered from coronary artery surgery or angioplasty, continues to require treatment, and has the symptoms described above.

Example 1: A 60-year-old family physician suffered from an acute anterior wall myocardial infarction six months ago. He had the classical history of chest pain, diaphoresis, and weakness, and typical ECG and enzyme changes. After discharge from the hospital, the patient entered a rehabilitation program, but even after three months he continued to experience fatigue and some breathlessness after a brisk walk of 20 to 30 minutes. The patient returned to work but limited his practice and accepted no new patients.

An ECG three months ago recorded a heart rate of 140 beats per minute after 10 minutes of exercise and ST segment elevation in leads 1, L, and V3 through V6. After exercising, the patient was tired but experienced no chest pain. A radioisotope angiogram revealed a large anterior aneurysm of the left ventricle and good function of the inferior wall of the left ventricle. The patient was placed on a regimen of a low salt diet, digoxin 0.25 mg daily, and hydrochlorothiazide 25 mg three times per week.

On physical examination, the patient is comfortable and there are no signs of heart failure. Blood pressure is 135/85 mm Hg and pulse is regular. Examination of the precordium reveals a large sustained impulse just above and lateral to the left nipple, centered in the third intercostal space at the anterior axillary line. A fourth heart sound is present.

The ECG shows a Q wave in leads 1, L, and V1 through V4. Chest radiograph shows cardiac enlargement and clear lung fields.

Diagnosis: Anterior left ventricular aneurysm secondary to coronary heart disease.

Impairment: 45% impairment of the whole person.

Example 2: A 62-year-old woman underwent quadruple coronary artery bypass surgery six months ago, but she continues to experience retrosternal chest discomfort if she hurries while doing usual activities. She is especially likely to experience discomfort in the morning and when outdoors in the cold. She enjoys walking but usually experiences discomfort if she hurries up a steep hill leading to her church. She is able to care for her house, and perform other activities without symptoms if she does not rush. She is on a diet, and she takes a beta adrenergic blocking agent and oral nitrates.

At the latest physical examination, she was comfortable and had no signs of congestive heart failure. Blood pressure was 110/70 mm Hg, and pulse was regular at 62 beats per minute. The apical impulse was normal and there were no gallops or murmurs.

An ECG showed low T waves in all leads, and the chest radiograph was normal. An exercise ECG recorded a heart rate of 118 beats per minute after 10 minutes of exercise. The patient experienced retrosternal discomfort during the last minute of exercise, and there was 1.5 mm of ST segment depression in leads V4 through V6 at one and two minutes after exercise. Thallium was injected during exercise, and a definite anterior wall filling defect was demonstrated that only partially refilled during redistribution study. A multigated blood pool radioisotope angiogram revealed reduction of movement of the anterior wall, and that part was akinetic during exercise.

A coronary angiogram revealed 90% or greater obstruction of all three coronary arteries. The grafts to the right, circumflex, and left anterior descending coronary arteries were patent, but the graft to the diagonal branch of the left anterior descending coronary artery could not be visualized.

Diagnosis: Coronary heart disease and continued chest discomfort following coronary artery bypass surgery.

Impairment: 45% impairment of the whole person.

Class 4—Impairment of the Whole Person, 55-100%: A patient belongs in Class 4 when (a) the patient has history of a myocardial infarction that is documented by appropriate laboratory studies, or angina pectoris that has been documented by changes on a resting ECG or radioisotope study that are highly suggestive of myocardial ischemia; *or* (b) the patient has either fixed or dynamic focal obstruction of at least 50% of one or more coronary arteries, demonstrated by angiography; *and* (c) moderate dietary adjustments or drugs are required to prevent angina or to remain free of symptoms and signs of congestive heart failure, but the patient continues to develop symptoms of angina pectoris or congestive heart failure during ordinary daily activities (functional Class 3 or 4), there are signs or laboratory evidence of cardiac enlargement and abnormal ventricular function; *or* (d) the patient has recovered from coronary artery bypass surgery or angioplasty and continues to require treatment and have symptoms as described above.

Example 1: A 42-year-old man suffered an anteroseptal myocardial infarction six months ago. Two years ago he had an inferior wall myocardial infarction. During the past six months he has continued to have episodes of retrosternal discomfort on minimal exertion and sometimes at rest, despite the use of adequate doses of beta adrenergic blocking agents, oral and sublingual nitrates, and more recently, a calcium channel blocking agent. He rarely goes a full day without an episode of chest discomfort lasting from 1 to 10 minutes.

On examination, the patient is comfortable at rest. His blood pressure is 120/80 mm Hg and his resting pulse rate is 54 beats per minute. There are no signs of congestive heart failure. The apical impulse is enlarged, sustained, and displaced laterally to the anterior axillary line at the fifth intercostal space. The first heart sound is soft and there is a prominent fourth heart sound. A grade 2/6 holosystolic murmur is present at the apex.

The resting ECG shows Q waves in leads 2, 3 and F, a QS pattern in V1 through V3 and a QR in V4; the T waves are low in all leads. The chest radiograph shows marked cardiomegaly and prominence of the vasculature in the upper lung fields. During exercise the patient develops pain and ST depression in 1, L, V5 and V6 after two minutes. The ejection fraction falls from 30% to 25% as measured by the multigated blood pool scan.

Diagnosis: Angina pectoris and left ventricular failure due to coronary heart disease.

Impairment: 90% impairment of the whole person.

Example 2: A 46-year-old woman had quadruple coronary artery bypass surgery six months ago but continues to have pain each day and to be weak and breathless after minimal exertion. She sleeps on three

Table 7. Impairment Classification for Coronary Heart Disease

Class 1 0-10% Impairment of Whole Person	**Class 2** 15-25% Impairment of Whole Person	**Class 3** 30-50% Impairment of Whole Person	**Class 4** 55-100% Impairment of Whole Person
Because of the serious implications of reduced coronary blood flow, it is not reasonable to classify the degree of impairment as 0% to 10% in any patient who has symptoms of coronary heart disease corroborated by physical examination or laboratory tests. This class of impairment should be reserved for the patient with an equivocal history of angina pectoris on whom coronary angiography is performed, or for a patient on whom coronary angiography is performed for other reasons and in whom is found less than 50% reduction in the cross sectional area of a coronary artery.	The patient has history of a myocardial infarction or angina pectoris that is documented by appropriate laboratory studies, but at the time of evaluation the patient has no symptoms while performing ordinary daily activities or even moderately heavy physical exertion (functional class 1); **and** The patient may require moderate dietary adjustment and/or medication to prevent angina or to remain free of signs and symptoms of congestive heart failure; **and** The patient is able to walk on the treadmill or bicycle ergometer and obtain a heart rate of 90% of his or her predicted maximum heart rate without developing significant ST segment shift, ventricular tachycardia, or hypotension; if the patient is uncooperative or unable to exercise because of disease affecting another organ system, this requirement may be omitted; **or** The patient has recovered from coronary artery surgery or angioplasty, remains asymptomatic during ordinary daily activities, and is able to exercise as outlined above. If the patient is taking a beta adrenergic blocking agent, he or she should be able to walk on the treadmill to a level estimated to cause an energy expenditure of at least 10 METS as a substitute for the heart rate target.	The patient has a history of myocardial infarction that is documented by appropriate laboratory studies, and/or angina pectoris that is documented by changes on a resting or exercise ECG or radioisotope study that are suggestive of ischemia; **or** The patient has either a fixed or dynamic focal obstruction of at least 50% of a coronary artery, demonstrated by angiography; **and** The patient requires moderate dietary adjustment or drugs to prevent frequent angina or to remain free of symptoms and signs of congestive heart failure, but may develop angina pectoris or symptoms of congestive heart failure after moderately heavy physical exertion (functional class 2); **or** The patient has recovered from coronary artery surgery or angioplasty, continues to require treatment, and has the symptoms described above.	The patient has history of a myocardial infarction that is documented by appropriate laboratory studies, or angina pectoris that has been documented by changes on a resting ECG or radioisotope study that are highly suggestive of myocardial ischemia; **or** The patient has either fixed or dynamic focal obstruction of at least 50% of one or more coronary arteries, demonstrated by angiography; **and** Moderate dietary adjustments or drugs are required to prevent angina or to remain free of symptoms and signs of congestive heart failure, but the patient continues to develop symptoms of angina pectoris or congestive heart failure during ordinary daily activities (functional class 3 or 4), or there are signs or laboratory evidence of cardiac enlargement and abnormal ventricular function; **or** The patient has recovered from coronary artery bypass surgery or angioplasty and continues to require treatment and have symptoms as described above.

pillows; often she awakens short of breath and must sit in a chair for the remainder of the night. These symptoms continue despite digitalis, diuretics, nitrates, calcium channel blocking agents, and hydralazine.

On examination, there is evidence of weight loss. The patient prefers the sitting position. Blood pressure is 110/70 mm Hg, and the heart rate is 92 beats per minute. The neck veins distend when hand pressure is applied to the abdomen, even when the head of the examining table is elevated 45 degrees. The apical impulse is enlarged, sustained, and displaced to the anterior axillary line, and a parasternal heave is present. There are rales at both lung bases and dullness at the right lung base. The first heart sound is soft and there is a prominent third heart sound. A grade 2/6 holosystolic murmur is present at the apex.

The ECG shows a QS pattern in V1 through V4, prominent Q waves in V5 and V6, and low R waves throughout. The T waves are inverted in 1, L and V1 through V5, and low elsewhere. Chest radiograph shows marked cardiomegaly, increased vascular markings in the upper lung fields, and a small, right-sided pleural effusion.

Coronary angiography shows total occlusion of the left anterior descending coronary artery and 90% blockage in both the right and circumflex coronary arteries. The graft to the right coronary artery and the graft to one of the branches of the circumflex artery are patent, but the graft to the other branch of the circumflex artery and the graft to the anterior descending artery are not visualized. The ventriculogram shows an ejection fraction of 20%; there is akinesis of the entire anterior wall and poor contraction elsewhere.

Diagnosis: Angina pectoris and left ventricular failure after coronary artery bypass surgery.

Impairment: 100% impairment of the whole person.

The criteria for permanent impairment due to coronary heart disease are found in Table 7.

6.3 Congenital Heart Disease

In recent years, surgical procedures designed to correct or improve the circulation of infants and children with congenital cardiac disorders have allowed many of these individuals to live to adulthood. Many of these surgically treated patients continue to have less than perfect functioning of the heart and circulation and are therefore impaired.

Congenital heart disease may be recognized by history and upon physical examination, but often the exact diagnosis and the patient's functional impairment require special studies, including ECG, chest radiograph, radioisotope studies, echocardiography, hemodynamic measurements, and angiography. A quantitation of limitations due to symptoms is found in Table 1.

Criteria for Evaluating Impairment Due to Congenital Heart Disease

Class 1—Impairment of the Whole Person, 0-10%:
A patient belongs in Class 1 when (a) the patient has evidence by physical examination or laboratory studies of congenital heart disease and has no symptoms in the performance of ordinary daily activities, or even upon moderately heavy physical exertion; *and* (b) continuous treatment is not required, although prophylactic antibiotics may be recommended after surgical procedures to reduce the risk of bacterial endocarditis; and the patient remains free of signs of congestive heart failure and cyanosis; *and* (c) there are no signs of cardiac chamber hypertrophy or dilation; the evidence of residual valvular stenosis or regurgitation is estimated to be mild; there is no evidence of left-to-right or right-to-left shunt; and the pulmonary vascular resistance is estimated to be normal; *or* (d) in the patient who has recovered from corrective heart surgery, all of the above criteria are met.

Example 1: A 22-year-old woman is known to have had a loud systolic murmur along the left sternal border since childhood. She underwent cardiac catheterization at the ages of 2 and 18 years, and on both occasions a 20 mm Hg gradient was noted between the right ventricle and the pulmonary artery. She also had normal pulmonary artery pressures, no evidence of shunts, and normal cardiac output. The patient has never had symptoms referable to the cardiovascular system.

At present, physical examination shows the patient to be comfortable without signs of heart failure or cyanosis. The precordium is without heaves, thrills, or taps. The first heart sound is normal and the second heart sound is widely split, and there is variation with respiration. There is a grade 3/6 systolic murmur that ends well short of the second heart sound; the murmur is loudest in the second left intercostal space. There are no diastolic murmurs or gallops. Chest radiograph and ECG are normal.

Diagnosis: Mild pulmonary valve stenosis.

Impairment: 10% impairment of the whole person.

Comment: If the gradient were greater than 40 mm Hg, or if the ECG were to show right ventricular hypertrophy, then the patient would be in a higher category of impairment, and should be considered for surgical treatment of the stenosis. An asymptomatic patient with a small ventricular septal defect also might be rated at the upper end of Class 1 impairment, but if bacterial endocarditis had ever been present, then the impairment rating would be higher. Also in this category might be a patient who has a small atrial septal defect with normal pressures in all cardiac chambers and great vessels, or a patient who has anomalous venous return of a small segment of the lung.

Example 2: A 25-year-old woman underwent repair of secundum atrial septal defect 10 years ago. There were no complications, and the patient remained asymptomatic and returned to a normally active life.

Physical examination at present shows a well healed wound over the sternum without tenderness. There are no abnormal precordial pulsations or signs of congestive heart failure. The first heart sound is normal. The second heart sound is widely split and there is some variation with respiration in the degree of splitting. A grade 2/6 early systolic ejection murmur is heard along the left sternal border.

The ECG shows an incomplete right bundle branch block pattern. The chest radiograph is normal. The echocardiogram shows enlargement of the right ventricle and reduced motion of the ventricular septum. Findings of cardiac catheterization and angiography are normal.

Diagnosis: Atrial septal defect with surgical closure.

Impairment: 0% impairment of the whole person.

Comment: If a very small left-to-right shunt were demonstrated postoperatively, then the degree of impairment might be raised to 5% to 10%. Echocardiogram, cardiac catheterization, and angiography are not necessary for evaluating the degree of impairment.

Class 2—Impairment of the Whole Person, 15-25%:
A patient belongs in Class 2 when (a) the patient has evidence by physical examination or laboratory studies of congenital heart disease, has no symptoms in the

performance of ordinary daily activities, and has symptoms with moderately heavy physical exertion (functional Class 2); or (b) the patient requires moderate dietary adjustments or drugs to prevent symptoms or to remain free of signs of congestive heart failure or other consequences of congenital heart disease, such as syncope, chest pain, emboli, or cyanosis; or (c) there are signs or laboratory evidence of cardiac chamber hypertrophy or dilation, or the severity of valvular stenosis or regurgitation is estimated to be moderate; or there is evidence of a small residual left-to-right or right-to-left shunt; or there is evidence of moderate elevation of the pulmonary vascular resistance, which should be less than one-half the systemic vascular resistance; or (d) the patient has recovered from surgery for the treatment of congenital heart disease and meets the above criteria for impairment.

Example 1: A 35-year-old woman had a systolic murmur and abnormal cardiac sounds for many years. She led a relatively normal life but avoided participation in sports at the advice of physicians. During the past year she noted becoming weak and tired more easily than usual and also noticed regular pounding of the heart with minimal exertion. The palpitations were not associated with symptoms of inadequate cerebral perfusion and were never sustained. There was no history of cyanosis, breathlessness, or peripheral edema.

On examination, the patient is comfortable and has no cyanosis. There are prominent V waves in the neck veins, and the liver is enlarged to a width of 12 cm. The lungs are clear. There are no thrills, taps or heaves in the precordium. The first heart sound is loud and is followed by a very loud, sharp sound in early systole that is heard best along the left sternal border. The second heart sound is loud, and there is an early diastolic sound heard best at the midprecordium. A holosystolic murmur is heard along the left sternal border that increases in intensity with inspiration.

The ECG demonstrates a right bundle branch block pattern, and the R wave in V1 is very low. There is a broad, notched P wave in leads 3 and F, and inverted T waves in V1 and V2. There are occasional premature atrial beats. The chest radiograph shows marked enlargement of the cardiac silhouette, particularly to the right of the sternum. The pulmonary vasculature is normal. Echocardiogram shows features suggesting Ebstein's anomaly of the tricuspid valve.

Cardiac catheterization and angiography demonstrate a mean right atrial pressure of 7 mm Hg with V waves of 15 mm Hg. Right ventricular and pulmonary artery pressures are normal. There is no evidence of left-to-right or right-to-left shunt.

Intracardiac electrograms show a right ventricular ECG pattern at the time the catheter lumen is recording right atrial pressures. Angiography reveals a markedly displaced tricuspid valve, an enormous right atrium, and a small right ventricle.

Diagnosis: Ebstein's anomaly of the tricuspid valve.

Impairment: 25% impairment of the whole person.

Comment: If the patient had a right-to-left shunt, then the rated degree of impairment would be considerably higher. Also, if the patient had cardiac arrhythmias causing symptoms, impairment would be rated according to the specific criteria for arrhythmias, and the impairment due to congenital heart disease and arrythmias would be combined using the Combined Values Chart.

Example 2: A 42-year-old male underwent open heart surgery 15 years ago for the treatment of tetralogy of Fallot. The procedure resulted in relief of pulmonary stenosis, placement of a pericardial bridge in the outflow tract of the right ventricle, and closure of the ventricular septal defect. After the operation, the patient did well without medication and achieved his present position as dispatcher for a trucking firm.

At examination, the man appears healthy. Blood pressure is 110/70 mm Hg and the pulse is regular at 70 beats per minute. There are no signs of congestive heart failure, and precordium is normal. The first heart sound is normal. The second heart sound is louder than normal and it is followed by a mid-diastolic, scratchy murmur heard in the second and third left intercostal spaces. There is also a short, grade 2/6 ejection systolic murmur heard in the same places.

The ECG shows right bundle branch block. Chest radiograph shows an apical prominence at the left side of the cardiac silhouette. Echocardiography shows thickening of the right ventricular wall and dilation of the right ventricular cavity with diminished ventricular septal motion. Cardiac catheterization and angiography demonstrate right ventricular pressure of 28 mm Hg in systole and 5 mm Hg in diastole, and a pulmonary artery pressure of 20 mm Hg in systole and 5 mm Hg in diastole. Cardiac output is normal and there is no evidence of a shunt.

Diagnosis: Tetralogy of Fallot with surgical relief of pulmonary valve stenosis and closure of the ventricular septal defect.

Impairment: 15% to 20% impairment of the whole person.

Comment: Had there been evidence of a shunt, the impairment rating would have been greater. Also, if a conduit or prosthesis had been placed in the pulmonary outflow tract, or if significant symptoms had been present, the rating would have been greater.

Class 3—Impairment of the Whole Person, 30-50%:
A patient belongs in Class 3 when (a) the patient has evidence by physical examination or laboratory studies of congenital heart disease and experiences symptoms during the performance of ordinary daily activities (functional Class 3); *and* (b) diet modifications and drugs do not completely control symptoms or prevent signs of congestive heart failure; *and* (c) there are signs or laboratory evidence of cardiac chamber hypertrophy or dilation; or the severity of valvular stenosis or regurgitation is estimated to be moderate or severe; or there is evidence of a right-to-left shunt; or there is evidence of a left-to-right shunt with the pulmonary flow being greater than two times the systemic flow; or the pulmonary vascular resistance is elevated to greater than one-half the systemic vascular resistance; *or* (d) the patient has recovered from surgery for the treatment of congenital heart disease but continues to have functional Class 3 symptoms; or continues to have signs of congestive failure or cyanosis, and there is evidence of cardiomegaly and significant residual valvular stenosis or regurgitation, left-to-right shunt, right-to-left shunt, or elevated pulmonary vascular resistance.

Example 1: A 52-year-old woman has Ebstein's anomaly of the tricuspid valve, the diagnosis having been made years ago with the aid of echocardiography, cardiac catheterization, and angiography. During the past several years, she has had increasing breathlessness during daily activities such as climbing stairs, mopping, or cleaning. Also, she has noticed ankle edema and increased abdominal girth. With the use of diuretics the edema and ascites have diminished. The patient restricts the salt in her diet and takes digitalis.

On examination, the patient appears well, but there is duskiness of the lips and the fingernails. The V wave in the neck veins is markedly elevated, and the liver is 14 cm wide and slightly pulsatile. The lungs are clear. A very active parasternal area without a distinct heave is found in the precordium. The first heart sound is loud and is followed by a loud early systolic sound along the left sternal border. The second heart sound is widely split and is followed by an early diastolic sound. There is a holosystolic murmur that increases with inspiration heard best at the left of the sternum. There is also a diastolic murmur heard best during inspiration

and along the left sternal border. There is no peripheral edema and no evidence of ascites at this time.

The ECG shows right bundle branch block with low R waves in V1 and prominent P waves. The chest radiograph shows a greatly enlarged cardiac silhouette especially to the right of the sternum. The pulmonary vasculature is normal. Echocardiogram shows typical changes of Ebstein's anomaly of the tricuspid valve. Previous cardiac catheterization showed changes of Ebstein's anomaly and a small atrial right-to-left shunt.

Diagnosis: Ebstein's anomaly of the tricuspid valve.

Impairment: 50% impairment of the whole person.

Example 2: A 20-year-old man underwent a Mustard procedure 10 years ago for treatment of transposition of the great vessels. In infancy he had a Blalock-Hanlon procedure. After the Mustard procedure, he did moderately well, but never developed satisfactory stamina, tiring easily and being unable to participate in activities such as tennis and hiking because of dyspnea and fatigue.

On examination, the patient appears healthy but underweight, and had no cyanosis. The neck veins are distended and show a prominent A wave. The liver is not enlarged and there is no peripheral edema. The lungs are clear. There are parasternal and apical heaves at the precordium. S1 and S2 are normal. There is a holosystolic murmur at the left sternal border, and a fourth heart sound is present.

The ECG shows tall R wave voltage in all of the precordial leads. The chest radiograph shows moderate cardiomegaly and clear lungs. The echocardiogram shows signs of a properly functioning intra-atrial baffle. Both ventricular cavities are enlarged, but there is good ventricular function. Cardiac catheterization and angiography demonstrate an elevated right mean atrial pressure of 12 mm Hg with A waves of 20 mm Hg. Right ventricular and pulmonary artery systolic pressures are 30 to 35 mm Hg.

Diagnosis: Transposition of the great vessels, with Mustard procedure.

Impairment: 40% to 50% impairment of the whole person.

Comment: If significant arrhythmias were to complicate the postoperative period, they would be evaluated according to the criteria in the section on arrythmias, and the two impairment ratings would be combined using the Combined Values Chart to determine impairment of the whole person due to cardiac disease.

Table 8. Impairment Classification for Congenital Heart Disease

Class 1 0-10% Impairment of Whole Person	Class 2 15-25% Impairment of Whole Person	Class 3 30-50% Impairment of Whole Person	Class 4 55-100% Impairment of Whole Person
The patient has evidence by physical examination or laboratory studies of congenital heart disease and has no symptoms in the performance of ordinary daily activities, or even upon moderately heavy physical exertion; **and** Continuous treatment is not required, although prophylactic antibiotics may be recommended after surgical procedures to reduce the risk of bacterial endocarditis; and the patient remains free of signs of congestive heart failure and cyanosis; **and** There are no signs of cardiac chamber hypertrophy or dilation; the evidence of residual valvular stenosis or regurgitation is estimated to be mild; there is no evidence of left-to-right or right-to-left shunt; and the pulmonary vascular resistance is estimated to be normal; **or** In the patient who has recovered from corrective heart surgery, all of the above criteria are met.	The patient has evidence by physical examination or laboratory studies of congenital heart disease, has no symptoms in the performance of ordinary daily activities, and has no symptoms with moderately heavy physical exertion (functional class 2); **or** The patient requires moderate dietary adjustments or drugs to prevent symptoms or to remain free of signs of congestive heart failure or other consequences of congenital heart disease, such as syncope, chest pain, emboli, or cyanosis; **or** There are signs or laboratory evidence of cardiac chamber hypertrophy or dilation, or the severity of valvular stenosis or regurgitation is estimated to be moderate; or there is evidence of a small residual left-to-right or right-to-left shunt; or there is evidence of moderate elevation of the pulmonary vascular resistance, which should be less than one-half the systemic vascular resistance; **or** The patient has recovered from surgery for the treatment of congenital heart disease and meets the above criteria for impairment.	The patient has evidence by physical examination or laboratory studies of congenital heart disease and experiences symptoms during the performance of ordinary daily activities (functional class 3); **and** Diet modification and drugs do not completely control symptoms or prevent signs of congestive heart failure; **and** There are signs or laboratory evidence of cardiac chamber hypertrophy or dilation; or the severity of valvular stenosis or regurgitation is estimated to be moderate or severe; or there is evidence of a right-to-left shunt; or there is evidence of a left-to-right shunt with the pulmonary flow being greater than two times the systemic flow; or the pulmonary vascular resistance is elevated to greater than one-half the systemic vascular resistance; **or** The patient has recovered from surgery for the treatment of congenital heart disease but continues to have functional class 3 symptoms; or continues to have signs of congestive failure or cyanosis, and there is evidence of cardiomegaly and significant residual valvular stenosis or regurgitation, left-to-right shunt, right-to-left shunt, or elevated pulmonary vascular resistance.	The patient has signs of congenital heart disease and experiences symptoms of congestive heart failure at less than ordinary daily activities (functional class 4); **and** Dietary therapy and drugs do not prevent symptoms or signs of congestive heart failure; **and** There is evidence from physical examination or laboratory studies of cardiac chamber hypertrophy or dilation, or the pulmonary vascular resistance remains elevated at greater than one-half of the systemic vascular resistance; or the severity of the valvular stenosis or regurgitation is estimated to be moderate to severe; or there is a left-to-right shunt with the pulmonary flow being greater than two times the systemic flow; or there is a left-to-right shunt with the pulmonary vascular resistance being elevated to greater than one-half the systemic vascular resistance; or there is a right-to-left shunt; **or** The patient has recovered from heart surgery for the treatment of congenital heart disease and continues to have symptoms or signs of congestive heart failure causing impairment as outlined above.

Class 4—Impairment of the Whole Person, 55-100%:
A patient belongs in Class 4 when (a) the patient has signs of congenital heart disease and experiences symptoms of congestive heart failure at less than ordinary daily activities (functional Class 4); *and* (b) dietary therapy and drugs do not prevent symptoms or signs of congestive heart failure; *and* (c) there is evidence from physical examination or laboratory studies of cardiac chamber hypertrophy or dilation, or the pulmonary vascular resistance remains elevated at greater than one-half of the systemic vascular resistance; or the severity of the valvular stenosis or regurgitation is estimated to be moderate to severe; or there is a left-to-right shunt with the pulmonary flow being greater than two times the systemic flow; or there is a left-to-right shunt with the pulmonary vascular resistance being elevated to greater than one-half the systemic vascular resistance; or there is a right-to-left shunt; *or* (d) the patient has recovered from heart surgery for the

treatment of congenital heart disease and continues to have symptoms or signs of congestive heart failure causing impairment as outlined above.

Example 1: A 23-year-old woman with Eisenmenger's complex, with a diagnosis made 10 years ago, has been followed regularly. She had cardiac catheterization and angiography, and a ventricular septal defect and pulmonary vascular resistance equal to systemic vascular resistance were found. Recently, she became markedly limited in her activities because of fatigue on minimal exertion. Peripheral edema of recent onset responded to diuretic therapy.

On examination, the woman has mild cyanosis that intensifies with exertion. There are prominent A waves in the neck veins, but there is no jugular venous distention when the patient is at a 45 degree angle. The liver is not enlarged and there is no peripheral edema.

The lungs are clear. There is a forceful, sustained parasternal heave. The first heart sound is normal and the second is narrowly split. There is a marked increase in the second component of the second sound. There is a short, early systolic ejection murmur along the left sternal border.

The ECG shows right ventricular hypertrophy and peaked P waves in leads 2, 3, and F. Chest radiograph shows evidence of right ventricular hypertrophy, marked prominence of the proximal portion of the pulmonary arteries, and greatly diminished pulmonary vascular markings in the periphery of the lung fields.

Diagnosis: Eisenmenger complex with ventricular septal defect and elevated pulmonary vascular resistance.

Impairment: 100% impairment of the whole person.

Example 2: A 35-year-old man with tetralogy of Fallot had a Blalock-Taussig systemic-to-pulmonary artery anastomosis as a child, which was ligated during a second operative procedure. At that time, pulmonary stenosis was relieved by removing muscle in the outflow area of the right ventricle, and the ventricular septal defect was closed. After the second operation the patient did not do well, continuing to tire easily. Significant peripheral edema and ascites responded to the use of diuretics. He was comfortable during light work activities about the home but became weak and breathless on more vigorous exertion.

At examination, the patient has no cyanosis. There is a prominent V wave in the neck veins. The liver is 14 cm across. There is palpable cardiac activity parasternally but no sustained heave. There is a grade 3/6 holosystolic murmur along the left sternal border and a mid-diastolic murmur in the second left interspace. The first heart sound is normal and the second heart sound is single and loud. The ECG shows right bundle branch block. The chest radiograph shows cardiomegaly and a right pleural effusion. The echocardiogram shows a dilated, poorly functioning right ventricle. Cardiac catheterization and angiography show severe tricuspid regurgitation and a dilated, poorly functioning right ventricle.

Diagnosis: Tetralogy of Fallot with surgical relief of the pulmonary stenosis and closure of the ventricular septal defect, followed by development of tricuspid regurgitation and heart failure.

Impairment: 90% impairment of the whole person.

Criteria for impairment due to congenital heart disease are found in Table 8.

6.4 Hypertensive Cardiovascular Disease

Elevated pressure within the systemic arterial system is known as hypertension. A transient elevation of arterial pressure is the normal physiologic response to exercise and excitement, but a sustained elevation of pressure is not normal and can lead to damage of arterial walls and of the organs supplied by these vessels, especially the brain and the kidneys. Also, sustained increased pressure may lead to a tearing of the intima of the aorta, and possibly to a dissection of the media and rupture. Elevated pressure in the arterial system, if sustained, greatly increases the work of the left ventricle. Initially this leads to compensatory hypertrophy, but eventually it causes failure of the left ventricle with all of the attendant complications including death.

The cause of hypertension in most patients is not understood, and the disorder is therefore called "essential" or "primary" hypertension. In some patients, the hypertension can be established as being due to other disorders, in which case the disorder is termed "secondary" hypertension. An organized approach to detect secondary disorders is warranted because their correction may lead to elimination of the hypertension. Secondary hypertension may be due to coarctation of the aorta, renal artery obstruction, renal parenchymal disease, hyperaldosteronism, Cushing's disease, rare endocrine disorders such as pheochromocytoma, and chronic nocturnal hypoxia due to the sleep apnea syndromes.

In the patient in whom a diagnosable disorder causes the hypertension, estimation of permanent impairment should not be undertaken until adequate time has elapsed after treatment of the disorder. If other organs are affected, as with the kidneys in chronic renal disease, then the degree of impairment due to the hypertension should be combined with that due to the other organ system, using the Combined Values Chart.

Drugs are now available with acceptable side effects that can maintain blood pressure in the normal range in most patients with primary hypertension and in most with secondary hypertension and no correctable cause. Ratings of impairment due to hypertension should be delayed until after the drugs have been prescribed and their doses have been adjusted to achieve maximum effect.

Before classifying a patient as having hypertensive cardiovascular disease, the physician should make several determinations of the arterial pressure. Hypertensive cardiovascular disease is not necessarily present when a patient exhibits transient or irregular episodes of elevated arterial pressure; these could be associated with an emotional or environmental stimulus or with signs or symptoms of cardiovascular system hyperactivity. Most authorities agree that hypertensive cardiovascular disease is present when the diastolic pressure is repeatedly in excess of 90 mm Hg.

Criteria for Evaluating Impairment Due to Hypertensive Cardiovascular Disease

Class 1—Impairment of the Whole Person, 0-10%:
A patient belongs in Class 1 when (1) the patient has no symptoms and the diastolic pressures are repeatedly in excess of 90 mm Hg; *and* (2) the patient is taking antihypertensive medications but has none of the following abnormalities: (a) abnormal urinalysis or renal function tests; (b) history of hypertensive cerebrovascular disease; (c) evidence of left ventricular hypertrophy; (d) hypertensive vascular abnormalities of the optic fundus, except minimal narrowing of arterioles.

Example: A 26-year-old ophthalmology resident was told when 18 years old that his blood pressure was high. This finding was confirmed by numerous determinations of blood pressure made during medical school. An employment examination at the beginning of his internship confirmed the elevated blood pressure, and he was sent for a diagnostic work-up and treatment. No cause for the elevated blood pressure was found. The patient was asymptomatic, and he was started on a regimen of restricted salt intake, weight control, and regular exercise. His blood pressure remained elevated and he was prescribed an antihypertensive medication.

At the latest series of examinations, the patient's blood pressure was 160/105 mm Hg in both arms and 170/105 mm Hg in the right leg. All arterial pulses were of good quality. A week later the pressures were the same. All other physical findings were normal.

The ECG and chest radiograph were normal. Serum electrolytes, including the BUN and serum creatinine, and urinanalysis were normal.

Diagnosis: Essential hypertension.

Impairment: 5% impairment of the whole person.

Comment: It may be necessary to alter the antihypertensive medication to effect a reduction in the blood pressure.

Class 2—Impairment of the Whole Person, 15-25%:
A patient belongs in Class 2 when (1) the patient has no symptoms and the diastolic pressures are repeatedly in excess of 90 mm Hg; *and* (2) the patient is taking antihypertensive medication and has any of the following abnormalities: (a) proteinuria and abnormalities of the urinary sediment, but no impairment of renal function as measured by blood urea nitrogen (BUN) and serum creatinine determinations; (b) history of hypertensive cerebrovascular damage; (c) definite hypertensive changes in the retinal arterioles, including crossing defects and/or old exudates.

Example: A 40-year-old woman had an elevated blood pressure during a pregnancy at age 32 years, but the pressure was normal three weeks and 12 months post partum. Recently she had bleeding between menstrual periods. Her gynecologist found her blood pressure to be in the range of 160/105 to 150/100 mm Hg on several occasions. Leg blood pressures were also elevated.

Findings on physical examination were normal, including the fundal vessels and the heart.

The ECG and chest radiograph were normal. Serum electrolytes were normal, including the BUN and creatinine levels. Urinalysis showed 2 + proteinuria, and the sediment showed one to three red blood cells per high power field. The proteinuria was confirmed on two occasions. A 24-hour urine collection yielded 1400 mg of protein.

Diagnosis: Essential hypertension with proteinuria.

Impairment: 15% impairment of the whole person.

Comment: If the pressure remains elevated after restricting dietary salt and beginning a regimen of weight control and exercise, an antihypertensive drug should be recommended.

Class 3—Impairment of the Whole Person, 30-50%:
A patient belongs in Class 3 when (1) the patient has no symptoms and the diastolic pressure readings are consistently in excess of 90 mm Hg; *and* (2) the patient is taking antihypertensive medication and has any of the following abnormalities: (a) diastolic pressure readings usually in excess of 120 mm Hg; (b) proteinuria or abnormalities in the urinary sediment, with evidence of impaired renal function as measured by elevated BUN and serum creatinine, or by creatinine clearance below 50%; (c) hypertensive cerebrovascular damage with permanent neurological residual; (d) left ventricular hypertrophy according to findings of physical examination, ECG, or chest radiograph, but no symptoms, signs, or evidence by chest radiograph of congestive heart failure; or (e) retinopathy, with definite hypertensive changes in the arterioles, such as "copper" or "silver wiring"; or A-V crossing changes, with or without hemorrhages and exudates.

Example: A 48-year-old man was admitted to the hospital eight months ago with headaches, blurred vision, and breathlessness of two weeks' duration. His blood pressure was 260/160 mm Hg in the arms and legs. He was drowsy, but he had no localizing neurological signs.

The patient's fundi showed arterial spasm, hemorrhages, and bilateral papilledema. Examination of the heart, lungs and abdomen, and chest radiograph were normal. The ECG showed low T waves in the lateral chest leads; the BUN was 40 mg/100 ml and serum creatinine 3.2 mg/100 ml. Urinalysis was abnormal, showing 3 + proteinuria, numerous red blood cells, and occasional white blood cells.

With treatment, the patient's symptoms cleared, and he remained asymptomatic. He took three antihypertensive drugs faithfully, but his diastolic blood pressures remained above 120 mm Hg.

Diagnosis: Essential hypertension with a history of hypertensive encephalopathy.

Impairment: 45% to 50% impairment of the whole person.

Comment: If any of the other findings had persisted, but the diastolic blood pressure had returned to normal, then the estimate of impairment would have been less.

Class 4—Impairment of the Whole Person, 55-100%: A patient belongs in Class 4 when (1) the patient has a diastolic pressure consistently in excess of 90 mm Hg; *and* (2) the patient is taking antihypertensive medication and has any two of the following abnormalities: (a) diastolic pressure readings usually in excess of 120 mm Hg; (b) proteinuria and abnormalities in the urinary sediment, with impaired renal function and evidence of nitrogen retention as measured by elevated BUN and serum creatinine or by creatinine clearance below 50%; (c) hypertensive cerebrovascular damage with permanent neurological deficits; (d) left ventricular hypertrophy; (e) retinopathy as manifested by hypertensive changes in the arterioles, retina, or optic nerve; (f) history of congestive heart failure; *or* (3) the patient has left ventricular hypertrophy with the persistence of congestive heart failure despite digitalis and diuretics.

Example 1: A 48-year-old man had a long history of severe hypertension and took drugs intermittently. He had no symptoms until a year ago, when he developed breathlessness on exertion, orthopnea, and occasional nocturnal dyspnea. These symptoms improved after the administration of digitalis and diuretics. However, he still became breathless on heavy exertion and occasionally awakened with breathlessness.

Examination reveals a comfortable patient with blood pressure of 170/95 mm Hg and a pulse rate of 84 beats per minute. There are no signs of congestive heart failure. In the fundus there are increased light reflex from the arterioles and A-V crossing depressions, but no hemorrhages or exudates; the disc is flat. The left ventricular impulse is enlarged and sustained but in the normal position. The first heart sound is normal and the second is increased in intensity. There is a fourth heart sound and no murmurs.

The ECG shows left ventricular hypertrophy as evidenced by tall R waves in the lateral chest leads and inverted T waves in the same leads. Chest radiograph shows mild cardiomegaly and normal pulmonary vasculature. The serum electrolytes and urinalysis are normal.

Diagnosis: Essential hypertension and hypertensive heart disease with history of congestive heart failure.

Impairment: 55% impairment of the whole person.

Example 2: A 62-year-old woman has received treatment for high blood pressure for 10 years. Despite taking drugs and following a restricted salt and weight control diet, she continued to have elevation of blood pressure. Two years ago she developed congestive heart failure that initially improved with the use of digitalis and diuretics. Six months ago she began to have marked tiredness and breathlessness on daily activities. Her ankles remained swollen.

Examination reveals a comfortable woman with blood pressure of 180/100 mm Hg in the arms and legs. There is edema of the ankles and lower legs. Fundal examination reveals increased light reflex of the arterioles with A-V crossing compressions and no hemorrhages or exudates; the discs are flat. There is no elevation of the neck veins. The apical impulse is enlarged, sustained, and displaced to the anterior axillary line. The first heart sound is normal, the second heart sound is increased, and there is a fourth heart sound. Rales are heard at both lung bases. There is edema of the ankles and pretibial area.

The ECG shows a deep S wave in V2, but the height of the R waves in V5 and V6 is normal. There are low T waves in 1, L, and V4 through V6. The chest radiograph shows cardiomegaly and prominence of the pulmonary vasculature in the upper lung fields. The serum electrolytes, BUN and creatinine, and urinalysis are normal.

Diagnosis: Essential hypertension with congestive heart failure.

Table 9. Impairment Classificaiton for Hypertensive Cardiovascular Disease

Class 1 0-10% Impairment of Whole Person	Class 2 15-25% Impairment of Whole Person	Class 3 30-50% Impairment of Whole Person	Class 4 55-100% Impairment of Whole Person
The patient has no symptoms and the diastolic pressures are repeatedly in excess of 90 mm Hg; **and** The patient is taking antihypertensive medications but has none of the following abnormalities: (1) abnormal urinalysis or renal function tests; (2) history of hypertensive cerebrovascular disease; (3) evidence of left ventricular hypertrophy; (4) hypertensive vascular abnormalities of the optic fundus, except minimal narrowing of arterioles.	The patient has no symptoms and the diastolic pressures are repeatedly in excess of 90 mm Hg; **and** The patient is taking antihypertensive medication and has any of the following abnormalities: (1) proteinuria and abnormalities of the urinary sediment, but no impairment of renal function as measured by blood urea nitrogen (BUN) and serum creatinine determinations; (2) history of hypertensive cerebrovascular damage; (3) definite hypertensive changes in the retinal arterioles, including crossing defects and old exudates.	The patient has no symptoms and the diastolic pressure readings are consistently in excess of 90 mm Hg; **and** The patient is taking antihypertensive medication and has any of the following abnormalities: (1) diastolic pressure readings usually in excess of 120 mm Hg; (2) proteinuria or abnormalities in the urinary sediment, with evidence of impaired renal function as measured by elevated BUN and serum creatinine, or by creatinine clearance below 50%; (3) hypertensive cerebrovascular damage with permanent neurological residual; (4) left ventricular hypertrophy according to findings of physical examination, ECG, or chest radiograph, but no symptoms, signs, or evidence by chest radiograph of congestive heart failure; or (5) retinopathy, with definite hypertensive changes in the arterioles, such as "copper" or "silver wiring," or A-V crossing changes, with or without hemorrhages and exudates.	The patient has a diastolic pressure consistently in excess of 90 mm Hg; **and** The patient is taking antihypertensive medication and has any two of the following abnormalities: (1) diastolic pressure readings usually in excess of 120 mm Hg; (2) proteinuria and abnormalities in the urinary sediment, with impaired renal function and evidence of nitrogen retention as measured by elevated BUN and serum creatinine or by creatinine clearance below 50%; (3) hypertensive cerebrovascular damage with permanent neurological deficits; (4) left ventricular hypertrophy; (5) retinopathy as manifested by hypertensive changes in the arterioles, retina, or optic nerve; (6) history of congestive heart failure; **or** The patient has left ventricular hypertrophy with the persistence of congestive heart failure despite digitalis and diuretics.

Impairment: 90% impairment of the whole person.

Criteria for impairment due to hypertensive cardiovascular diseases are found in Table 9.

6.5 Cardiomyopathies

Cardiomyopathies result in impairment of the whole person by causing abnormal ventricular function. Abnormal ventricular function may not result in abnormal hemodynamics, or it may result in pulmonary and/or systemic organ congestion and decreased cardiac output. Abnormal ventricular function related to coronary heart disease, valvular heart disease and hypertensive heart disease are covered in their respective sections. Cardiomyopathies may also cause arrhythmias; these are considered in a different section of this chapter. Some cardiomyopathies are reversible. Every effort should be made to identify the reversible forms and to treat them appropriately over an adequate period of time before estimating any suspected permanent impairment.

There are many mechanisms by which the cardiomyopathies arise, but they can be divided conveniently into three major types: (1) dilated or congestive; (2) hypertrophic; and (3) restrictive. These disorders can be recognized in most patients by taking careful histories and performing careful physical examinations.

In most patients, it also is appropriate to supplement these procedures with selected laboratory studies.

Criteria for Evaluating Impairment Due to Cardiomyopathy

Class 1—Impairment of the Whole Person, 0-10%:
A patient belongs in Class 1 when (a) the patient is asymptomatic and there is evidence of impaired left ventricular function from clinical examination or laboratory studies; *and* (b) there is no evidence of congestive heart failure or cardiomegaly from physical examination or laboratory studies.

Example: One year ago a 26-year-old woman delivered a normal child, but three days post partum she developed signs of pulmonary congestion. She was normotensive. There was no evidence of valvular heart disease, and the ECG was within normal limits except for sinus tachycardia. She was treated successfully with digitalis and diuretics. Over the next several months, the woman returned to full activities and had no symptoms. Six months ago the digitalis and diuretics were discontinued. She was advised to avoid subsequent pregnancies. She led a normal life caring for three children and her home.

At present, the woman has no signs of congestive failure. Blood pressure is 110/70 mm Hg, and pulse is regular at 70 beats per minute. The precordium is quiet without ventricular heaves. The heart sounds are normal. The ECG is normal. The chest radiograph demonstrates slight cardiomegaly without specific chamber enlargement. Echocardiography shows an ejection fraction of 55%. Exercise testing demonstrates no ECG change; echo-measured ejection fraction falls to 50%.

Diagnosis: Postpartum cardiomyopathy.

Impairment: 10% impairment of the whole person.

Comment: If the woman had symptoms, she would be rated as having considerably greater impairment. If the heart size were normal, and the ejection fraction were normal at rest and increased on exercise, then the estimate of impairment would be less than 10%.

Class 2—Impairment of the Whole Person, 15-25%:
A patient belongs in Class 2 when (a) the patient is asymptomatic and there is evidence of impaired left ventricular function from physical examination or laboratory studies; *and* (b) moderate dietary adjustment or drug therapy is necessary for the patient to be free of symptoms and signs of congestive heart failure; *or* (c) the patient has recovered from surgery for the treatment of hypertrophic cardiomyopathy and meets the criteria in (a) and (b) above.

Example 1: A 59-year-old man consumed excessive amounts of alcohol over a period of many years and probably had a poor diet most of that time. He was admitted to the hospital a year ago with severe pulmonary congestion. A thorough evaluation indicated that this was probably due to left ventricular failure attributable to a combination of excessive alcohol intake and poor nutrition. The man responded promptly to nutritional treatment, digitalis, and diuretics. He avoided alcohol and returned to a fully active life, working as greens keeper on a golf course. During the past year he was seen regularly by his physician, who elected to maintain him on digitalis and moderate salt restriction because of a persisting gallop rhythm.

On examination, the patient appears comfortable and has no signs of congestive heart failure. Blood pressure is 120/80 mm Hg, and pulse is regular at 70 beats per minute. At the precordium, the apical impulse is larger than normal, slightly sustained, and displaced to the anterior axillary line. There is no parasternal heave. The first and second heart sounds are normal. A third heart sound is present at the apex. There are no murmurs.

The ECG shows small R waves in the lateral chest leads and low T waves in the same leads. The chest radiograph shows moderate cardiomegaly with no specific chamber enlargement. There is no pulmonary congestion. The echocardiogram at rest has an ejection fraction of 40%, and this remains at 40% following exercise. There are no ECG changes during exercise.

Diagnosis: Cardiomyopathy, probably alcoholic and nutritional.

Impairment: 25% impairment of the whole person.

Example 2: An 18-year-old man, whose father has hypertrophic cardiomyopathy, was examined by his physician and found to have evidence of hypertrophic cardiomyopathy. The patient had no heart-related symptoms and was an active participant in sports.

On examination, the man appears healthy and has no evidence of congestive heart failure. Blood pressure is 130/70 mm Hg and the pulse is regular at 70 beats per minute. Carotid pulses are brisk and the apical impulse is normal. The first and second heart sounds are normal, and there is a grade 2/6 midsystolic murmur heard best along the left sternal border; there is no gallop.

The ECG shows prominent Q waves and low T waves in the lateral chest leads. Chest radiograph shows a normal-sized heart and no pulmonary congestion. Echocardiogram shows marked thickening of the ventricular septum and some thickening of the posterior ventricular wall. The mitral valve motion is normal, and ejection fraction is 80%.

Diagnosis: Hypertrophic cardiomyopathy.

Impairment: 20% impairment of the whole person.

Comment: The patient was advised to avoid strenuous physical exertion, and the importance of follow-up evaluation was stressed.

Class 3—Impairment of the Whole Person, 30-50%:
A patient belongs in Class 3 when (a) the patient develops symptoms of congestive heart failure on greater than ordinary daily activities (functional Class 3) and there is evidence of abnormal ventricular function from physical examination or laboratory studies; *and* (b) moderate dietary restriction or the use of drugs is necessary to minimize the patient's symptoms, or to prevent the appearance of signs of congestive heart failure or evidence of it by laboratory study; *or* (c) the patient has recovered from surgery for the treatment of hypertrophic cardiomyopathy and meets the criteria described above.

Example: A 54-year-old woman has been treated by her physician for the past three years for symptoms of congestive heart failure and inadequate cardiac output.

Two years ago she underwent cardiac catheterization and cineangiography, the studies demonstrating no evidence of coronary artery or valvular disease. Ventricular function then was poor; the end diastolic pressure was elevated to 18 mm Hg and the ejection fraction was 30%. During the past year the patient's condition has been stable; and she has been able to do kitchen work, go shopping, and drive an automobile. She becomes breathless on climbing a flight of stairs and prefers to sleep on two pillows.

At examination, the patient's blood pressure is 110/70 mm Hg, and the pulse is regular at 70 beats per minute. The neck veins are not distended, there is no peripheral edema, and the lungs are clear. There is a markedly enlarged apical impulse, which is sustained and displaced laterally to the anterior axillary line. An early diastolic impulse is palpable following the systolic impulse. The first heart sound is diminished, the second heart sound is normal, and there is a prominent third heart sound. There are no murmurs.

The ECG shows low T waves in all leads. There is a QS pattern in V1 and V2. The chest radiograph shows marked cardiomegaly with some distention of the pulmonary vessels in the upper lobes. Echocardiography shows a moderately dilated left ventricle with an ejection fraction of 30% and an enlarged left atrium.

Diagnosis: Idiopathic cardiomyopathy.

Impairment: 50% impairment of the whole person.

Class 4—Impairment of the Whole Person, 55-100%: A patient belongs in Class 4 when (a) the patient is symptomatic during ordinary daily activities despite the appropriate use of dietary adjustment and drugs, and there is evidence of abnormal ventricular function from physical examination or laboratory studies; *or* (b) there are persistent signs of congestive heart failure despite the use of dietary adjustment and drugs; *or* (c) the patient has recovered from surgery for the treatment of hypertrophic cardiomyopathy and meets the above criteria.

Example: A 38-year-old woman had the diagnosis made of hypertrophic cardiomyopathy at age 30 years. For a number of years she frequently experienced chest pain despite the use of beta adrenergic blocking agents. Nitrates were not effective and seemed to worsen her pain. Because of the angina, the woman underwent cardiac surgery to remove a large portion of the ventricular septum. There were no postoperative complications. She continued to experience angina almost on a daily basis. Many of the episodes occurred at rest, but they could also be provoked by sexual intercourse, by running up stairs, or by other activities. She also experienced several syncopal spells in the past two months.

Examination discloses that the patient is comfortable at rest. Her blood pressure is 140/80 mm Hg, and the pulse is regular at 52 beats per minute. The carotid pulse is quick and "jerky" in quality bilaterally. The venous pressure is normal and the lungs are clear. There is no peripheral edema. There is a sustained apical impulse that is moderately enlarged and displaced laterally to the anterior axillary line. A grade 3/6 long, almost holosystolic murmur is heard best at the left mid-precordium and poorly transmitted to the left axilla. The first and second heart sounds are normal and a fourth heart sound is present.

The ECG shows a sinus rhythm with Q waves in leads 1, L, and V1 through V3, and low T waves in the lateral chest leads as well as in leads 1 and L. Chest radiograph shows moderate cardiomegaly with normal pulmonary vasculature. Exercise ECG shows ST segment depression in 1, L, and V4 through V6, at a heart rate of 75 beats per minute that is low because the patient is receiving beta adrenergic blocking agents. The resting 201 Thallium perfusion scan shows the ventricular septum to be thick. No new perfusion defect develops following exercise.

Echocardiography shows a thick ventricular septum and a reduced ventricular ejection fraction of 35%. Mitral valve motion is slightly abnormal in that there is evidence of impaired left ventricular filling. The left atrium is enlarged.

Diagnosis: Hypertrophic cardiomyopathy, with resection of a portion of the left ventricular septum.

Impairment: 100% impairment of the whole person.

The criteria for permanent impairment due to cardiomyopathies are found in Table 10.

6.6 Pericardial Heart Disease

Diseases of the pericardium include inflammation (1) associated with systemic illnesses such as lupus erythematosis; (2) in reaction to mechanical forces such as trauma or irradiation; (3) with no obvious cause (idiopathic pericarditis); and (4) associated with infections caused by viruses or bacteria. The pericardium may also be affected by tumors.

The most common pericardial disorder leading to permanent impairment is constrictive pericarditis. Surgical removal of the thickened pericardium may significantly reduce symptoms and improve the overall condition of the patient with constrictive pericarditis.

Table 10. Impairment Classification for Cardiomyopathies

Class 1 0-10% Impairment of Whole Person	Class 2 15-25% Impairment of Whole Person	Class 3 30-50% Impairment of Whole Person	Class 4 55-100% Impairment of Whole Person
The patient is asymptomatic and there is evidence of impaired left ventricular function from clinical examination or laboratory studies; **and** There is no evidence of congestive heart failure or cardiomegaly from physical examination or laboratory studies.	The patient is asymptomatic and there is evidence of impaired left ventricular function from physical examination or laboratory studies; **and** Moderate dietary adjustment or drug therapy is necessary for the patient to be free of symptoms and signs of congestive heart failure; **or** The patient has recovered from surgery for the treatment of hypertrophic cardiomyopathy and meets the criteria in (a) and (b) above.	The patient develops symptoms of congestive heart failure on greater than ordinary daily activities (functional class 3) and there is evidence of abnormal ventricular function from physical examination or laboratory studies; **and** Moderate dietary restriction or the use of drugs is necessary to minimize the patient's symptoms, or to prevent the appearance of signs of congestive heart failure or evidence of it by laboratory study; **or** The patient has recovered from surgery for the treatment of hypertrophic cardiomyopathy and meets the criteria described above.	The patient is symptomatic during ordinary daily activities despite the appropriate use of dietary adjustment and drugs, and there is evidence of abnormal ventricular function from physical examination or laboratory studies; **or** There are persistent signs of congestive heart failure despite the use of dietary adjustment and drugs; **or** The patient has recovered from surgery for the treatment of hypertrophic cardiomyopathy and meets the above criteria.

It is imperative to allow sufficient time for the patient to recover from the surgical before assessing permanent impairment.

While pain and compromise of cardiac function because of tamponade can cause some impairment, they are rare as causes of permanent impairment, although chronic pericarditis with recurring episodes of tamponade, or pericardial disease related to tumors, may lead to permanent impairment. It is important to allow adequate time for resolution of an acute illness, and for medical or surgical therapy to be effective, before assessing permanent impairment.

Diagnosis of pericardial disease can be made by history, identifying a pericardial friction rub or early diastolic pericardial knock, by demonstrating pericardial effusion, thickening or calcification on an echocardiogram, or by hemodynamic or angiographic findings at cardiac catheterization.

Criteria for Evaluating Impairment Due to Pericardial Heart Disease

Class 1—Impairment of the Whole Person, 0-10%:

A patient belongs in Class 1 when (a) the patient has no symptoms in the performance of ordinary daily activities or moderately heavy physical exertion, but does have evidence from either physical examination or laboratory studies of pericardial heart disease; *and* (b) continuous treatment is not required, and there are no signs of cardiac enlargement, or of congestion of lungs or other organs; *or* (c) in the patient who has had surgical removal of the pericardium, there are no adverse consequences of the surgical removal and the patient meets the criteria above.

Example: A 28-year-old male postal clerk experienced an acute, self-limited, febrile illness three months ago, associated with anterior chest pain and a pericardial friction rub, diagnosed as acute pericarditis. His echocardiogram at that time showed a small pleural effusion. The illness resolved with curtailed physical activities and the taking of aspirin over a period of three weeks. The patient returned to work and led a normal life without symptoms. Evaluation for the presence of tuberculosis and for systemic illnesses was negative.

Diagnosis: Acute benign idiopathic pericarditis.

Impairment: 0% impairment of the whole person.

Comment: Though it is possible that constrictive pericarditis might develop later, most patients such as the one described above would experience no long-term disorder that would increase the permanent impairment rating above 0%.

Class 2—Impairment of the Whole Person, 15-25%:

A patient belongs in Class 2 when (a) the patient has no symptoms in the performance of ordinary daily activities, but does have evidence from either physical examination or laboratory studies of pericardial heart disease; *but* (b) moderate dietary adjustment or drugs are required to keep the patient free from symptoms and signs of congestive heart failure; *or* (c) the patient has signs or laboratory evidence of cardiac chamber hypertrophy or dilation; *or* (d) the patient has recovered from surgery to remove the pericardium and meets the criteria above.

Table 11. Impairment Classification for Pericardial Disease

Class 1 0-10% Impairment of Whole Person	Class 2 15-25% Impairment of Whole Person	Class 3 30-50% Impairment of Whole Person	Class 4 55-100% Impairment of Whole Person
The patient has no symptoms in the performance of ordinary daily activities or moderately heavy physical exertion, but does have evidence from either physical examination or laboratory studies of pericardial heart disease; **and** Continuous treatment is not required, and there are no signs of cardiac enlargement, or of congestion of lungs or other organs; **or** In the patient who has had surgical removal of the pericardium, there are no adverse consequences of the surgical removal and the patient meets the criteria above.	The patient has no symptoms in the performance of ordinary daily activities, but does have evidence from either physical examination or laboratory studies of pericardial heart disease; **but** Moderate dietary adjustment or drugs are required to keep the patient free from symptoms and signs of congestive heart failure; **or** The patient has signs or laboratory evidence of cardiac chamber hypertrophy or dilation; **or** The patient has recovered from surgery to remove the pericardium and meets the criteria above.	The patient has slight to moderate discomfort in the performance of greater than ordinary daily activities (functional class 2) despite dietary or drug therapy, and the patient has evidence from physical examination or laboratory studies of pericardial heart disease; **and** Physical signs are present, or there is laboratory evidence of cardiac chamber enlargement or there is evidence of significant pericardial thickening and calcification; **or** The patient has recovered from surgery to remove the pericardium but continues to have the symptoms, signs and laboratory evidence described above.	The patient has symptoms on performance of ordinary daily activities (functional class 3 or 4) in spite of using appropriate dietary restrictions or drugs, and evidence from physical examination or laboratory studies of pericardial heart disease; **and** The patient has signs or laboratory evidence of congestion of the lungs or other organs; **or** The patient has recovered from surgery to remove the pericardium and continues to have symptoms, signs, and laboratory evidence described above.

Example: A 52-year-old man was treated for tuberculous pericarditis one year ago with good response to chemotherapy. The diagnosis was established by a pericardial biopsy demonstrating acid fast bacilli. After the initiation of therapy, the patient remained asymptomatic and fully active.

At present, the patient is comfortable and has no signs of congestive heart failure. The heart sounds are of good quality and there are no abnormal sounds or rubs.

The ECG shows flat T waves in leads 1, L, V5 and V6. The chest radiograph is normal. The echocardiogram shows some thickening of the pericardium posteriorly and normal ventricular and valvular function.

Diagnosis: Inactive tuberculous pericarditis.

Impairment: 15% impairment of the whole person.

Class 3—Impairment of the Whole Person, 30-50%: A patient belongs in Class 3 when (a) the patient has slight to moderate discomfort in the performance of greater than ordinary daily activities (functional Class 2) despite dietary or drug therapy, and the patient has evidence from physical examination or laboratory studies of pericardial heart disease; *and* (b) physical signs are present, or there is laboratory evidence of cardiac chamber enlargement or there is evidence of significant pericardial thickening and calcification; *or* (c) the patient has recovered from surgery to remove the pericardium but continues to have the symptoms, signs and laboratory evidence described above.

Example: A 45-year-old real estate broker and school teacher had a pericardiectomy for constrictive pericarditis 10 years ago and had a good recovery. He continued to have some limitation of activity characterized by weakness and breathlessness on heavy physical exertion but worked regularly.

The venous pressure is normal and there is no edema. His blood pressure is normal and his pulse is regular on examination. There are no ventricular heaves, thrills, or taps. The first heart sound is normal and the second heart sound is diminished. There are no extra sounds or rubs.

The ECG demonstrates low voltage QRS and T waves in all leads. The chest radiograph shows considerable cardiomegaly and some calcification at the posterior aspect of the heart. The lung fields are clear. Echocardiography shows thickening of the pericardium and moderate diminution of right and left ventricular contraction; the left ventricular ejection fraction is 50%.

Diagnosis: Constrictive pericarditis with pericardiectomy.

Impairment: 30% impairment of the whole person.

Comment: If the patient had even more limitation of activities, a level of impairment beyond the 30% might be assigned.

Class 4—Impairment of the Whole Person, 55-100%: A patient belongs in Class 4 when (a) the patient has symptoms on performance of ordinary daily activities (functional Class 3 or 4) in spite of using appropriate dietary restriction or drugs, and evidence from physical examination or laboratory studies of pericardial heart disease; *and* (b) the patient has signs or laboratory evidence of congestion of the lungs or other organs; *or* (c) the patient has recovered from surgery to remove the pericardium and continues to have the symptoms, signs, and laboratory evidence described above.

Example: One year ago a 62-year-old man had profound ascites, peripheral edema, weight loss, and signs of pulmonary congestion that were attributed to constrictive pericarditis. Pericardiectomy relieved the severe ascites and peripheral edema. However, the man continued to have fatigue and breathlessness on ordinary daily activities and was unable because of weakness to climb a flight of stairs without resting. He was relatively comfortable when walking on the level and doing light household activities.

On examination, the man is comfortable. The neck veins are normal and there is no peripheral edema or ascites. Evidence of marked weight loss remains. There are no ventricular heaves, thrills, or taps in the precordium. The heart sounds are diminished, and there are no murmurs or extra sounds.

An ECG shows low voltage of the QRS and the T waves. The chest radiograph shows marked cardiomegaly and some distention of pulmonary vasculature in the upper lobes. The echocardiogram demonstrates reduction of ventricular function and left ventricular ejection fraction of 40%.

Diagnosis: Constrictive pericarditis with pericardiectomy.

Impairment: 75% impairment of the whole person.

Comment: If the patient had symptoms with minimal daily activities, or if he had signs of overt congestion at the time of evaluation, then the degree of impairment might be as high as 100%.

The criteria for impairment due to pericardial disease are found in Table 11.

6.7 Arrhythmias

Arrhythmias may occur in patients with structurally and functionally normal hearts or in patients with any type of organic heart disease. An arrhythmia is defined as one or more heart beats generated at a site other than the sinus node. An impulse that is generated in the sinus node but is not transmitted normally through the conducting system is considered an arrhythmia of the conduction defect type.

Arrhythmias tend to fluctuate remarkably in the frequency with which they occur. Thus, adequate

documentation of the arrhythmia and estimation of the frequency with which it occurs must be made. The associated symptoms may be considerably different from the symptoms of other forms of heart disease. Arrhythmias may cause syncope, palpitation, dizziness, light headedness, chest heaviness, or shortness of breath, or combinations of these symptoms.

The degree of impairment from cardiac arrhythmias often will have to be combined with the degree of impairment due to an underlying heart disease; this combining should be done according to the Combined Values Chart. After instituting therapy for the arrhythmias, one should allow an appropriate amount of time to pass before estimating the extent of the permanent impairment.

Criteria for Evaluating Impairment Due to Arrhythmias

Class 1–Impairment of the Whole Person, 0-10%: A patient belongs in Class 1 when (a) the patient is asymptomatic during ordinary activities and a cardiac arrhythmia is documented by ECG; *and* (b) there is no documentation of three or more consecutive ectopic beats or periods of asystole greater than 1.5 seconds, and both the atrial and ventricular rates are maintained between 50 and 100 beats per minute; *and* (c) there is no evidence of organic heart disease.

Example: A 56-year-old man without symptoms had frequent premature beats during an annual physical examination. The remainder of the examination was normal. An ECG showed frequent premature complexes. Chest radiograph was normal.

Diagnosis: Atrial premature complexes.

Impairment: 0% impairment of the whole person.

Class 2–Impairment of the Whole Person, 15-25%: A patient belongs in Class 2 when (a) the patient is asymptomatic during ordinary daily activities and a cardiac arrhythmia is documented by ECG; *and* (b) moderate dietary adjustment, or the use of drugs, or an artificial pacemaker, is required to prevent symptoms related to the cardiac arrhythmia; *or* (c) the arrhythmia persists and there is organic heart disease.

Example 1: A 62-year-old man without symptoms during an annual examination had atrial fibrillation with an irregular ventricular response of about 85 beats per minute. The remainder of the examination was normal, including ECG, chest radiograph, and echocardiogram.

Diagnosis: Atrial fibrillation.

Impairment: 15% impairment of the whole person.

Comment: If it were necessary for the patient to take digitalis to maintain the ventricular response between 50 and 100 per minute, the estimated impairment would be slightly greater.

Example 2: A 52-year-old plumber had recurring syncope a year ago and was treated with insertion of a permanent artificial pacemaker. After treatment, the patient felt well and continued to work.

On examination, the man appears well and shows no signs of congestive heart failure. His pulse is regular at 72 beats per minute, and blood pressure is 120/80 mm Hg. There are no ventricular heaves, thrills, or taps in the precordium. The heart sounds are of good quality and there are no murmurs.

The ECG shows complete capture of the heart by the artificial pacemaker running at 72 beats per minute. A rare premature ventricular beat is sensed by the pacemaker, and the pacemaker is properly inhibited.

Diagnosis: Adams-Stokes attacks in a patient with complete heart block, managed with a properly functioning artificial pacemaker.

Impairment: 20% impairment of the whole person.

Class 3—Impairment of the Whole Person, 30-50%:
A patient belongs in Class 3 when (a) the patient has symptoms despite the use of dietary therapy or drugs or of an artificial pacemaker and a cardiac arrhythmia is documented with ECG; *but* (b) the patient is able to lead an active life and the symptoms due to the arrhythmia are limited to infrequent palpitations and episodes of light-headedness, or other symptoms of temporarily inadequate cardiac output.

Example: A 44-year-old airline ground crew member experienced recurrent episodes of a sensation of rapid heart action accompanied by light-headedness or "swimming" in the head. The episodes lasted five to fifteen minutes. While vagal-type maneuvers occasionally terminated an episode, usually they stopped for no obvious reason. During the episodes the patient felt weak and could not perform any type of physical activity. Usually he would lie down and try breathholding and other maneuvers. He never experienced frank syncope.

The patient underwent Holter monitoring and was found to have atrial tachycardia of 155 beats per minute during one of the symptomatic episodes. The ECG showed typical patterns of the Wolff-Parkinson-White syndrome. The patient was started on quinidine sulfate 300 mg every six hours, but he continued to have an occasional episode. After the dose was increased to 400 mg, the patient became symptom-free. He was

on that regimen for eight months. His stools were loose, he had no severe diarrhea, and he has experienced no abdominal pain.

Diagnosis: Wolff-Parkinson-White syndrome with atrial tachycardia, adequately controlled by quinidine.

Impairment: 30% impairment of the whole person.

Comment: If the patient were to continue to have palpitations, or even a rare episode associated with symptoms of inadequate cerebral perfusion, then the degree of estimated impairment might be as high as 50%.

Class 4—Impairment of the Whole Person, 55-100%:
A patient belongs in Class 4 when (a) the patient has symptoms due to documented cardiac arrhythmia that are constant and interfere with ordinary daily activities (functional Class 3 or 4); *or* (b) the patient has frequent symptoms of inadequate cardiac output documented by ECG to be due to frequent episodes of cardiac arrhythmia; *or* (c) the patient continues to have episodes of syncope that are either due to, or have a high probability of being related to, the arrhythmia. To fit into this category of impairment, the symptoms must be present despite the use of dietary therapy, drugs, or artificial pacemakers.

Example: A 28-year-old mother of three has experienced episodes of rapid heart action for over 10 years. These are associated with an uncomfortable retrosternal pressure, a fainting sensation, and general weakness. She has had several spells of unconsciousness, during which her husband has had to use cardiopulmonary resuscitation. During all episodes the tachyarrhythmia has ended spontaneously within 30 minutes, and external electrical conversion has not been necessary.

The patient has had a number of antiarrhythmic medications, and for the past six months she has been taking quinidine sulfate 300 mg every six hours, procainamide 750 mg every four hours, and propranalol 160 mg twice daily. This program had controlled the arrhythmia fairly well. However, the patient continues to have episodes about once a month, none associated with loss of consciousness. She has developed serological abnormalities characteristic of lupus erythematosis and has had occasional swelling of the small joints in the hands, which has responded to low doses of corticosteroids.

A thorough evaluation of the patient's cardiovascular system has revealed no evidence of valvular or myocardial disease. An interval ECG shows a normal pattern and rhythm; ECGs taken during the episodes of the palpitations have shown a rapid regular rhythm at about 220 to 250 beats per minute. Electrophysiological studies have demonstrated no abnormal conduc-

Table 12. Impairment Classification for Cardiac Arrhythmias*

Class 1 0-10% Impairment of Whole Person	Class 2 15-25% Impairment of Whole Person	Class 3 30-50% Impairment of Whole Person	Class 4 55-100% Impairment of Whole Person
The patient is asymptomatic during ordinary activities and a cardiac arrhythmia is documented by ECG; **and** There is no documentation of three or more consecutive ectopic beats or periods of asystole greater than 1.5 seconds, and both the atrial and ventricular rates are maintained between 50 and 100 beats per minute; **and** There is no evidence of organic heart disease.	The patient is asymptomatic during ordinary daily activities and a cardiac arrhythmia is documented by ECG; **and** Moderate dietary adjustment, or the use of drugs, or an artificial pacemaker, is required to prevent symptoms related to the cardiac arrhythmia; **or** The arrhythmia persists and there is organic heart disease.	The patient has symptoms despite the use of dietary therapy or drugs or of an artificial pacemaker and a cardiac arrhythmia is documented with ECG; **but** The patient is able to lead an active life and the symptoms due to the arrhythmia are limited to infrequent palpitations and episodes of light-headedness, or other symptoms of temporarily inadequate cardiac output.	The patient has symptoms due to documented cardiac arrhythmia that are constant and interfere with ordinary daily activities (functional class 3 or 4); **or** The patient has frequent symptoms of inadequate cardiac output documented by ECG to be due to frequent episodes of cardiac arrhythmia; **or** The patient continues to have episodes of syncope that are either due to, or have a high probability of being related to, the arrhythmia. To fit into this category of impairment, the symptoms must be present despite the use of dietary therapy, drugs, or artificial pacemakers.

*If an arrhythmia is a result of organic heart disease, the arrhythmia should be evaluated separately and its impairment rating should be combined with the impairment rating for the organic heart disease using the Combined Values Chart.

tion problems. Ventricular tachycardia has been easily induced, its pattern being similar to that recorded during one of her spontaneous episodes.

Diagnosis: Recurrent ventricular tachycardia.

Impairment: 90% impairment of the whole person.

Comment: The degree of impairment would depend upon how often the patient has episodes and the nature of the systemic symptoms that these episodes produced.

The criteria for permanent impairment due to arrhythmias are found in Table 12.

6.8 Vascular Diseases Affecting the Extremities

Permanent impairment due to peripheral vascular disorders most commonly results from (1) diseases of the arteries that reduce blood flow and lead to one or more of the following: intermittent claudication, pain at rest, minor trophic changes, ulceration, gangrene, loss of extremity, Raynaud's phenomenon; (2) diseases of the veins resulting in one or more of the following: pain, edema, induration, stasis dermatitis, ulceration; or (3) disorders of the lymphatics, leading to chronic lymphedema that may be complicated by recurrent acute infection.

The etiological factors most commonly encountered in patients with arterial disorders are arteriosclerosis, trauma, and inflammatory processes as with thromboangiitis obliterans. The venous system is most frequently affected by varicose veins, thrombosis, and chronic deep venous insufficiency. Diseases of the lymphatic system that most frequently cause impairment are obstructive lesions of an inflammatory or neoplastic origin.

Prior to evaluation of impairment, a specific diagnosis of vascular disease should be established. The estimated amount of the impairment depends on the severity and extent of the lesions, however, rather than on the specific diagnosis. The criteria for evaluating impairment due to vascular disease of the upper extremity are found in Table 15, Section 3.1; of Chapter 3; the criteria for the lower extremity are found in Table 48, Section 3.2g of Chapter 3.

References

1. American Heart Association Committee on Exercise: *Exercise Testing and Training of Individuals with Heart Disease or at High Risk for its Development.* Dallas, American Heart Association, 1973.

2. Sheffield LT, Roitman D: Stress testing methodology. *Progress in Cardiovascular Diseases* 1976; 19:33-49.

3. Fox SM III, Naughton JP, Haskell WL: Physical activity and the prevention of coronary heart disease. *Annals of Clinical Research* 1971; 3:404-432.

4. Bruce RA: Exercise testing for evaluation of ventricular functions. *N Engl J Med* 1977; 296:671-675.

Chapter 7

The Hematopoietic System

7.0 Introduction

The hematopoietic system deals with red cells, white cells, platelets and coagulation factors, and it includes the immune defense system. Cellular elements and proteins are manufactured in the bone marrow, lymph nodes, spleen, and liver. Abnormalities may be quantitative, with too few or too many elements being produced, as in aplastic anemia and polycythemia, or they may be qualitative, with faulty production, as in congenital hemolytic anemia and hemophilia.

Hereditary defects frequently involve only a single cell line, as with the red cells in hereditary spherocytosis, or a single protein, as with factor VIII in hemophilia. Acquired disorders are more likely to involve several cell lines, as with leukemia, or several proteins, as with disseminated intravascular coagulation. Neither quantitative nor qualitative disorders necessarily imply impairment. Rather, impairment depends on the severity of the defect and the mode of clinical expression.

Within this chapter, general reference is made to symptomatology and to limitations of the patient's daily activities. The physician should determine whether these fit into one of the following categories: (a) NONE—there are no complaints or evidence of disease, and the usual activities of daily living can be performed; (b) MINIMAL—some signs or symptoms of disease are present, and there is some difficulty in performing the usual activities of daily living; (c) MODERATE—signs and symptoms of disease are present, and difficulty is experienced in performing the usual activities of daily living that now require varying amounts of assistance from others; or (d) MARKED—signs and symptoms of disease are present, and assistance is needed in performing most to all activities of daily living.

Before using the information in this chapter, the reader is urged to review Chapters 1 and 2, which provide a general discussion of the purpose of the *Guides* and of the situations in which they are useful; and which discuss techniques for the evaluation of the subject and for preparation of a report. The report should include the information found in the following outline, which is developed more fully in Chapter 2.

A. Medical Evaluation
1. Narrative history of medical conditions
2. Results of the most recent clinical evaluation
3. Assessment of current clinical status and statement of future plans
4. Diagnoses and clinical impressions
5. Expected date of full or partial recovery

B. Analysis of Findings
1. Impact of medical condition(s) on life activities
2. Explanation for concluding that the medical condition(s) has or has not become static or well-stabilized
3. Explanation for concluding that the individual is or is not likely to suffer from sudden or subtle incapacitation
4. Explanation for concluding that the individual is or is not likely to suffer injury or further impairment by engaging in life activities or by attempting to meet personal, social, and occupational demands
5. Explanation for concluding that accommodations and/or restrictions are or are not warranted

C. Comparison of Results of Analysis with Impairment Criteria

1. Description of clinical findings, and how these findings relate to specific criteria in the chapter
2. Explanation of each percent of impairment rating
3. Summary list of all impairment ratings
4. Overall rating of impairment of the whole person

7.1 Permanent Impairment Related to Anemia

The effects of chronic anemia on function depend upon the degree of compensatory response by the cardiovascular system. Regardless of the pathogenesis of the anemia, impairment is related to inability to deliver adequate oxygen to tissues. The heart compensates for the anemia by increasing cardiac output through an increase in heart rate, and there is further compensation through increased extraction of O_2 by the tissues, that is, an increased arteriovenous difference. Therefore, mild anemia with a hemoglobin level of about 10 gm/100 ml is associated with little impairment in a patient who has a normal cardiovascular system.

Greater degrees of anemia may be associated with increasing impairment that leads, in succession, to lack of stamina, fatigue upon exertion, fatigue at rest, and finally, dyspnea at rest. Thus, there are no specific concentrations of hemoglobin that determine impairment in a given patient. Impairment is measured instead in terms of the limitations of cardiovascular response. Because anemia can be treated by transfusion, impairment may be lessened by that therapy.

Iron deficiency anemia and the megaloblastic anemias are usually reversible with proper management, and they would not feature impairment upon recovery. The same is true for many hemolytic anemias. An important exception is the patient with combined system disease, who has neurologic symptoms that become irreversible because proper therapy was given too late. Gait disturbance may render such an individual severely impaired. Persistent refractory anemia may cause impairment, regardless of etiology; the degree of impairment is related to the severity of the anemia and the need for transfusions.

Under the best of circumstances, with normal survival of transfused red cells, the beneficial effects of transfusions last 6 to 8 weeks. In patients with hemolytic anemias due to serum factors, and in some patients who have been transfused many times, the survival of transfused cells becomes shortened and transfusions must be repeated at shorter intervals of 1 to 5 weeks. As hemolysis becomes more severe, impairment increases.

Table 1 provides criteria for rating permanent impairment due to anemia.

Table 1. Criteria For Evaluating Permanent Impairment Related to Anemia

Symptoms	Hemoglobin Level (gm/100 ml)	Transfusion Requirement	Impairment (%)
None	10-12	None	0
Minimal	8-10	None	30
Moderate-Marked	5-8*	2-3 units every 4-6 weeks	70
Moderate-Marked	5-8*	2-3 units every 2 weeks**	70-100

*Level before transfusion
**Implies hemolysis of transfused blood

7.2 Permanent Impairment Related to Polycythemia

Polycythemia vera is manifested by elevated hematocrit values above 52% in men and above 49% in women, and by red cell volumes above 36 ml/kg in men and above 32 ml/kg in women. Normal arterial oxygen tension, an enlarged spleen, slight elevation of the white cell and platelet counts, and increased leukocyte alkaline phosphatase are frequently seen.

Erythrocytosis and increased red cell volume may be seen in subjects who do not have true polycythemia but who smoke more than two packs of cigarettes a day; increased carbon monoxide levels are characteristic of this so-called "smoker's polycythemia."

Polycythemia vera is usually well controlled by phlebotomy and/or the administration of radioactive phosphorus. Patients in remission on appropriate therapy have no impairment and may remain this way for many years. Eventually, myelofibrosis may develop. This is manifested by the gradual development of anemia in patients who are no longer being treated with phlebotomy or radioactive phosphorus. In addition, the spleen enlarges, the peripheral blood smear shows "tearshaped" red cells, nucleated red cells, and giant platelets, and there is a slight "shift to the left" in the white cell population. Many patients with myelofibrosis complain of fatigue, lack of energy, low grade fever, and bone pain. Impairment may vary from moderate to marked, even in the absence of severe anemia. Most of these clinical findings are subjective, and it may be very difficult to assess objectively the degree of impairment. Weight loss, fever, perspiration, increasing serum lactic dehydrogenase (LDH), and increased reticulin and fibroblasts seen upon bone marrow biopsy may be of help in evaluation.

Currently, no therapy exists to relieve the symptoms of myelofibrosis. Transfusions may be needed for severe anemia. Patients who develop acute leukemia after years of polycythemia are, of course, totally impaired. This particular leukemia tends to be resistant to chemotherapy.

7.3 Permanent Impairment Related to White Blood Cell Diseases or Abnormalities

The primary function of the white blood cells (leukocytes) is to provide protection against invading organisms, foreign proteins and particles. Three separate white cell "families" interact to provide this protection. In addition to the cells in the circulation, each white cell family has a fixed tissue component that not only provides the renewal or precursor pool, but also functions at fixed sites, such as the bone marrow, spleen, and lymph nodes. The white cell families are the granulocytes, lymphocytes, and monocytes-macrophages. Abnormalities in the white cell families are expressed both in terms of numbers and of alterations in function.

Granulocytes:
The major function of the granulocytes is to protect against infection through the phagocytosis of invading organisms. Thus, granulocytes function primarily at the site of tissue invasion, and the observation or enumeration of granulocytes in the circulation is in reality a view of traffic to tissues. Survival of granulocytes in the circulation is brief, the half-life being approximately 6 hours. When granulocytes leave the circulation, they generally do not return. The granulocyte precursor pool is in the bone marrow, where a very large production capacity exists.

Granulocyte abnormalities of function are most commonly congenital, although acquired functional abnormalities may result from drugs and toxins. Defective granulocyte function is recognized by the occurrence of frequent infections. The evaluation of impairment under such circumstances is based on the type, frequency, and severity of the recurring infections. These may vary from furunculosis, which has no impact on functional capacity, to recurring septicemias with death. The variety of potential lesions makes a tight formula for impairment unworkable. In general, an affected individual will have a reasonably consistent pattern of infection that makes characterization on clinical grounds reliable.

Quantitative granulocyte abnormalities are of two different forms. The first is agranulocytosis, in which a loss of the granulocyte precursor pool or a markedly accelerated destruction of the granulocytes results in a reduction in circulating granulocytes. Since granulocytes in the circulation are really in transit to the tissues, there is normally a large excess or reserve of available granulocytes. Indeed, significant infections due to low numbers are uncommon, unless the circulating granulocytes are less than $500/\mu l$. Such decreases may be seen with anti-inflammatory and anti-thyroid drugs, anti-convulsants, toxins, Felty's syndrome, cancer therapy with ionizing radiation or drugs, and occasionally without recognizable cause. In the absence of reversibility, chronic neutropenia with counts below $500/\mu l$ is associated with substantially increased risk of infection, and impairment is defined in terms of the infections.

A second type of granulocyte impairment due to altered numbers is leukemic transformation. Both acute granulocytic leukemia and chronic granulocytic leukemia result in impaired function and limited life expectancy, even with currently available therapy. The evaluation of the degree of impairment is based upon the presence of symptoms and physical findings, the requirement for, and frequency of, therapy, and the ability to carry out the activities of daily living. In general, the granulocytic leukemias are less amenable to successful therapy than are the other forms of leukemia.

Lymphocytes:
The major function of the lymphocytes is to provide humoral and cellular defense mechanisms. The circulating lymphocytes have their origin in lymphoid tissues, that is, the bone marrow, spleen, lymph nodes and thymus, and two-way traffic between the circulation and these tissues is known. Lymphocytes are cell types with heterogeneous functions.

Of the two major subgroups, the "T," or thymus-derived, lymphocytes, are primarily responsible for cellular immunity and are involved in delayed hypersensitivity reactions, tissue grafts, etc. The "B," or bursal-derived, lymphocytes, are primarily responsible for humoral immunity related to their production of immunoglobulins and biologically active kinins. Each of these subgroups is heterogeneous, but the exact extent of the functional heterogeneity is not yet clear. Methods have not yet been developed to identify completely all subsets of these cells, such as memory cells, natural killer cells, and helper cells.

Lymphocyte abnormalities of function and number occur. In general, congenital abnormalities of function have been seen in the formation of parts of the lymphoid system. Acquired defects in function have been identified in Hodgkin's disease, in connective tissue diseases, and in cases following exposure to ionizing radiation. In general, the clinical clue to altered function is the presence of recurrent infections. Since the lymphoid precursor mass is large and extensive, and since there are not yet good methods of quantifying the subsets of lymphocytes, simple enumeration in the circulation has not been effective.

Determining failure of end-functions, such as generalized deficiencies of immunoglobulins or failure of delayed hypersensitivity reactions, has provided the best documentation of defective lymphocyte function or numbers. The evaluation of impaired function due to lymphopenia must be based upon the severity of the impairment because of recurrent infections. Finally, it should be emphasized that some diseases that are called "auto-immune" may be due to functionally altered or numerically predominant subsets of lymphocytes.

Abnormalities of lymphocyte numbers are associated with two forms of neoplastic transformation. The first form is the leukemias, either acute lymphocytic leukemia or chronic lymphocytic leukemia. The second form is the malignant lymphoid lesions that include Hodgkin's disease, malignant lymphoma, and mycosis fungoides. Evaluation of impairment due to these neoplasms follows the same parameters as expressed above.

Infection by the Human Immunodeficiency Virus (HIV) has presented a new set of diseases and syndromes whose full expression is not fully known. Since the virus causes a depletion of the T4 helper lymphocytes, the diseases with which HIV is associated, acquired immunodeficiency syndrome (AIDS) and AIDS-related complex (ARC), may be considered diseases of the hematopoietic system. However, the clinical presentation of the infection ranges from no abnormal signs or symptoms (and therefore no impairment) to disorders of the respiratory system, gastrointestinal system, central nervous system, peripheral nervous system, and skin, as well as other abnormalities of the hematopoietic system (anemia, thrombocytopenia, hypergammaglobulinemia). Furthermore, the progression of the HIV infection from its asymptomatic state to AIDS in any given individual is not fully understood. Thus, evaluating persons with HIV infection for impairment may require numerous examinations, and requires use of the information in this chapter as well as information in Chapter 4 (The Nervous System), Chapter 5 (The Respiratory System), Chapter 10 (The Digestive System), Chapter 13 (The Skin), Chapter 14 (Mental and Behavioral Disorders), and possible other chapters, depending upon the presentation of the disease.

Monocytes-Macrophages:

The major function of the monocyte-macrophage family is to ingest foreign proteins, remove cellular debris and particulate material, and modulate immune responses. This functional unit of circulating monocytes and fixed macrophages, or "histiocytes," is structurally associated with endothelial cells and fibroblasts in the reticuloendothelial system. Recognition of this system is based primarily upon the phagocytic capacity of monocytes and macrophages.

Although these cells have their origin in bone marrow precursors, their traffic, potential for circulation and recirculation, and mode of activation are not yet clearly understood. It appears that a true "reserve pool" does not exist, and that mature monocytes are released randomly to circulate for an approximate survival of 72 hours, at which time they enter the tissues to become part of the macrophage pool; however, their subsequent history is not known. This system is known to require a state of "enhanced cellular metabolism," which is called "activation," in order to function. Thus, impairment could result from either a functional defect or from altered numbers.

At present, knowledge of functional defects in the monocyte-macrophage system is limited, and the degree of impairment of the system can be correlated with the nature, type, and extent of infection.

A second abnormality of the system is seen in the lipid storage diseases (Niemann-Pick's, Fabry's, and Gaucher's diseases, and gangliosidosis type I or sea-blue histiocytosis), in which the macrophages become repositories for lipids, and cellular and organ hyperplasia occurs in the spleen, lymph nodes, bone marrow, and elsewhere. Impairment from these disorders depends upon the nature of the lipid and the rate of deposition.

Neoplastic transformation of the family occurs primarily as acute monocytic leukemia, a relatively rare form of acute leukemia. A more chronic variant, leukemic reticuloendotheliosis, is a recently recognized variant. The exact cell of origin is not clear, but the condition behaves as a form of chronic neoplastic transformation.

7.4 Criteria for Evaluating Permanent Impairment of the White Cell Systems

Class 1—Impairment of the Whole Person, 0-10%: A patient belongs in Class 1 when (a) there are symptoms or signs of leukocyte abnormality; *and* (b) no or infrequent treatment is needed; *and* (c) all or most of the activities of daily living can be performed.

Example 1: A 50-year-old man with no previous symptoms was admitted to the hospital after a work injury. Routine examination of the blood disclosed a leukocyte count of 18,000/cu mm, of which 82% were lymphocytes. Erythrocyte and platelet counts were within normal limits. Diagnosis was leukemia, but treatment was not given. The patient recovered from the injury and resumed normal activities.

Diagnosis: Chronic lymphocytic leukemia, stage O-I.

Impairment: 0% impairment of the whole person.

Example 2: A healthy 21-year-old man suffered a ruptured spleen in an automobile crash. A splenectomy was performed. The postoperative course was uneventful. The patient returned to his normal activities of living.

Diagnosis: Splenectomy for splenic rupture.

Impairment: 0% impairment of the whole person.

Class 2—Impairment of the Whole Person, 15-25%:
A patient belongs in Class 2 when (a) there are symptoms and signs of leukocyte abnormality; *and* (b) although continuous treatment is required, most of the activities of daily living can be performed.

Example: A 40-year-old man complained of pain and tightness in the left upper abdominal quadrant, and of an 8 lb weight loss. He was found to have splenomegaly, the spleen extending 12 cm below the costal margin, and a leukocyte count of 150,000/cu mm, with many myelocytes and progranulocytes. With treatment, the spleen regressed to 4 cm, and the leukocyte count fell to the normal range. On daily medication, the patient remains in remission. Periodic adjustment of the dosage, based on laboratory values, is required.

Diagnosis: Chronic granulocytic leukemia.

Impairment: 15% impairment of the whole person.

Class 3—Impairment of the Whole Person, 30-50%:
A patient belongs in Class 3 when (a) there are symptoms and signs of leukocyte abnormality; *and* (b) continuous treatment is required; *and* (c) there is interference with the performance of daily activities that requires occasional assistance from others.

Example 1: A boy, age six, was admitted to the hospital with bacterial pneumonia. He first had suffered from pneumonia at six months of age. Since then, he has had repeated hospitalizations for three episodes of bacterial meningitis, and several episodes of septicemia, purulent sinusitis, exudative pharyngitis, and otitis media. Between episodes of infections, he was asymptomatic and experienced few limitations in his daily activities; however, there was need for regular medical supervision, and intercurrent infections occurred frequently.

At present, there is absence of gamma globulin in the patient's electrophoretic pattern. He has a younger brother with decreased gamma globulin levels.

Diagnosis: Agammaglobulinemia.

Impairment: 50% impairment of the whole person.

Example 2: A 55-year-old woman complained of weakness and dyspnea. The patient was found to have a hemoglobin of 7 gm/100 ml of blood, a hematocrit of 21%, leukocyte count of 82,000/cu mm, reticulocytes of 13%, and a positive Coombs' antiglobulin test. Although the anemia responded well to treatment, the patient developed progressive cachexia, extreme weight loss, profound weakness, and fever.

Diagnosis: Chronic lymphocytic leukemia with autoimmune hemolytic anemia.

Impairment: 40% impairment due to the leukemia and 0% impairment due to the anemia controlled by therapy, which combine to give 40% impairment of the whole person.

Example 3: A 28-year-old man was found by lymph node biopsy to have Hodgkin's disease. Although he responded at first to treatment with ionizing radiation, recurrence of generalized lymphadenopathy below and above the diaphragm, pruritus, chills, and fever made necessary the employment of continuous chemotherapy. He became profoundly weak due to anemia that responded temporarily to drug treatment and transfusions.

Diagnosis: Hodgkin's disease, recurrent, active.

Impairment: 50% impairment from the advanced Hodgkin's disease, which is to be combined with an appropriate value for impairment from anemia, to determine impairment of the whole person.

Class 4—Impairment of the Whole Person, 55-90%:
A patient belongs in Class 4 when (a) there are symptoms and signs of leukocyte abnormality; *and* (b) continuous treatment is required; *and* (c) difficulty is experienced in the performance of the activities of daily living that requires continuous care from others.

Example: A 55-year-old man developed profound weakness, chills, night sweats, and fever. He had gingival hypertrophy, nosebleeds, splenomegaly such that the spleen extended 4 cm below the costal margin, and ecchymoses. Hematologic values included hemoglobin, 4 gm/100 ml; white blood cell count, 12,000/cu mm, with 80% blast forms; and platelet count, 18,000/cu mm. He responded partially to treatment but required continuous observation, frequent blood transfusions, and continuing assistance with the activities of daily living.

Diagnosis: Acute leukemia.

Impairment: 90% impairment of the whole person.

7.5 Hemorrhagic Disorders and Platelets

There are several different types of bleeding disorders. In general, they may be categorized as hereditary or acquired, and as caused primarily by defects affecting platelets or blood clotting protein. Occasionally, inherited or acquired disorders, such as von Willebrand's disease and disseminated intravascular coagulation, may have both types of defects.

The initial tests useful for the diagnosis of platelet defects are the platelet count and the template bleeding time. A specific diagnosis requires further testing that involves platelet aggregation studies and various tests for the factor VIII complex.

The laboratory tests that are useful for the diagnosis of blood clotting disorders are the partial thromboplastin time, prothrombin time, thrombin time and fibrinogen level, and plasma protamine paracoagulation tests and tests for fibrin degradation products. Making a specific diagnosis frequently requires specific functional assays for clotting factor activity and occasionally measurement of the protein level in the blood, usually by immunologic assay.

In the great majority of hereditary disorders, with the notable exception of von Willebrand's disease, the basic hemostatic defect remains unchanged throughout the patient's life. The latter disorder may be mild, with bleeding occurring only after trauma or surgery, or may be severe, with bleeding occurring spontaneously. Patients with severe hereditary blood coagulation disorders may require prophylactic therapy; this may help them participate in activities such as bicycling, that they might otherwise have to avoid because of the threat of trauma. Moreover, there are many patients who require frequent home treatment to control bleeding that interferes with their daily activities. Patients with such severe hereditary blood coagulation disorders would have 15% to 50% impairment of the whole person, depending on the frequency of treatment and the extent of interference with their normal activities.

Patients with an inherited bleeding disorder may develop complications from recurrent hemorrhage, such as joint dysfunction. Impairment from such a complica-

tion should be evaluated in accordance with criteria in the appropriate chapter of the *Guides.* Percentage values of several impairments should be combined using the Combined Values Chart.

Example: A 21-year-old man has severe factor VIII deficiency, or hemophilia A. He frequently has spontaneous bleeding into large joints and muscles that requires home therapy with intravenous factor VIII concentrate two times per week. In addition, because of past joint hemorrhages, he has significant chronic dysfunction of his left knee, right ankle, and both elbows. The frequent joint and muscle hemorrhages and the need for continuous medical treatment interfere with his usual daily activities.

Diagnosis: Severe hemophilia A with permanent joint dysfunction secondary to recurrent bleeding.

Impairment: 40% impairment for the underlying bleeding disorder, combined using the Combined Values Chart with whatever percentages of impairment deemed appropriate for the joint dysfunction.

Acquired bleeding disorders may be due to platelet defects, blood clotting protein disorders, or a combination of both. Platelet defects may be due to either a decrease in the number of platelets or to an abnormality in their function. Since patients with these disorders need to avoid activities that may lead to trauma, or may need constant endocrine therapy to avoid heavy menstrual flow, a patient with a platelet disorder would have 0% to 10% impairment of the whole person. Complications that may ensue as a result of blood platelet disorders, such as hemorrhage or thrombosis, should be evaluated in accordance with the criteria for evaluating impairment of the particular body system or organ affected, and should be combined using the Combined Values Chart with the rating for the blood platelet disorders.

Similarly, persons with autoimmune thrombocytopenia may require long-term immunosuppressive therapy, which in itself can lead to a variety of organ dysfunctions that hamper the activities of daily living. Complications resulting from therapy should be evaluated according to the criteria for evaluating impairment of the particular body system or organ affected, and combined with the rating for the appropriate blood platelet disorder, using the Combined Values Chart.

Acquired blood clotting defects are usually secondary to severe underlying conditions, such as chronic liver disease. But many patients with venous or arterial thromboembolic disease receive anticoagulant therapy with a vitamin K antagonist such as warfarin, and they need to avoid activities that might lead to trauma. In these patients there is a 0% to 10% impairment of the whole person.

Example: A 49-year-old woman has chronic idiopathic autoimmune thrombocytopenia of five years duration. She had a splenectomy, and during four of the past five years, she received corticosteroids and other immuno-suppressive drugs. She is not on any medication, and her platelet count is 30,000/μl. Except for bruising eas-ily, she has no significant bleeding problem. The patient also has severe osteoporosis and compression fractures of T12 and L1 vertebrae, and these cause her to have chronic low back pain that interferes significantly with her daily activities.

Diagnosis: Chronic idiopathic autoimmune thrombo-cytopenic purpura.

Impairment: 0% impairment for the underlying bleed-ing disorder, combined with whatever percentage of impairment is deemed appropriate for her back prob-lem, to arrive at the estimated impairment of the whole person.

References

1. Cecil R: *Cecil's Textbook of Medicine,* ed 17, Wyngaarden JB, Smith LH, Jr (eds). Philadelphia, WB Saunders Co, 1985.

2. Harrison TR: *Harrison's Principles of Internal Medicine,* ed 11, Braunwald E, Isselbacher KJ, Petersdorf RG, et al (eds). New York, McGraw Hill, 1987.

3. Fishman MC, Hoffman AR, Klausner RD, Thaler MS: *Medicine,* ed 2. Philadelphia, JB Lippincott, 1985.

4. Krupp MA, Schroeder SA, Tierney LM, Jr (eds): *Cur-rent Medical Diagnosis and Treatment,* ed 26. Norwalk, CT, Appleton and Lange, 1987.

5. American Medical Association Council on Scientific Affairs: Information on AIDS for the Practicing Physi-cian. Chicago, American Medical Association, 1987.

Chapter 8

The Visual System

8.0 Introduction

The purpose of this chapter is to provide criteria for use in evaluating permanent impairment resulting from dysfunction of the visual system, which consists of the eyes, ocular adnexa, and the visual pathways. A simplified method is provided for quantitating visual impairment, which can then be translated into impairment of the whole person.

Visual impairment in varying degrees occurs in the presence of a deviation from normal in one or more functions of the eye, including (1) corrected visual acuity for objects at distance and near; (2) visual fields; and (3) ocular motility with diplopia. Evaluation of visual impairment is based on these three functions. Although they are not equally important, vision is imperfect without the coordinated function of all three.

Other ocular functions and disturbances are considered to the extent that they are reflected in one or more of the three coordinated functions. These other functions include color perception, adaptation to light and dark contrast sensitivity, accommodation, metamorphopsia, and stereoscopic vision. Ocular disturbances include paresis of accommodation, iridoplegia, entropion, ectropion, epiphora, lagophthalmos, and scarring. To the extent that any ocular disturbance causes impairment not reflected in visual acuity, visual fields, or ocular motility with diplopia, the impairment must be evaluated by the physician and be added to the impairment of the visual system.

One or more other ocular impairments, such as vitreous opacities, a nonreactive pupil, and light scattering disturbances of the cornea or other media, may be calculated as an additional 5% to 10% impairment of the involved eye. Permanent deformities of the orbit, scars, and cosmetic defects that may not alter ocular function should be considered individually as an additional factor that can cause up to 10% impairment of the whole person. If facial disfigurement due to scarring above the upper lip is evaluated using the criteria in Chapter 9, then any overlapping percentage of impairment due to ocular scarring should be subtracted from the larger percentage.

The following equipment is necessary to test the functions of the eyes:

1. Visual acuity test charts for distance and near vision. For distance vision, the Snellen test chart with nonserif block letters* or numbers, or the illiterate E chart, or Landolt's broken-ring chart is desirable. For near vision, many charts are available, such as those with print similar to that of the Snellen chart, with Revised Jaeger Standard print, or with American point-type notation for use at 35 cm or 14 inches.

2. An arc, bowl, or other validated perimeter with standard radius of 30 cm to 33 cm, or with a larger radius, if an appropriately larger target is used.

3. Refraction equipment.

Before using the information in this chapter, the reader is urged to review Chapters 1 and 2, which provide a general discussion of the purpose of the *Guides* and of

---

*The 10 equally difficult letters (D, K, R, H, V, C, N, Z, S, O) of Louise L. Sloan are recommended for uniformity. Each letter subtends a visual angle of 5 minutes and a stroke width of 1 minute.

the situations in which they are useful; and which discuss techniques for the evaluation of the subject and for preparation of a report. The report should include the information found in the following outline, which is developed more fully in Chapter 2.

A. Medical Evaluation
1. Narrative history of medical conditions
2. Results of the most recent clinical evaluation
3. Assessment of current clinical status and statement of future plans
4. Diagnoses and clinical impressions
5. Expected date of full or partial recovery

B. Analysis of Findings
1. Impact of medical condition(s) on life activities
2. Explanation for concluding that the medical condition(s) has or has not become static or well-stabilized
3. Explanation for concluding that the individual is or is not likely to suffer from sudden or subtle incapacitation
4. Explanation for concluding that the individual is or is not likely to suffer injury or further impairment by engaging in life activities or by attempting to meet personal, social and occupational demands
5. Explanation for concluding that accommodations and/or restrictions are or are not warranted

C. Comparison of Results of Analysis with Impairment Criteria
1. Description of clinical findings, and how these findings relate to specific criteria in the chapter
2. Explanation of each percent of impairment rating
3. Summary list of all impairment ratings
4. Overall rating of impairment of the whole person

Criteria and Methods for Evaluating Permanent Impairment

8.1 Central Visual Acuity

Test chart illumination of at least 5 foot-candles is recommended to attain a distinct contrast of .85 or greater and a comfortable luminance of approximately 85±5 candelas per square meter. The chart or reflecting surface should not be dirty or discolored. The far test distance simulates infinity at 6 m (20 ft) or at no less than 4 m (13 ft 1 in). The near test distance should be fixed at 35 cm (14 in) in keeping with the Revised Jaeger Standard. Adequate and comfortable illumination must be diffused onto the test card at a level about three times greater than that of usual room illumination.

Table 1. Visual Acuity Notations With Corresponding Percentages of Loss of Central Vision

For Distance

English	Snellen Notations Metric 6	Metric 4	% Loss
20/15	6/5	4/3	0
20/20	6/6	4/4	0
20/25	6/7.5	4/5	5
20/30	6/10	4/6	10
20/40	6/12	4/8	15
20/50	6/15	4/10	25
20/60	6/20	4/12	35
20/70	6/22	4/14	40
20/80	6/24	4/16	45
20/100	6/30	4/20	50
20/125	6/38	4/25	60
20/150	6/50	4/30	70
20/200	6/60	4/40	80
20/300	6/90	4/60	85
20/400	6/120	4/80	90
20/800	6/240	4/160	95

For Near

Near Snellen Inches	Centimeters	Revised Jaeger Standard	American point-type	% Loss
14/14	35/35	1	3	0
14/18	35/45	2	4	0
14/21	35/53	3	5	5
14/24	35/60	4	6	7
14/28	35/70	5	7	10
14/35	35/88	6	8	50
14/40	35/100	7	9	55
14/45	35/113	8	10	60
14/60	35/150	9	11	80
14/70	35/175	10	12	85
14/80	35/200	11	13	87
14/88	35/220	12	14	90
14/112	35/280	13	21	95
14/140	35/350	14	23	98

Measurements of visual acuity at near have less intertest reproducibility than those made of visual acuity at distance. Many occupational needs depend disproportionately on acuity of near vision.

Central vision should be measured and recorded for distance and for near objects, with and without wearing conventional spectacles. The use of contact lenses may further improve vision reduced by irregular astigmatism due to corneal injury or disease. However, practical problems related to fitting, expense, development of tolerance, and the fact that contact lenses are at times medically contraindicated, are sufficient at present to justify the recommendation that conventional ophthalmic lenses be used to obtain best corrected vision. In the absence of contraindications, if the patient is well adapted to contact lenses and wishes to wear them, correction by contact lenses is acceptable.

Visual acuity for distance should be recorded in the Snellen notation, using a fraction, in which the numerator is the test distance in feet or meters and the denominator is the distance at which the smallest letter discriminated by the patient would subtend 5 minutes of arc, that is, the distance at which an eye with 20/20 vision would see that letter. The fraction notation is one of convenience that does not imply percentage of visual acuity. A similar Snellen notation using centimeters or inches, or a comparable Revised Jaeger Standard or American point-type notation, may be used in designating near visual acuity.

The notations for acuity of distance and near vision that appear in Table 1, with corresponding percentages of loss of central vision, are included only to indicate the basic values used in developing Table 2. Simply adding two percentages of loss, corresponding to appropriate notations for distance and near vision, does not provide the true percentage of loss of central vision. Rather, the functional loss of central vision is the mean of the two percentages.

Monocular aphakia or monocular pseudophakia is considered to be an additional visual impairment, and if it is present, it is weighted by an additional 50% decrease in the value for remaining corrected central vision, as noted in Table 2.

The procedure for determining loss of central vision in one eye is:

1. Measure and record best central visual acuity for distance and for near, with and without conventional corrective spectacles or contact lenses.

Table 2. Loss of Central Vision* In Percentage

Snellen Rating for Distance in Feet	Approximate Snellen Rating for Near in Inches													
	$\frac{14}{14}$	$\frac{14}{18}$	$\frac{14}{21}$	$\frac{14}{24}$	$\frac{14}{28}$	$\frac{14}{35}$	$\frac{14}{40}$	$\frac{14}{45}$	$\frac{14}{60}$	$\frac{14}{70}$	$\frac{14}{80}$	$\frac{14}{88}$	$\frac{14}{112}$	$\frac{14}{140}$
$\frac{20}{15}$	0 / 50	0 / 50	3 / 52	4 / 52	5 / 53	25 / 63	27 / 64	30 / 65	40 / 70	43 / 72	44 / 72	45 / 73	48 / 74	49 / 75
$\frac{20}{20}$	0 / 50	0 / 50	3 / 52	4 / 52	5 / 53	25 / 63	27 / 64	30 / 65	40 / 70	43 / 72	44 / 72	46 / 73	48 / 74	49 / 75
$\frac{20}{25}$	3 / 52	3 / 52	5 / 53	6 / 53	8 / 54	28 / 64	30 / 65	33 / 67	43 / 72	45 / 73	46 / 73	48 / 74	50 / 75	52 / 76
$\frac{20}{30}$	5 / 53	5 / 53	8 / 54	9 / 54	10 / 55	30 / 65	32 / 66	35 / 68	45 / 73	48 / 74	49 / 74	50 / 75	53 / 76	54 / 77
$\frac{20}{40}$	8 / 54	8 / 54	10 / 55	11 / 56	13 / 57	33 / 67	35 / 68	38 / 69	48 / 74	50 / 75	51 / 76	53 / 77	55 / 78	57 / 79
$\frac{20}{50}$	13 / 57	13 / 57	15 / 58	16 / 58	18 / 59	38 / 69	40 / 70	43 / 72	53 / 77	55 / 78	56 / 78	58 / 79	60 / 80	62 / 81
$\frac{20}{60}$	16 / 58	16 / 58	18 / 59	20 / 60	22 / 61	41 / 70	44 / 72	46 / 73	56 / 78	59 / 79	60 / 80	61 / 81	64 / 82	65 / 83
$\frac{20}{80}$	20 / 60	20 / 60	23 / 62	24 / 62	25 / 63	45 / 73	47 / 74	50 / 75	60 / 80	63 / 82	64 / 82	65 / 83	68 / 84	69 / 85
$\frac{20}{100}$	25 / 63	25 / 63	28 / 64	29 / 64	30 / 65	50 / 75	52 / 76	55 / 78	65 / 83	68 / 84	69 / 84	70 / 85	73 / 87	74 / 87
$\frac{20}{125}$	30 / 65	30 / 65	33 / 67	34 / 67	35 / 68	55 / 78	57 / 79	60 / 80	70 / 85	73 / 87	74 / 87	75 / 88	78 / 89	79 / 90
$\frac{20}{150}$	34 / 67	34 / 67	37 / 68	38 / 69	39 / 70	59 / 80	61 / 81	64 / 82	74 / 87	77 / 88	78 / 89	79 / 90	82 / 91	83 / 92
$\frac{20}{200}$	40 / 70	40 / 70	43 / 72	44 / 72	45 / 73	65 / 83	67 / 84	70 / 85	80 / 90	83 / 91	84 / 92	85 / 93	88 / 94	89 / 95
$\frac{20}{300}$	43 / 72	43 / 72	45 / 73	46 / 73	48 / 74	68 / 84	70 / 85	73 / 87	83 / 91	85 / 93	86 / 93	88 / 94	90 / 95	92 / 96
$\frac{20}{400}$	45 / 73	45 / 73	48 / 74	49 / 74	50 / 75	70 / 85	72 / 86	75 / 88	85 / 93	88 / 94	89 / 94	90 / 95	93 / 97	94 / 97
$\frac{20}{800}$	48 / 74	48 / 74	50 / 75	51 / 76	53 / 77	73 / 87	75 / 88	78 / 89	88 / 94	90 / 95	91 / 96	93 / 97	95 / 98	97 / 99

*Upper figure = % loss of central vision without allowance for monocular aphakia or monocular pseudophakia; lower figure = % loss of central vision with allowance for monocular aphakia or monocular pseudophakia.

2. Consult Table 2 to derive the percentage loss by combining best corrected near and distance acuities, and to calculate the additional loss of central vision that results from the presence of aphakia or pseudophakia.

Example: Without allowance for monocular aphakia, 14/70 for near vision and 20/200 for distance produce 83% loss of central vision. With allowance for monocular aphakia, which is applicable to corrected vision only, 14/70 for near vision and 20/200 for distance produce 91% loss of central vision.

8.2 Visual Fields

For the purposes of these *Guides,* one level suprathreshold screening is acceptable. The standard reference for visual field measurement is the Goldmann kinetic outer isopter of the III/4e stimulus. This is approximately equivalent to the arc perimeter examination using a 3 mm white test target at a radius of 330 mm, which is also acceptable under these *Guides.* Automated programs cannot be used to quantify visual field impairments between the outer limit of their radii (usually 30° or 60° and, less frequently 70° or 80° from fixation) and the normal outer extent of the functional visual field.

Current and widely available automated perimeters, such as the Allergan-Humphrey 635 or the Techna

Vision, Inc (formerly Coopervision) Dicon, can test only those points of the visual field that are within the radius of the bowl or radius of the specific programmed test sequence used. Thus, the Allergan-Humphrey Field Analyzer with its 30-1 or 30-2 program tests only within a field radius of 30°. At the 10 decibel level this provides an equivalent stimulus to the Goldmann III/4e but no direct test of the visual field between 30° from fixation and the outer limit or normal extent of the visual field. The Humphrey "full field 81-point program" tests only within the radius of 60° from fixation; however, threshold peripheral tests from 30° to 60° from fixation are available. The Squid (Synemed, Inc) provides a peripheral field program covering the outer ring from 30° to 70° from fixation. Techna Vision offers a 30-2 program with two peripheral isopters at 30° and 80° plus Esterman monocular and binocular grid programs at a suitable target intensity of 2500 apostilbs. Software packages are available to deliver Esterman monocular and binocular scores.

If the ocular history and examination are essentially normal and suggest no lesions involving the outer extent of the visual fields, then normal central visual fields produced by automated programs within 30° or 60° may be submitted to confirm a report of normal visual fields. Alternatively, if the history and examination indicate circumferential impairment of the peripheral fields extending within the programmed test radius of 30° or 60° from fixation, then automated programs may be used to report visual field loss of such

Figure 1. Example of Perimetric Charts Used to Plot Extent or Outline of Visual Field Along the Eight Principal Meridians that are Separated by 45° Intervals.

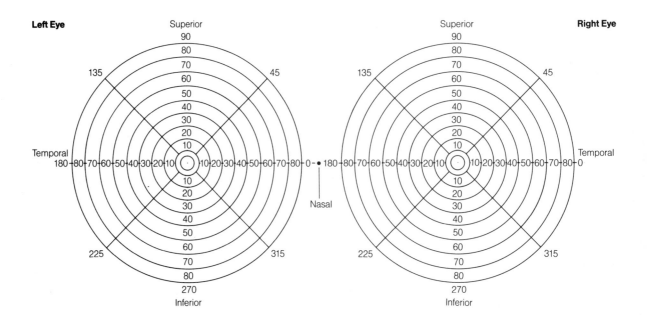

a greater extent. This will be based on findings transferred to an Esterman Grid or plotted as loss from the normal extent of visual field from point of fixation (Figure 1).

The examiner should use preferentially a binocular test of the functional visual field in distinction to the monocular visual field test, which is done for diagnostic purposes and may be assessed with a wide range of instruments. For binocular field testing the patient should have two eyes, proper alignment of the eyes, and no diplopia. If the patient has only one eye, if there is deviation (heterotropia) of either eye, or diplopia, then monocular visual field testing must be done. The binocular or functional field is derived from the usual use of the two eyes together and involves an overlapping area in the nasal portion of each field. This produces some enhancement of object awareness in the overlapping areas, although apparently not in the patient with advanced glaucoma. The chin rest must be positioned in the midline for suitable candidates so that the two eyes are evenly to the right and to the left of the central fixation target. Both eyes are kept open and the seeing field outline (isopter) is recorded on an Esterman Grid or similar chart (Figure 2A). A normal or standard outer isopter for the binocular field has been validated in studies of more than 2,000 individuals.

Accordingly, an outer limit (isopter) of functional awareness must be established from examination by arc perimeter, bowl perimeter, or other validated instrument and transferred as a line to the Esterman 120 unit binocular grid. A simple count of all the printed dots seen to be entirely outside of or falling on the line (isopter) marking the extent of the visual field provides for the scoring of functional loss to a maximum of 120 units. This is multiplied by 5/6 to yield the percentage loss of the binocular functional field.

For the one-eyed patient or the individual with diplopia or with apparent deviation of either eye (heterotropia), the Esterman 100 unit monocular field is preferably used (Figure 2B). A simple count of all the printed dots seen to be entirely outside of or falling on the line (isopter) marking the extent of the visual field provides an immediate percentage of field loss. (Conversely, a simple count of the printed dots within each grid square which fall within or do not touch the contour line gives the percentage of visual field retention for that eye.)

For an examination with an arc perimeter, the examiner should use a white disc that is 6 mm in diameter, at a distance of 33 cm, to test an aphakic patient whose eye is uncorrected, that is, not adapted to a contact lens or to an intraocular (pseudophake) implant, or whose eye is fitted with aphakic spectacles.

Figure 2A. Esterman 120-unit Binocular Scoring Grid for Use with Both Eyes Open.

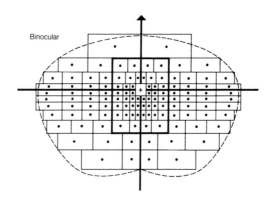

Figure 2B. Esterman 100-unit Monocular Scoring Grid for Arc or Bowl Perimeter or Similar Automated Instrument Providing Full Monocular Field Analysis.

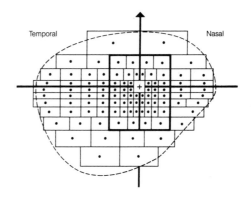

(Grids may be obtained from the Manhattan Eye, Ear and Throat Hospital, 210 East 64th Street, NY, NY 10021)

Table 3. Minimal Normal Extent of Monocular Visual Field from Point of Fixation

Direction of Vision	Degrees of Field
Temporally	85
Down temporally	85
Direct down	65
Down nasally	50
Nasally	60
Up nasally	55
Direct up	45
Up temporally	55
Total	500

If in these instances a Goldmann bowl perimeter is used, the target should be IV/4e in the kinetic mode. If the aphakic patient is well adapted to a contact lens or an intraocular lens, then the examiner should use the 3 mm diameter white target at 33 cm, or the Goldmann III/4e target, or equivalent.

In kinetic testing, the object is brought from the periphery to the seeing area. At least two peripheral fields should be obtained that agree within 15° in each meridian. The reliability of the patient's responses should be noted. The result is plotted on a visual field chart for each of the eight principal meridians that are separated by 45° intervals (Figure 1). The minimal normal extent of the visual field from the point of fixation is indicated in Table 3 above. The figures represent somewhat less than average normal performance, which allows for poor or delayed subjective responses or for unusual prominence of brow or nose.

The percentage of retained visual field in one eye is obtained by adding to the number of degrees remaining along the eight principal meridians given in Table 3 for the 3/330 white isopter, which normally sum to 500 degrees, and dividing the total by 5. Conversely, the percentage loss of visual field is obtained by adding the number of degrees lost along each of the eight meridians, and dividing the total by 5. Where there is loss of a quadrant or of half a field, one-half of the value of each of the two boundary meridians should be added to the calculated loss. Visual field losses of other amounts and from other conditions can be calculated in a similar manner.

Although the extent of loss of visual fields cannot be determined accurately for a scotoma, an approximation can be obtained by subtracting the width of the scotoma from the peripheral visual field value at the same meridians. A similar estimation of visual field loss can be applied to enlargement of the blind spot, with the use of a 2 mm test object at a distance of 1 m from the tangent screen while the patient is wearing corrective lenses. For example, a general enlargement of the blind spot of 5° would result in a visual field loss of $8 \times 5 \div 5 = 8\%$ loss. Because a central scotoma directly affects central visual acuity, which is evaluated first, such visual field loss is not used again in the final calculation of visual loss.

8.3 Determining Loss of Monocular Visual Fields

The following steps are taken to determine the loss of monocular visual fields in each eye:

1. The nontested eye is occluded, and the patient is positioned on the chin rest so that the tested eye is centered on the fixation target.

2. Plot the extent of the visual fields on each of the eight principal meridians of a visual field chart. (See Figure 1.)

3. (a) Determine the degrees lost by adding the degrees of visual field lost in each of the principal meridians. (See Table 3.)

(b) If half of a field is lost, include the two boundary meridians at a value equal to one half their total degrees value. (See Table 3.)

4. Consult Table 4 to ascertain corresponding percentage of visual field loss.

5. Because the inferior visual field is occupationally more significant than the superior visual field, lower quadrant defects are weighted by an additional 5% loss of the visual field. Correspondingly, an inferior hemianopic loss is weighted by an additional 10% loss of the visual field.

6. When the monocular Esterman scale (Figure 2B) is used, count all the printed dots seen to be entirely outside of or falling on the line (isopter) marking the extent of the visual field. This number is the final percent of visual field loss for that eye and automatically takes into account the additional weighting for lower field defects.

Example 1: A patient has a concentric contraction to 30°:

Loss	Degrees
Temporally	55
Down temporally	55
Direct down	35
Down nasally	20
Nasally	30
Up nasally	25
Direct up	15
Up temporally	25
Total loss	260

The loss of 260° is equivalent to 52% loss of visual field.

Table 4. Loss of Monocular Visual Field

Total Degrees		% of Loss	Total Degrees		% of Loss	Total Degrees		% of Loss
Lost	Retained		Lost	Retained		Lost	Retained	
0	500*	0	170	330	34	340	160	68
5	495	1	175	325	35	345	155	69
10	490	2	180	320	36	350	150	70
15	485	3	185	315	37	355	145	71
20	480	4	190	310	38	360	140	72
25	475	5	195	305	39	365	135	73
30	470	6	200	300	40	370	130	74
35	465	7	205	295	41	375	125	75
40	460	8	210	290	42	380	120	76
45	455	9	215	285	43	385	115	77
50	450	10	220	280	44	390	110	78
55	445	11	225	275	45	395	105	79
60	440	12	230	270	46	400	100	80
65	435	13	235	265	47	405	95	81
70	430	14	240	260	48	410	90	82
75	425	15	245	255	49	415	85	83
80	420	16	250	250	50	420	80	84
85	415	17	255	245	51	425	75	85
90	410	18	260	240	52	430	70	86
95	405	19	265	235	53	435	65	87
100	400	20	270	230	54	440	60	88
105	395	21	275	225	55	445	55	89
110	390	22	280	220	56	450	50	90
115	385	23	285	215	57	455	45	91
120	380	24	290	210	58	460	40	92
125	375	25	295	205	59	465	35	93
130	370	26	300	200	60	470	30	94
135	365	27	305	195	61	475	25	95
140	360	28	310	190	62	480	20	96
145	355	29	315	185	63	485	15	97
150	350	30	320	180	64	490	10	98
155	345	31	325	175	65	495	5	99
160	340	32	330	170	66	500	0	100
165	335	33	335	165	67			

*Or more.

Example 2: A patient has an entire temporal field loss:

Loss	Degrees
Up temporally	55
Temporally	85
Down temporally	85
Half of direct up and direct down (45 & 65)	55
Total loss	280

The loss of 280° is equivalent to 56% loss of visual field.

8.4 Abnormal Ocular Motility and Binocular Diplopia

Unless a patient has diplopia within 30° of the center of fixation, the diplopia rarely causes significant visual impairment. An exception is diplopia upon looking downward. The extent of diplopia in the various directions of gaze is determined on an arc perimeter at 33 cm, or at an equivalent bowl perimeter radius, from the patient's eyes. Examination is made in each of the eight major meridians by using a small test light, or the projected light of approximately Goldmann III/4e without adding colored lenses or correcting prisms.

To determine the impairment of ocular motility the patient is seated with both eyes open and the chin resting in the chin rest, approximately centered so that the eyes are equidistant to either side of the central fixation target.

1. Plot the presence of diplopia along the meridians of a suitable visual field chart.

2. Add the percentages for loss of ocular motility due to diplopia in the meridian of maximum impairment as indicated in Figure 3.

3. In the patient with one eye, with profound amblyopia or with profound loss of vision, individual evaluation of motility will be made by the examiner.

Example: Diplopia within the central 20° is equivalent to 100% impairment of ocular motility.

Example: Diplopia on looking horizontally off center from 20° to 30° is equivalent to 20% loss of ocular motility; 30° to 40° is equivalent to 10% loss of ocular motility, for a total of 30% loss of ocular motility.

8.5 Steps To Determine Impairment of the Visual System and of the Whole Person Contributed by the Visual System

Calculate and record:

· percentage loss of central vision (CV) for each eye separately,

· percentage loss of visual field (VF) for each eye separately (monocular) or for both eyes together (binocular), and

· percentage loss of ocular motility (OM).

A. If the percentage loss of VF is calculated for each eye separately (monocular), using the Combined Values Chart, combine the percentage loss of central vision with the percentage loss of visual field in each eye and record these values.

Example:

Right eye

loss of central vision (both near and distance)	56%
loss of visual field	32%
56% combined with 32%	70%

Left eye

loss of central vision (both near and distance)	46%
loss of visual field	32%
46% combined with 32%	63%

Again using the Combined Values Chart, combine the percentage loss of ocular motility with the combined value for central vision and visual field in the eye manifesting greater impairment. Disregard the loss of ocular motility in the other eye.

Example:

Right eye

combined value of CV and VF	70%
loss of ocular motility	25%
70% combined with 25%	78%

Consult Table 5 to ascertain impairment of the visual system.

Figure 3. Percentage/loss of ocular motility of one eye in diplopia fields.

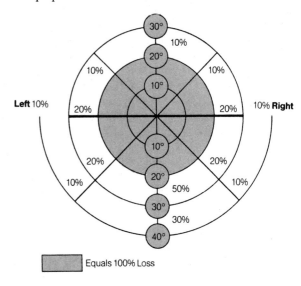

Equals 100% Loss

Example:

impairment of right (worse) eye	78%
impairment of left (better) eye	63%
impairment of visual system	67%

Consult Table 6 to ascertain the impairment of the whole person that is contributed by impairment of the visual system.

Example:
67% impairment of the visual system is equivalent to 63% impairment of the whole person.

B. If the percentage loss of VF is calculated for both eyes together (using the Esterman binocular grid), consult Table 5 to ascertain impairment of the visual system due to loss of central vision.

Using a similar example:

Right eye

loss of CV (both near and distance)	56%

Left eye

loss of CV (both near and distance)	46%
impairment due to loss of CV of both eyes	49%

Using the Combined Values Chart combine the impairment due to loss of CV with the impairment due to binocular visual field loss. *Note:* No value for loss of ocular motility is provided since binocular VF testing is not recommended when loss of ocular motility is present.

Table 5. Visual System

The values in this table are based on the following formula:

$$\frac{3 \times \text{impairment value of better eye} + \text{impairment value of worse eye}}{4} = \text{impairment of visual system}$$

The guides to the table are percentage impairment values for each eye. The percentage for the worse eye is read at the side of the table. The percentage for the better eye is read at the bottom of the table. At the intersection of the column for the worse eye and the column for the better eye is the impairment of visual system value.

For example, when there is 60% impairment of one eye and 30% impairment of the other eye, read down the side of the table until you come to the larger value (60%). Then follow across the row until it is intersected by the column headed by 30% at the bottom of the page. At the intersection of these two columns is printed the number 38. This number (38) represents the percentage impairment of the visual system when there is 60% impairment of one eye and 30% impairment of the other eye.

If bilateral aphakia is present and corrected central vision has been used in evaluation, impairment of the visual system is weighted by an additional 25% decrease in the value of the remaining corrected vision. For example, a 38% impairment (62% remaining) would be increased to 38% + (25%)(62%) = 54%.

% Impairment Worse Eye (rows) × **% Impairment Better Eye** (columns)

W\B	0	1	2	3	4	5	6	7	8	9	10	11	12	13	14	15	16	17	18	19	20	21	22	23	24	25	26	27	28	29	30	31	32	33	34	35	36	37	38	39	40	41	42	43	44	45	46	47	48	49
0	0																																																	
1	0	1																																																
2	1	1	2																																															
3	1	2	2	3																																														
4	1	2	3	3	4																																													
5	1	2	3	4	4	5																																												
6	2	2	3	4	5	5	6																																											
7	2	3	3	4	5	6	6	7																																										
8	2	3	4	4	5	6	7	7	8																																									
9	2	3	4	5	5	6	7	8	8	9																																								
10	3	3	4	5	6	6	7	8	9	9	10																																							
11	3	4	4	5	6	7	7	8	9	10	10	11																																						
12	3	4	5	5	6	7	8	8	9	10	11	11	12																																					
13	3	4	5	6	6	7	8	9	9	10	11	12	12	13																																				
14	4	4	5	6	7	7	8	9	10	10	11	12	13	13	14																																			
15	4	5	5	6	7	8	8	9	10	11	11	12	13	14	14	15																																		
16	4	5	6	6	7	8	9	9	10	11	12	12	13	14	15	15	16																																	
17	4	5	6	7	7	8	9	10	10	11	12	13	13	14	15	16	16	17																																
18	5	5	6	7	8	8	9	10	11	11	12	13	14	14	15	16	17	17	18																															
19	5	6	6	7	8	9	9	10	11	12	12	13	14	15	15	16	17	18	18	19																														
20	5	6	7	7	8	9	10	10	11	12	13	13	14	15	16	16	17	18	19	19	20																													
21	5	6	7	8	8	9	10	11	11	12	13	14	14	15	16	17	17	18	19	20	20	21																												
22	6	6	7	8	9	9	10	11	12	12	13	14	15	15	16	17	18	18	19	20	21	21	22																											
23	6	7	7	8	9	10	10	11	12	13	13	14	15	16	16	17	18	19	19	20	21	22	22	23																										
24	6	7	8	8	9	10	11	11	12	13	14	14	15	16	17	17	18	19	20	20	21	22	23	23	24																									
25	6	7	8	9	9	10	11	12	12	13	14	15	15	16	17	18	18	19	20	21	21	22	23	24	24	25																								
26	7	7	8	9	10	10	11	12	13	13	14	15	16	16	17	18	19	19	20	21	22	22	23	24	25	25	26																							
27	7	8	8	9	10	11	11	12	13	14	14	15	16	17	17	18	19	20	20	21	22	23	23	24	25	26	26	27																					
28	7	8	9	9	10	11	12	12	13	14	15	15	16	17	18	18	19	20	21	21	22	23	24	24	25	26	27	27	28																				
29	7	8	9	10	10	11	12	13	13	14	15	16	16	17	18	19	19	20	21	22	22	23	24	25	25	26	27	28	28	29																			
30	8	8	9	10	11	11	12	13	14	14	15	16	17	17	18	19	20	20	21	22	23	23	24	25	26	26	27	28	29	29	30																		
31	8	9	9	10	11	12	12	13	14	15	15	16	17	18	18	19	20	21	21	22	23	24	24	25	26	27	27	28	29	30	30	31																	
32	8	9	10	10	11	12	13	13	14	15	16	16	17	18	19	19	20	21	22	22	23	24	25	25	26	27	28	28	29	30	31	31	32																
33	8	9	10	11	11	12	13	14	14	15	16	17	17	18	19	20	20	21	22	23	23	24	25	26	26	27	28	29	29	30	31	32	32	33															
34	9	9	10	11	12	12	13	14	15	15	16	17	18	18	19	20	21	21	22	23	24	24	25	26	27	27	28	29	30	30	31	32	33	33	34														
35	9	10	10	11	12	13	13	14	15	16	16	17	18	19	19	20	21	22	22	23	24	25	25	26	27	28	28	29	30	31	31	32	33	34	34	35													
36	9	10	11	11	12	13	14	14	15	16	17	17	18	19	20	20	21	22	23	23	24	25	26	26	27	28	29	29	30	31	32	32	33	34	35	35	36												
37	9	10	11	12	12	13	14	15	15	16	17	18	18	19	20	21	21	22	23	24	24	25	26	27	27	28	29	30	30	31	32	33	33	34	35	36	36	37											
38	10	10	11	12	13	13	14	15	16	16	17	18	19	19	20	21	22	22	23	24	25	25	26	27	28	28	29	30	31	31	32	33	34	34	35	36	37	37	38										
39	10	11	11	12	13	14	14	15	16	17	17	18	19	20	20	21	22	23	23	24	25	26	26	27	28	29	29	30	31	32	32	33	34	35	35	36	37	38	38	39									
40	10	11	12	12	13	14	15	15	16	17	18	18	19	20	21	21	22	23	24	24	25	26	27	27	28	29	30	30	31	32	33	33	34	35	36	36	37	38	39	39	40								
41	10	11	12	13	13	14	15	16	16	17	18	19	19	20	21	22	22	23	24	25	25	26	27	28	28	29	30	31	31	32	33	34	34	35	36	37	37	38	39	40	40	41							
42	11	11	12	13	14	14	15	16	17	17	18	19	20	20	21	22	23	23	24	25	26	26	27	28	29	29	30	31	32	32	33	34	35	35	36	37	38	38	39	40	41	41	42						
43	11	12	12	13	14	15	15	16	17	18	18	19	20	21	21	22	23	24	24	25	26	27	27	28	29	30	30	31	32	33	33	34	35	36	36	37	38	39	39	40	41	42	42	43					
44	11	12	13	13	14	15	16	16	17	18	19	19	20	21	22	22	23	24	25	25	26	27	28	28	29	30	31	31	32	33	34	34	35	36	37	37	38	39	40	40	41	42	43	43	44				
45	11	12	13	14	14	15	16	17	17	18	19	20	20	21	22	23	23	24	25	26	26	27	28	29	29	30	31	32	32	33	34	35	35	36	37	38	38	39	40	41	41	42	43	44	44	45			
46	12	12	13	14	15	15	16	17	18	18	19	20	21	21	22	23	24	24	25	26	27	27	28	29	30	30	31	32	33	33	34	35	36	36	37	38	39	39	40	41	42	42	43	44	45	45	46		
47	12	13	13	14	15	16	16	17	18	19	19	20	21	22	22	23	24	25	25	26	27	28	28	29	30	31	31	32	33	34	34	35	36	37	37	38	39	40	40	41	42	43	43	44	45	46	46	47	
48	12	13	14	14	15	16	17	17	18	19	20	20	21	22	23	23	24	25	26	26	27	28	29	29	30	31	32	32	33	34	35	35	36	37	38	38	39	40	41	41	42	43	44	44	45	46	47	47	48
49	12	13	14	15	15	16	17	18	18	19	20	21	21	22	23	24	24	25	26	27	27	28	29	30	30	31	32	33	33	34	35	36	36	37	38	39	39	40	41	42	42	43	44	45	45	46	47	48	48	49

% Impairment Better Eye

Combined value chart — % Impairment Worse Eye (rows) combined with % Impairment Better Eye (columns 0–100).

Worse\Better	0	1	2	3	4	5	6	7	8	9	10	11	12	13	14	15	16	17	18	19	20	21	22	23	24	25	26	27	28	29	30	31	32	33	34	35	36	37	38	39	40	41	42	43	44	45	46	47	48	49	50	51	52	53	54	55	56	57	58	59	60	61	62	63	64	65	66	67	68	69	70	71	72	73	74	75	76	77	78	79	80	81	82	83	84	85	86	87	88	89	90	91	92	93	94	95	96	97	98	99	100
50	13	13	14	15	16	16	17	18	19	19	20	21	22	22	23	24	25	25	26	27	28	28	29	30	31	31	32	33	34	34	35	36	37	37	38	39	40	40	41	42	43	43	44	45	46	46	47	48	49	49	50																																																			
51	13	14	14	15	16	17	17	18	19	20	20	21	22	23	23	24	25	26	26	27	28	29	29	30	31	32	32	33	34	35	35	36	37	38	38	39	40	41	41	42	43	44	44	45	46	47	47	48	49	50	50	51																																																	
52	13	14	15	15	16	17	18	18	19	20	21	21	22	23	24	24	25	26	27	27	28	29	30	30	31	32	33	33	34	35	36	36	37	38	39	39	40	41	42	42	43	44	45	45	46	47	48	48	49	50	51	51	52																																														
53	13	14	15	16	16	17	18	19	19	20	21	22	22	23	24	25	25	26	27	28	28	29	30	31	31	32	33	34	34	35	36	37	37	38	39	40	40	41	42	43	43	44	45	46	46	47	48	49	49	50	51	52	52	53																																												
54	14	14	15	16	17	17	18	19	20	20	21	22	23	23	24	25	26	26	27	28	29	29	30	31	32	32	33	34	35	35	36	37	38	38	39	40	41	41	42	43	44	44	45	46	47	47	48	49	50	50	51	52	53	53	54																																										
55	14	15	15	16	17	18	18	19	20	21	21	22	23	24	24	25	26	27	27	28	29	30	30	31	32	33	33	34	35	36	36	37	38	39	39	40	41	42	42	43	44	45	45	46	47	48	48	49	50	51	51	52	53	54	54	55																																									
56	14	15	16	16	17	18	19	19	20	21	22	22	23	24	25	25	26	27	28	28	29	30	31	31	32	33	34	34	35	36	37	37	38	39	40	40	41	42	43	43	44	45	46	46	47	48	49	49	50	51	52	52	53	54	55	55	56																																								
57	14	15	16	17	17	18	19	20	20	21	22	23	23	24	25	26	26	27	28	29	29	30	31	32	32	33	34	35	35	36	37	38	38	39	40	41	41	42	43	44	44	45	46	47	47	48	49	50	50	51	52	53	53	54	55	56	56	57																																							
58	15	15	16	17	18	18	19	20	21	21	22	23	24	24	25	26	27	27	28	29	30	30	31	32	33	33	34	35	36	36	37	38	39	39	40	41	42	42	43	44	45	45	46	47	48	48	49	50	51	51	52	53	54	54	55	56	57	57	58																																						
59	15	16	16	17	18	19	19	20	21	22	22	23	24	25	25	26	27	28	28	29	30	31	31	32	33	34	34	35	36	37	37	38	39	40	40	41	42	43	43	44	45	46	46	47	48	49	49	50	51	52	52	53	54	55	55	56	57	58	58	59																																					
60	15	16	17	17	18	19	20	20	21	22	23	23	24	25	26	26	27	28	29	29	30	31	32	32	33	34	35	35	36	37	38	38	39	40	41	41	42	43	44	44	45	46	47	47	48	49	50	50	51	52	53	53	54	55	56	56	57	58	59	59	60																																					
61	15	16	17	18	18	19	20	21	21	22	23	24	24	25	26	27	27	28	29	30	30	31	32	33	33	34	35	36	36	37	38	39	39	40	41	42	42	43	44	45	45	46	47	48	48	49	50	51	51	52	53	54	54	55	56	57	57	58	59	60	60	61																																				
62	16	16	17	18	19	19	20	21	22	22	23	24	25	25	26	27	28	28	29	30	31	31	32	33	34	34	35	36	37	37	38	39	40	40	41	42	43	43	44	45	46	46	47	48	49	49	50	51	52	52	53	54	55	55	56	57	58	58	59	60	61	61	62																																			
63	16	17	17	18	19	20	20	21	22	23	23	24	25	26	26	27	28	29	29	30	31	32	32	33	34	35	35	36	37	38	38	39	40	41	41	42	43	44	44	45	46	47	47	48	49	50	50	51	52	53	53	54	55	56	56	57	58	59	59	60	61	62	62	63																																		
64	16	17	18	18	19	20	21	21	22	23	24	24	25	26	27	27	28	29	30	30	31	32	33	33	34	35	36	36	37	38	39	39	40	41	42	42	43	44	45	45	46	47	48	48	49	50	51	51	52	53	54	54	55	56	57	57	58	59	60	60	61	62	63	63	64																																	
65	16	17	18	19	19	20	21	22	22	23	24	25	25	26	27	28	28	29	30	31	31	32	33	34	34	35	36	37	37	38	39	40	40	41	42	43	43	44	45	46	46	47	48	49	49	50	51	52	52	53	54	55	55	56	57	58	58	59	60	61	61	62	63	64	64	65																																
66	17	17	18	19	20	20	21	22	23	23	24	25	26	26	27	28	29	29	30	31	32	32	33	34	35	35	36	37	38	38	39	40	41	41	42	43	44	44	45	46	47	47	48	49	50	50	51	52	53	53	54	55	56	56	57	58	59	59	60	61	62	62	63	64	65	65	66																															
67	17	18	18	19	20	21	21	22	23	24	24	25	26	27	27	28	29	30	30	31	32	33	33	34	35	36	36	37	38	39	39	40	41	42	42	43	44	45	45	46	47	48	48	49	50	51	51	52	53	54	54	55	56	57	57	58	59	60	60	61	62	63	63	64	65	66	66	67																													
68	17	18	19	19	20	21	22	22	23	24	25	25	26	27	28	28	29	30	31	31	32	33	34	34	35	36	37	37	38	39	40	40	41	42	43	43	44	45	46	46	47	48	49	49	50	51	52	52	53	54	55	55	56	57	58	58	59	60	61	61	62	63	64	64	65	66	67	67	68																												
69	17	18	19	20	20	21	22	23	23	24	25	26	26	27	28	29	29	30	31	32	32	33	34	35	35	36	37	38	38	39	40	41	41	42	43	44	44	45	46	47	47	48	49	50	50	51	52	53	53	54	55	56	56	57	58	59	59	60	61	62	62	63	64	65	65	66	67	68	68	69																											
70	18	18	19	20	21	21	22	23	24	24	25	26	27	27	28	29	30	30	31	32	33	33	34	35	36	36	37	38	39	39	40	41	42	42	43	44	45	45	46	47	48	48	49	50	51	51	52	53	54	54	55	56	57	57	58	59	60	60	61	62	63	63	64	65	66	66	67	68	69	69	70																										
71	18	19	19	20	21	22	22	23	24	25	25	26	27	28	28	29	30	31	31	32	33	34	34	35	36	37	37	38	39	40	40	41	42	43	43	44	45	46	46	47	48	49	49	50	51	52	52	53	54	55	55	56	57	58	58	59	60	61	61	62	63	64	64	65	66	67	67	68	69	70	70	71																									
72	18	19	20	20	21	22	23	23	24	25	26	26	27	28	29	29	30	31	32	32	33	34	35	35	36	37	38	38	39	40	41	41	42	43	44	44	45	46	47	47	48	49	50	50	51	52	53	53	54	55	56	56	57	58	59	59	60	61	62	62	63	64	65	65	66	67	68	68	69	70	71	71	72																								
73	18	19	20	21	21	22	23	24	24	25	26	27	27	28	29	30	30	31	32	33	33	34	35	36	36	37	38	39	39	40	41	42	42	43	44	45	45	46	47	48	48	49	50	51	51	52	53	54	54	55	56	57	57	58	59	60	60	61	62	63	63	64	65	66	66	67	68	69	69	70	71	72	72	73																							
74	19	19	20	21	22	22	23	24	25	25	26	27	28	28	29	30	31	31	32	33	34	34	35	36	37	37	38	39	40	40	41	42	43	43	44	45	46	46	47	48	49	49	50	51	52	52	53	54	55	55	56	57	58	58	59	60	61	61	62	63	64	64	65	66	67	67	68	69	70	70	71	72	73	73	74																						
75	19	20	20	21	22	23	23	24	25	26	26	27	28	29	29	30	31	32	32	33	34	35	35	36	37	38	38	39	40	41	41	42	43	44	44	45	46	47	47	48	49	50	50	51	52	53	53	54	55	56	56	57	58	59	59	60	61	62	62	63	64	65	65	66	67	68	68	69	70	71	71	72	73	74	74	75																					
76	19	20	21	21	22	23	24	24	25	26	27	27	28	29	30	30	31	32	33	33	34	35	36	36	37	38	39	39	40	41	42	42	43	44	45	45	46	47	48	48	49	50	51	51	52	53	54	54	55	56	57	57	58	59	60	60	61	62	63	63	64	65	66	66	67	68	69	69	70	71	72	72	73	74	75	75	76																				
77	19	20	21	22	22	23	24	25	25	26	27	28	28	29	30	31	31	32	33	34	34	35	36	37	37	38	39	40	40	41	42	43	43	44	45	46	46	47	48	49	49	50	51	52	52	53	54	55	55	56	57	58	58	59	60	61	61	62	63	64	64	65	66	67	67	68	69	70	70	71	72	73	73	74	75	76	76	77																			
78	20	20	21	22	23	23	24	25	26	26	27	28	29	29	30	31	32	32	33	34	35	35	36	37	38	38	39	40	41	41	42	43	44	44	45	46	47	47	48	49	50	50	51	52	53	53	54	55	56	56	57	58	59	59	60	61	62	62	63	64	65	65	66	67	68	68	69	70	71	71	72	73	74	74	75	76	77	77	78																		
79	20	21	21	22	23	24	24	25	26	27	27	28	29	30	30	31	32	33	33	34	35	36	36	37	38	39	39	40	41	42	42	43	44	45	45	46	47	48	48	49	50	51	51	52	53	54	54	55	56	57	57	58	59	60	60	61	62	63	63	64	65	66	66	67	68	69	69	70	71	72	72	73	74	75	75	76	77	78	78	79																	
80	20	21	22	22	23	24	25	25	26	27	28	28	29	30	31	31	32	33	34	34	35	36	37	37	38	39	40	40	41	42	43	43	44	45	46	46	47	48	49	49	50	51	52	52	53	54	55	55	56	57	58	58	59	60	61	61	62	63	64	64	65	66	67	67	68	69	70	70	71	72	73	73	74	75	76	76	77	78	79	79	80																
81	20	21	22	23	23	24	25	26	26	27	28	29	29	30	31	32	32	33	34	35	35	36	37	38	38	39	40	41	41	42	43	44	44	45	46	47	47	48	49	50	50	51	52	53	53	54	55	56	56	57	58	59	59	60	61	62	62	63	64	65	65	66	67	68	68	69	70	71	71	72	73	74	74	75	76	77	77	78	79	80	80	81															
82	21	21	22	23	24	24	25	26	27	27	28	29	30	30	31	32	33	33	34	35	36	36	37	38	39	39	40	41	42	42	43	44	45	45	46	47	48	48	49	50	51	51	52	53	54	54	55	56	57	57	58	59	60	60	61	62	63	63	64	65	66	66	67	68	69	69	70	71	72	72	73	74	75	75	76	77	78	78	79	80	81	81	82														
83	21	22	22	23	24	25	25	26	27	28	28	29	30	31	31	32	33	34	34	35	36	37	37	38	39	40	40	41	42	43	43	44	45	46	46	47	48	49	49	50	51	52	52	53	54	55	55	56	57	58	58	59	60	61	61	62	63	64	64	65	66	67	67	68	69	70	70	71	72	73	73	74	75	76	76	77	78	79	79	80	81	82	82	83													
84	21	22	23	23	24	25	26	26	27	28	29	29	30	31	32	32	33	34	35	35	36	37	38	38	39	40	41	41	42	43	44	44	45	46	47	47	48	49	50	50	51	52	53	53	54	55	56	56	57	58	59	59	60	61	62	62	63	64	65	65	66	67	68	68	69	70	71	71	72	73	74	74	75	76	77	77	78	79	80	80	81	82	83	83	84												
85	21	22	23	24	24	25	26	27	27	28	29	30	30	31	32	33	33	34	35	36	36	37	38	39	39	40	41	42	42	43	44	45	45	46	47	48	48	49	50	51	51	52	53	54	54	55	56	57	57	58	59	60	60	61	62	63	63	64	65	66	66	67	68	69	69	70	71	72	72	73	74	75	75	76	77	78	78	79	80	81	81	82	83	84	84	85											
86	22	22	23	24	25	25	26	27	28	28	29	30	31	31	32	33	34	34	35	36	37	37	38	39	40	40	41	42	43	43	44	45	46	46	47	48	49	49	50	51	52	52	53	54	55	55	56	57	58	58	59	60	61	61	62	63	64	64	65	66	67	67	68	69	70	70	71	72	73	73	74	75	76	76	77	78	79	79	80	81	82	82	83	84	85	85	86										
87	22	23	23	24	25	26	26	27	28	29	29	30	31	32	32	33	34	35	35	36	37	38	38	39	40	41	41	42	43	44	44	45	46	47	47	48	49	50	50	51	52	53	53	54	55	56	56	57	58	59	59	60	61	62	62	63	64	65	65	66	67	68	68	69	70	71	71	72	73	74	74	75	76	77	77	78	79	80	80	81	82	83	83	84	85	86	86	87									
88	22	23	24	24	25	26	27	27	28	29	30	30	31	32	33	33	34	35	36	36	37	38	39	39	40	41	42	42	43	44	45	45	46	47	48	48	49	50	51	51	52	53	54	54	55	56	57	57	58	59	60	60	61	62	63	63	64	65	66	66	67	68	69	69	70	71	72	72	73	74	75	75	76	77	78	78	79	80	81	81	82	83	84	84	85	86	87	87	88								
89	22	23	24	25	25	26	27	28	28	29	30	31	31	32	33	34	34	35	36	37	37	38	39	40	40	41	42	43	43	44	45	46	46	47	48	49	49	50	51	52	52	53	54	55	55	56	57	58	58	59	60	61	61	62	63	64	64	65	66	67	67	68	69	70	70	71	72	73	73	74	75	76	76	77	78	79	79	80	81	82	82	83	84	85	85	86	87	88	88	89							
90	23	23	24	25	26	26	27	28	29	29	30	31	32	32	33	34	35	35	36	37	38	38	39	40	41	41	42	43	44	44	45	46	47	47	48	49	50	50	51	52	53	53	54	55	56	56	57	58	59	59	60	61	62	62	63	64	65	65	66	67	68	68	69	70	71	71	72	73	74	74	75	76	77	77	78	79	80	80	81	82	83	83	84	85	86	86	87	88	89	89	90						
91	23	24	24	25	26	27	27	28	29	30	30	31	32	33	33	34	35	36	36	37	38	39	39	40	41	42	42	43	44	45	45	46	47	48	48	49	50	51	51	52	53	54	54	55	56	57	57	58	59	60	60	61	62	63	63	64	65	66	66	67	68	69	69	70	71	72	72	73	74	75	75	76	77	78	78	79	80	81	81	82	83	84	84	85	86	87	87	88	89	90	90	91					
92	23	24	25	25	26	27	28	28	29	30	31	31	32	33	34	34	35	36	37	37	38	39	40	40	41	42	43	43	44	45	46	46	47	48	49	49	50	51	52	52	53	54	55	55	56	57	58	58	59	60	61	61	62	63	64	64	65	66	67	67	68	69	70	70	71	72	73	73	74	75	76	76	77	78	79	79	80	81	82	82	83	84	85	85	86	87	88	88	89	90	91	91	92				
93	23	24	25	26	26	27	28	29	29	30	31	32	32	33	34	35	35	36	37	38	38	39	40	41	41	42	43	44	44	45	46	47	47	48	49	50	50	51	52	53	53	54	55	56	56	57	58	59	59	60	61	62	62	63	64	65	65	66	67	68	68	69	70	71	71	72	73	74	74	75	76	77	77	78	79	80	80	81	82	83	83	84	85	86	86	87	88	89	89	90	91	92	92	93			
94	24	24	25	26	27	27	28	29	30	30	31	32	33	33	34	35	36	36	37	38	39	39	40	41	42	42	43	44	45	45	46	47	48	48	49	50	51	51	52	53	54	54	55	56	57	57	58	59	60	60	61	62	63	63	64	65	66	66	67	68	69	69	70	71	72	72	73	74	75	75	76	77	78	78	79	80	81	81	82	83	84	84	85	86	87	87	88	89	90	90	91	92	93	93	94			
95	24	25	25	26	27	28	28	29	30	31	31	32	33	34	34	35	36	37	37	38	39	40	40	41	42	43	43	44	45	46	46	47	48	49	49	50	51	52	52	53	54	55	55	56	57	58	58	59	60	61	61	62	63	64	64	65	66	67	67	68	69	70	70	71	72	73	73	74	75	76	76	77	78	79	79	80	81	82	82	83	84	85	85	86	87	88	88	89	90	91	91	92	93	94	94	95		
96	24	25	26	26	27	28	29	29	30	31	32	32	33	34	35	35	36	37	38	38	39	40	41	41	42	43	44	44	45	46	47	47	48	49	50	50	51	52	53	53	54	55	56	56	57	58	59	59	60	61	62	62	63	64	65	65	66	67	68	68	69	70	71	71	72	73	74	74	75	76	77	77	78	79	80	80	81	82	83	83	84	85	86	86	87	88	89	89	90	91	92	92	93	94	95	95	96	
97	24	25	26	27	27	28	29	30	30	31	32	33	33	34	35	36	36	37	38	39	39	40	41	42	42	43	44	45	45	46	47	48	48	49	50	51	51	52	53	54	54	55	56	57	57	58	59	60	60	61	62	63	63	64	65	66	66	67	68	69	69	70	71	72	72	73	74	75	75	76	77	78	78	79	80	81	81	82	83	84	84	85	86	87	87	88	89	90	90	91	92	93	93	94	95	96	96	97
98	25	25	26	27	28	28	29	30	31	31	32	33	34	34	35	36	37	37	38	39	40	40	41	42	43	43	44	45	46	46	47	48	49	49	50	51	52	52	53	54	55	55	56	57	58	58	59	60	61	61	62	63	64	64	65	66	67	67	68	69	70	70	71	72	73	73	74	75	76	76	77	78	79	79	80	81	82	82	83	84	85	85	86	87	88	88	89	90	91	91	92	93	94	94	95	96	97	97	98
99	25	26	26	27	28	29	29	30	31	32	32	33	34	35	35	36	37	38	38	39	40	41	41	42	43	44	44	45	46	47	47	48	49	50	50	51	52	53	53	54	55	56	56	57	58	59	59	60	61	62	62	63	64	65	65	66	67	68	68	69	70	71	71	72	73	74	74	75	76	77	77	78	79	80	80	81	82	83	83	84	85	86	86	87	88	89	89	90	91	92	92	93	94	95	95	96	97	98	98	99
100	25	26	27	27	28	29	30	30	31	32	33	33	34	35	36	36	37	38	39	39	40	41	42	42	43	44	45	45	46	47	48	48	49	50	51	51	52	53	54	54	55	56	57	57	58	59	60	60	61	62	63	63	64	65	66	66	67	68	69	69	70	71	72	72	73	74	75	75	76	77	78	78	79	80	81	81	82	83	84	84	85	86	87	87	88	89	90	90	91	92	93	93	94	95	96	96	97	98	99	99	100

% Impairment Worse Eye

% Impairment Better Eye

% Impairment Worse Eye / % Impairment Better Eye

% Impairment Worse Eye	50	51	52	53	54
50	50				
51	50	51			
52	51	51	52		
53	51	52	52	53	
54	51	52	53	53	54
55	51	52	53	54	54
56	52	52	53	54	55
57	52	53	53	54	55
58	52	53	54	54	55
59	52	53	54	55	55
60	53	53	54	55	56
61	53	54	54	55	56
62	53	54	55	55	56
63	53	54	55	56	56
64	54	54	55	56	57
65	54	55	55	56	57
66	54	55	56	56	57
67	54	55	56	57	57
68	55	55	56	57	58
69	55	56	56	57	58
70	55	56	57	57	58
71	55	56	57	58	58
72	56	56	57	58	59
73	56	57	57	58	59
74	56	57	58	58	59
75	56	57	58	59	59
76	57	57	58	59	60
77	57	58	58	59	60
78	57	58	59	59	60
79	57	58	59	60	60
80	58	58	59	60	61
81	58	59	59	60	61
82	58	59	60	60	61
83	58	59	60	61	61
84	59	59	60	61	62
85	59	60	60	61	62
86	59	60	61	61	62
87	59	60	61	62	62
88	60	60	61	62	63
89	60	61	61	62	63
90	60	61	62	62	63
91	60	61	62	63	63
92	61	61	62	63	64
93	61	62	62	63	64
94	61	62	63	63	64
95	61	62	63	64	64
96	62	62	63	64	65
97	62	63	63	64	65
98	62	63	64	64	65
99	62	63	64	65	65
100	63	63	64	65	66

% Impairment Worse Eye	55	56	57	58	59
55	55				
56	55	56			
57	56	56	57		
58	56	57	57	58	
59	56	57	58	58	59
60	56	57	58	59	59
61	57	57	58	59	60
62	57	58	58	59	60
63	57	58	59	59	60
64	57	58	59	60	60
65	58	58	59	60	61
66	58	59	59	60	61
67	58	59	60	60	61
68	58	59	60	61	61
69	59	59	60	61	62
70	59	60	60	61	62
71	59	60	61	61	62
72	59	60	61	62	62
73	60	60	61	62	63
74	60	61	61	62	63
75	60	61	62	62	63
76	60	61	62	63	63
77	61	61	62	63	64
78	61	62	62	63	64
79	61	62	63	63	64
80	61	62	63	64	64
81	62	62	63	64	65
82	62	63	63	64	65
83	62	63	64	64	65
84	62	63	64	65	65
85	63	63	64	65	66
86	63	64	64	65	66
87	63	64	65	65	66
88	63	64	65	66	66
89	64	64	65	66	67
90	64	65	65	66	67
91	64	65	66	66	67
92	64	65	66	67	67
93	65	65	66	67	68
94	65	66	66	67	68
95	65	66	67	67	68
96	65	66	67	68	68
97	66	66	67	68	69
98	66	67	67	68	69
99	66	67	68	68	69
100	66	67	68	69	69

% Impairment Worse Eye	60	61	62	63	64
60	60				
61	60	61			
62	61	61	62		
63	61	62	62	63	
64	61	62	63	63	64
65	61	62	63	64	64
66	62	62	63	64	65
67	62	63	63	64	65
68	62	63	64	64	65
69	62	63	64	65	65
70	63	63	64	65	66
71	63	64	64	65	66
72	63	64	65	65	66
73	63	64	65	66	66
74	64	64	65	66	67
75	64	65	65	66	67
76	64	65	66	66	67
77	64	65	66	67	67
78	65	65	66	67	68
79	65	66	66	67	68
80	65	66	67	67	68
81	65	66	67	68	68
82	66	66	67	68	69
83	66	67	67	68	69
84	66	67	68	68	69
85	66	67	68	69	69
86	67	67	68	69	70
87	67	68	68	69	70
88	67	68	69	69	70
89	67	68	69	70	70
90	68	68	69	70	71
91	68	69	69	70	71
92	68	69	70	70	71
93	68	69	70	71	71
94	69	69	70	71	72
95	69	70	70	71	72
96	69	70	71	71	72
97	69	70	71	72	72
98	70	70	71	72	73
99	70	71	71	72	73
100	70	71	72	72	73

% Impairment Worse Eye	65	66	67	68	69
65	65				
66	65	66			
67	66	66	67		
68	66	67	67	68	
69	66	67	68	68	69
70	66	67	68	69	69
71	67	67	68	69	70
72	67	68	68	69	70
73	67	68	69	69	70
74	67	68	69	70	70
75	68	68	69	70	71
76	68	69	69	70	71
77	68	69	70	70	71
78	68	69	70	71	71
79	69	69	70	71	72
80	69	70	70	71	72
81	69	70	71	71	72
82	69	70	71	72	72
83	70	70	71	72	73
84	70	71	71	72	73
85	70	71	72	72	73
86	70	71	72	73	73
87	71	71	72	73	74
88	71	72	72	73	74
89	71	72	73	73	74
90	71	72	73	74	74
91	72	72	73	74	75
92	72	73	73	74	75
93	72	73	74	74	75
94	72	73	74	75	75
95	73	73	74	75	76
96	73	74	74	75	76
97	73	74	75	75	76
98	73	74	75	76	76
99	74	74	75	76	77
100	74	75	75	76	77

% Impairment Worse Eye	70	71	72	73	74
70	70				
71	70	71			
72	71	71	72		
73	71	72	72	73	
74	71	72	73	73	74
75	71	72	73	74	74
76	72	72	73	74	75
77	72	73	73	74	75
78	72	73	74	74	75
79	72	73	74	75	75
80	73	73	74	75	76
81	73	74	74	75	76
82	73	74	75	75	76
83	73	74	75	76	76
84	74	74	75	76	77
85	74	75	75	76	77
86	74	75	76	76	77
87	74	75	76	77	77
88	75	75	76	77	78
89	75	76	76	77	78
90	75	76	77	77	78
91	75	76	77	78	78
92	76	76	77	78	79
93	76	77	77	78	79
94	76	77	78	78	79
95	76	77	78	79	79
96	77	77	78	79	80
97	77	78	78	79	80
98	77	78	79	79	80
99	77	78	79	80	80
100	78	78	79	80	81

% Impairment Worse Eye	75	76	77	78	79
75	75				
76	75	76			
77	76	76	77		
78	76	77	77	78	
79	76	77	78	78	79
80	76	77	78	79	79
81	77	77	78	79	80
82	77	78	78	79	80
83	77	78	79	79	80
84	77	78	79	80	80
85	78	78	79	80	81
86	78	79	79	80	81
87	78	79	80	80	81
88	78	79	80	81	81
89	79	79	80	81	82
90	79	80	80	81	82
91	79	80	81	81	82
92	79	80	81	82	82
93	80	80	81	82	83
94	80	81	81	82	83
95	80	81	82	82	83
96	80	81	82	83	83
97	81	81	82	83	84
98	81	82	82	83	84
99	81	82	83	83	84
100	81	82	83	84	84

% Impairment Worse Eye	80	81	82	83	84
80	80				
81	80	81			
82	81	81	82		
83	81	82	82	83	
84	81	82	83	83	84
85	81	82	83	84	84
86	82	82	83	84	85
87	82	83	83	84	85
88	82	83	84	84	85
89	82	83	84	85	85
90	83	83	84	85	86
91	83	84	84	85	86
92	83	84	85	85	86
93	83	84	85	86	86
94	84	84	85	86	87
95	84	85	85	86	87
96	84	85	86	86	87
97	84	85	86	87	87
98	85	85	86	87	88
99	85	86	86	87	88
100	85	86	87	87	88

% Impairment Worse Eye	85	86	87	88	89
85	85				
86	85	86			
87	86	86	87		
88	86	87	87	88	
89	86	87	88	88	89
90	86	87	88	89	89
91	87	87	88	89	90
92	87	88	88	89	90
93	87	88	89	89	90
94	87	88	89	90	90
95	88	88	89	90	91
96	88	89	89	90	91
97	88	89	90	90	91
98	88	89	90	91	91
99	89	89	90	91	92
100	89	90	90	91	92

% Impairment Worse Eye	90	91	92	93	94
90	90				
91	90	91			
92	91	91	92		
93	91	92	92	93	
94	91	92	93	93	94
95	91	92	93	94	94
96	92	92	93	94	95
97	92	93	93	94	95
98	92	93	94	94	95
99	92	93	94	95	95
100	93	93	94	95	96

% Impairment Worse Eye	95	96	97	98	99	100
95	95					
96	95	96				
97	96	96	97			
98	96	97	97	98		
99	96	97	98	98	99	
100	96	97	98	99	99	100

% Impairment Better Eye

Table 6. Impairment of the Visual System as it Relates to Impairment of the Whole Person

% Impairment of		% Impairment of		% Impairment of		% Impairment of		% Impairment of		% Impairment of	
Visual System	Whole Person	Visual System	Whole Person	Visual System	Whole Person	Visual System	Whole Person	Visual System	Whole Person	Visual System	Whole Person
0	0	15	14	30	28	45	42	60	57	75	71
1	1	16	15	31	29	46	43	61	58	76	72
2	2	17	16	32	30	47	44	62	59	77	73
3	3	18	17	33	31	48	45	63	59	78	74
4	4	19	18	34	32	49	46	64	60	79	75
5	5	20	19	35	33	50	47	65	61	80	76
6	6	21	20	36	34	51	48	66	62	81	76
7	7	22	21	37	35	52	49	67	63	82	77
8	8	23	22	38	36	53	50	68	64	83	78
9	8	24	23	39	37	54	51	69	65	84	79
10	9	25	24	40	38	55	52	70	66	85	80
11	10	26	25	41	39	56	53	71	67	86	81
12	11	27	25	42	40	57	54	72	68	87	82
13	12	28	26	43	41	58	55	73	69	88	83
14	13	29	27	44	42	59	56	74	70	89	84
										90-100	85

	% Impairment Visual System	% Impairment Whole Person
Total loss of vision one eye	25	24
Total loss of vision both eyes	100	85

Example:

impairment due to loss of CV of both eyes	49%
impairment due to binocular VF loss	20%
impairment of visual system	59%

Consult Table 6 to ascertain the impairment of the whole person that is contributed by the visual system.

Example:
59% impairment of the visual system is equivalent to 56% impairment of the whole person.

8.6 Other Conditions

Up to an additional 10% impairment may be combined with the impairment of the whole person caused by the visual system for such conditions as permanent deformities of the orbit, scars, and other cosmetic deformities that do not otherwise alter ocular function.

References

1. Sloan LL: New test charts for the measurement of visual acuity. *Am J Ophthalmol* 1959;48:807-813.

2. Report of Working Group 39, Committee on Vision, National Academy of Sciences: Recommended Standard Procedures for the Clinical Measurement and Specification of Visual Acuity. *Adv Ophthalmol* 1980; 41:103-143.

3. Esterman B: Grid for scoring visual fields, II perimeter. *Arch Ophthalmol* 1968;79:400-406.

4. Keeney AH, Duerson HL, Jr: Collated near-vision test card. *Am J Ophthalmol* 1958;46(4):592-594.

5. Keeney AH: *Ocular Examination: Basis and Technique* (ed 2). St. Louis, CV Mosby Co, 1976.

6. Newell FW: *Ophthalmology: Principles and Concepts* (ed 5). St. Louis, CV Mosby Co, 1982.

7. Esterman B: Functional scoring of the binocular visual field. *Ophthalmol* 1982;89:1226-1234.

8. Esterman B, Blanche E, Wallach M, Bonelli A: Computerized scoring of the functional field: Preliminary report. *Doc Ophthalmol Proc Ser* 1985;42:333-339.

9. Keltner JC, Johnson CA: Comparative materials on automated and semi-automated perimeters in 1985. *Opthalmol* 1985; 92:34-37.

10. Anderson DR: *Perimetry: With and Without Automation* (ed 2). St. Louis, CV Mosby Co, 1987.

Chapter 9

Ear, Nose, Throat and Related Structures

9.0 Introduction

The purpose of this chapter is to provide criteria for use in evaluating permanent impairment resulting from the principal dysfunctions of the ear, nose, throat, and related structures, and thereby to determine the corresponding percentage of permanent impairment of the whole person. Although the ear, nose, throat, and related structures each have multiple functions, some of which are closely allied, permanent impairment usually results from a clinically established deviation from normal in one or more of the following functions: (1) hearing; (2) equilibrium; (3) respiration; (4) mastication and deglutition; (5) olfaction and taste; (6) speech; and (7) facial features and movement.

Before using the information in this chapter, the reader is urged to review Chapters 1 and 2, which provide a general discussion of the purpose of the *Guides* and of the situations in which they are useful; and which discuss techniques for the evaluation of the subject and for preparation of a report. The report should include the information found in the following outline, which is developed more fully in Chapter 2.

A. Medical Evaluation
1. Narrative history of medical conditions
2. Results of the most recent clinical evaluation
3. Assessment of current clinical status and statement of future plans
4. Diagnoses and clinical impressions
5. Expected date of full or partial recovery

B. Analysis of Findings
1. Impact of medical condition(s) on life activities
2. Explanation for concluding that the medical condition(s) has or has not become static or well-stabilized
3. Explanation for concluding that the individual is or is not likely to suffer from sudden or subtle incapacitation
4. Explanation for concluding that the individual is or is not likely to suffer injury or further impairment by engaging in life activities or by attempting to meet personal, social, and occupational demands
5. Explanation for concluding that accommodations and/or restrictions are or are not warranted

C. Comparison of Results of Analysis with Impairment Criteria
1. Description of clinical findings, and how these findings relate to specific criteria in the chapter
2. Explanation of each percent of impairment rating
3. Summary list of all impairment ratings
4. Overall rating of impairment of the whole person

9.1 The Ear

The ear consists of the auricle, the external canal, the tympanum, the eustachian tube, the mastoid, the internal ear, the central pathways, and the auditory cortex.

The functions of the ear are hearing and equilibrium, which are considered separately in the following sections. The criteria for evaluating hearing impairment are relatively specific. In contrast, providing rather general criteria for disturbances of equilibrium is necessary. Such disturbances of the ear as chronic otorrhea, otalgia, and tinnitus are not measurable and, therefore, the physician should assign a degree of impairment that is based on severity and importance, and is consistent with established values.

9.1a Hearing

The following criteria have been adapted from information provided by the American Academy of Otolaryngology—Head and Neck Surgery, and the American Council of Otolaryngology—Head and Neck Surgery. For the purpose of this chapter, impairment of the whole person is determined from the calculation of permanent binaural hearing impairment. In using these criteria, certain abbreviations and definitions should be kept in mind:

1. Permanent hearing impairment: This is reduced hearing sensitivity that is outside the range of normal. Hearing should be evaluated after maximum rehabilitation has been achieved and when the impairment is nonprogressive. The determination of impairment is basic to the evaluation of permanent handicap and disability.

2. Permanent binaural hearing impairment: This is the disadvantage caused by a binaural hearing impairment sufficient to affect the individual's efficiency in the activities of daily living.

3. Intensity: This is measured in decibels, abbreviated *dB*.

4. Frequency: This is measured in hertz, abbreviated *Hz*.

5. Hearing threshold level for pure tones: This is defined as the number of decibels (dB) above a standard audiometric zero for a given frequency at which the listener's threshold of hearing lies. It is the reading on the hearing level (HL) dial of an audiometer that is calibrated according to the American National Standards Institute (ANSI) specifications for Audiometers S3.6-1969, which were reaffirmed in 1973. This chapter provides for the rating of hearing impairment using audiometers calibrated according to the ANSI standard. Hearing levels obtained from audiometers calibrated to the older ASA-1951 standard should be corrected using Table 1.

It is common practice to add 10 dB to the average of hearing threshold levels at these four frequencies when correcting from the ASA to ANSI values.

6. Estimated hearing level for speech: This is the simple average of hearing threshold levels at the four frequencies of 500, 1,000, 2,000, and 3,000 Hz. Because of present limitations of speech audiometry, the hearing loss for speech is estimated from measurements made

Table 1. Correction Factors for ASA—1951 Standards

Frequency (Hz)	Correction Factor
500	+14 dB
1,000	+10 dB
2,000	+8.5 dB
3,000	+8.5 dB

with a pure tone audiometer. The hearing threshold level at 3,000 Hz is included to provide an accurate assessment of hearing impairment in a variety of everyday listening conditions.

7. Evaluation of monaural hearing impairment: If the average hearing level at 500, 1,000, 2,000, and 3,000 Hz is 25 dB (ANSI-1969) or less, no impairment is presumed to exist in the ability to hear everyday sounds under everyday listening conditions. At the other extreme, however, if the average hearing level at 500, 1,000, 2,000, and 3,000 Hz is over 91.7 dB, the impairment for hearing everyday speech should be considered total, that is, 100%. For every decibel that the estimated hearing level for speech exceeds 25 dB (ANSI-1969), 1.5% of monaural impairment is assigned, to a maximum of 100%. This maximum is reached at 91.7 dB (see Table 2).

This method of computation should be applied only to adults who have acquired language. The child who has not acquired language does not benefit from the redundancy of language enjoyed by the comprehending adult. Evidence suggests that material impairment for the prelingual child may exist when the average hearing level is in the range of 15.25 dB.

8. Evaluation of binaural hearing impairment: The evaluation of binaural hearing impairment of adults is derived from the pure tone audiogram and is always based upon the functional state of both ears. The range of binaural hearing impairment is not as wide as the audiometric range of human hearing. Audiometric zero, which is presumably the average normal threshold level, is not the point at which impairment begins. Binaural hearing impairment is determined using the following formula:

$$\text{Binaural Hearing Impairment, (\%)} = \frac{5 \times \%\text{ hearing impairment of better ear} + \%\text{ hearing impairment of poorer ear}}{6}$$

A purely monaural hearing impairment should be converted to binaural hearing impairment using the formula above, with 0% hearing impairment for the better ear.

Table 3 is derived from this formula.

Table 4 converts binaural hearing impairment to impairment of the whole person.

9.1b Objective Techniques To Determine Hearing Impairment

To determine impairment, the following steps should be taken:

1. Test each ear separately with a pure-tone audiometer and record the hearing levels at (a) 500 Hz; (b) 1,000 Hz; (c) 2,000 Hz; and (d) 3,000 Hz. It is necessary that the hearing level for each frequency be determined in every patient. The following rules apply for extreme values:

a. If the hearing level at a given frequency is greater than 100 dB or is beyond the range of the audiometer, the level shall be taken as 100 dB.

b. If the hearing level for a given frequency is better than normal, the level shall be taken as 0 dB.

2. Total these four decibel values for each ear separately. In the examples below, hearing levels are determined in dB according to ANSI-1969 standards.

Example a:

Right Ear		Left Ear
15	500 Hz	30
25	1,000 Hz	45
45	2,000 Hz	60
55	3,000 Hz	85
140		220

Example b:

Right Ear		Left Ear
80	500 Hz	75
90	1,000 Hz	80
100	2,000 Hz	90
100	3,000 Hz	95
370		340

3. Consult Table 2 for percentage of monaural hearing impairment(s). "DSHL" is the decibel sum of the hearing threshold levels at 500, 1,000, 2,000, and 3,000 Hz, and is equated to percentage of monaural hearing impairment.

Example a: Right ear: DSHL is 140, resulting in 15% hearing impairment. Left ear: DSHL is 220, resulting in 45% hearing impairment.

Example b: Right ear: DSHL is 370, resulting in 100% hearing impairment. Left ear: DSHL is 340, resulting in 90% hearing impairment.

4. Consult Table 3 to determine percentage of binaural hearing impairment.

Example a: 140 DSHL (better ear) + 220 DSHL (poorer ear) = 20% binaural hearing impairment.

Table 2. Monaural Hearing Impairment (%)*

DSHL†	%	DSHL	%	DSHL	%
100	0.0	190	33.8	285	69.3
		195	35.6	290	71.2
105	1.9	200	37.5	295	73.1
110	3.8			300	75.0
115	5.6	205	39.4		
120	7.5	210	41.2	305	76.9
		215	43.1	310	78.8
125	9.4	220	45.0	315	80.6
130	11.2			320	82.5
135	13.1	225	46.9		
140	15.0	230	48.9	325	84.4
		235	50.6	330	86.2
145	16.9	240	52.5	335	88.1
150	18.8			340	90.0
155	20.6	245	54.4		
160	22.5	250	56.2	345	90.9
		255	58.1	350	93.8
165	24.4	260	60.0	355	95.6
170	26.2			360	97.5
175	28.1	265	61.9		
180	30.0	270	63.8	365	99.4
		275	65.6	368	100.0
185	31.9	280	67.5	or greater	

*Audiometers are calibrated to ANSI-1969 standard reference levels.
†Decibel sum of the hearing threshold levels at 500, 1,000, 2,000, and 3,000 Hz.

Example b: 340 DSHL (better ear) + 370 DSHL* (poorer ear) = 92% binaural hearing impairment. *Note: Use a maximum value of 368 DSHL.

5. Consult Table 4 to determine impairment of whole person.

Example a: 20% binaural hearing impairment results in 7% impairment of the whole person.

Example b: 92% binaural hearing impairment results in 32% impairment of the whole person.

9.1c Equilibrium

Equilibrium or orientation in space is maintained by the visual, kinesthetic, and vestibular mechanisms.

Vertigo, or vestibular dysequilibrium, is a sense of movement that is perceived by the patient as "subjective," in the case of movement of self, or as "objective," in the case of movement of the environment. The movements may be described as a sense of spinning, pulsion, or tilting of the visual environment with change of head position.

Disturbances of equilibrium may be classified clinically as: (1) abnormalities of gait not associated with vertigo; (2) giddiness or light-headedness that is distinguished from vertigo by the absence of feelings of movement; and (3) vertigo produced by disorders of the vestibular mechanism and its central nervous system components, including cerebral cortex, cerebellum, and brain stem, and by eye movements.

Table 3. Computation Of Binaural Hearing Impairment

Worse Ear	100	105	110	115	120	125	130	135	140	145	150	155	160	165	170	175	180	185	190	195	200	205	210	215	220	225	230
100	0																										
105	.3	1.9																									
110	.6	2.2	3.8																								
115	.9	2.5	4.1	5.6																							
120	1.3	2.8	4.4	5.9	7.5																						
125	1.6	3.1	4.7	6.3	7.8	9.4																					
130	1.9	3.4	5	6.6	8.1	9.7	11.3																				
135	2.2	3.8	5.3	6.9	8.4	10	11.6	13.1																			
140	2.5	4.1	5.6	7.2	8.8	10.3	11.9	13.4	15																		
145	2.8	4.4	5.9	7.5	9.1	10.6	12.2	13.8	15.3	16.9																	
150	3.1	4.7	6.3	7.8	9.4	10.9	12.5	14.1	15.6	17.2	18.8																
155	3.4	5	6.6	8.1	9.7	11.3	12.8	14.4	15.9	17.5	19.1	20.6															
160	3.8	5.3	6.9	8.4	10	11.6	13.1	14.7	16.3	17.8	19.4	20.9	22.5														
165	4.1	5.6	7.2	8.8	10.3	11.9	13.4	15	16.6	18.1	19.7	21.3	22.8	24.4													
170	4.4	5.9	7.5	9.1	10.6	12.2	13.8	15.3	16.9	18.4	20	21.6	23.1	24.7	26.3												
175	4.7	6.3	7.8	9.4	10.9	12.5	14.1	15.6	17.2	18.8	20.3	21.9	23.4	25	26.6	28.1											
180	5	6.6	8.1	9.7	11.3	12.8	14.4	15.9	17.5	19.1	20.6	22.2	23.8	25.3	26.9	28.4	30										
185	5.3	6.9	8.4	10	11.6	13.1	14.7	16.3	17.8	19.4	20.9	22.5	24.1	25.6	27.2	28.8	30.3	31.9									
190	5.6	7.2	8.8	10.3	11.9	13.4	15	16.6	18.1	19.7	21.3	22.8	24.4	25.9	27.5	29.1	30.6	32.2	33.8								
195	5.9	7.5	9.1	10.6	12.2	13.8	15.3	16.9	18.4	20	21.6	23.1	24.7	26.3	27.8	29.4	30.9	32.5	34.1	35.6							
200	6.3	7.8	9.4	10.9	12.5	14.1	15.6	17.2	18.8	20.3	21.9	23.4	25	26.6	28.1	29.7	31.3	32.8	34.4	35.9	37.5						
205	6.6	8.1	9.7	11.3	12.8	14.4	15.9	17.5	19.1	20.6	22.2	23.8	25.3	26.9	28.4	30	31.6	33.1	34.7	36.3	37.8	39.4					
210	6.9	8.4	10	11.6	13.1	14.7	16.3	17.8	19.4	20.9	22.5	24.1	25.6	27.2	28.8	30.3	31.9	33.4	35	36.6	38.1	39.7	41.3				
215	7.2	8.8	10.3	11.9	13.4	15	16.6	18.1	19.7	21.3	22.8	24.4	25.9	27.5	29.1	30.6	32.2	33.8	35.3	36.9	38.4	40	41.6	43.1			
220	7.5	9.1	10.6	12.2	13.8	15.3	16.9	18.4	20	21.6	23.1	24.7	26.3	27.8	29.4	30.9	32.5	34.1	35.6	37.2	38.8	40.3	41.9	43.4	45		
225	7.8	9.4	10.9	12.5	14.1	15.6	17.2	18.8	20.3	21.9	23.4	25	26.6	28.1	29.7	31.3	32.8	34.4	35.9	37.5	39.1	40.6	42.2	43.8	45.3	46.9	
230	8.1	9.7	11.3	12.8	14.4	15.9	17.5	19.1	20.6	22.2	23.8	25.3	26.9	28.4	30	31.6	33.1	34.7	36.3	37.8	39.4	40.9	42.5	44.1	45.6	47.2	48.8
235	8.4	10	11.6	13.1	14.7	16.3	17.8	19.4	20.9	22.5	24.1	25.6	27.2	28.8	30.3	31.9	33.4	35	36.6	38.1	39.7	41.3	42.8	44.4	45.9	47.5	49.1
240	8.8	10.3	11.9	13.4	15	16.6	18.1	19.7	21.3	22.8	24.4	25.9	27.5	29.1	3.06	32.2	33.8	35.3	36.9	38.4	40	41.6	43.1	44.7	46.3	47.8	49.4
245	9.1	10.6	12.2	13.8	15.3	16.9	18.4	20	21.6	23.1	24.7	26.3	27.8	29.4	30.9	32.5	34.1	35.6	37.2	38.8	40.3	41.9	43.4	45	46.6	48.1	49.7
250	9.4	10.9	12.5	14.1	15.6	17.2	18.8	20.3	21.9	23.4	25	26.6	28.1	29.7	31.3	32.8	34.4	35.9	37.5	39.1	40.6	42.2	43.8	45.3	46.9	48.4	50
255	9.7	11.3	12.8	14.4	15.9	17.5	19.1	20.6	22.2	23.8	25.3	26.9	28.4	30	31.6	33.1	34.7	36.3	37.8	39.4	40.9	42.5	44.1	45.6	47.2	48.8	50.3
260	10	11.6	13.1	14.7	16.3	17.8	19.4	20.9	22.5	24.1	25.6	27.2	28.8	30.3	31.9	33.4	35	36.6	38.1	39.7	41.3	42.8	44.4	45.9	47.5	49.1	50.6
265	10.3	11.9	13.4	15	16.6	18.1	19.7	21.3	22.8	24.4	25.9	27.5	29.1	30.6	32.2	33.8	35.3	36.9	38.4	40	41.6	43.1	44.7	46.3	47.8	49.4	50.9
270	10.6	12.2	13.8	15.3	16.9	18.4	20	21.6	23.1	24.7	26.3	27.8	29.4	30.9	32.5	34.1	35.6	37.2	38.8	40.3	41.9	43.4	45	46.6	48.1	49.7	51.3
275	10.9	12.5	14.1	15.6	17.2	18.8	20.3	21.9	23.4	25	26.6	28.1	29.7	31.3	32.8	34.4	35.9	37.5	39.1	40.6	42.2	43.8	45.3	46.9	48.4	50	51.6
280	11.3	12.8	14.4	15.9	17.5	19.1	20.6	22.2	23.8	25.3	26.9	28.4	30	31.6	33.1	34.7	36.3	37.8	39.4	40.9	42.5	44.1	45.6	47.2	48.8	50.3	51.9
285	11.6	13.1	14.7	16.3	17.8	19.4	20.9	22.5	24.1	25.6	27.2	28.8	30.3	31.9	33.4	35	36.6	38.1	39.7	41.3	42.8	44.4	45.9	47.5	49.1	50.6	52.2
290	11.9	13.4	15	16.6	18.1	19.7	21.3	22.8	24.4	25.9	27.5	29.1	30.6	32.2	33.8	35.3	36.9	38.4	40	41.6	43.1	44.7	46.3	47.8	49.4	50.9	52.5
295	12.2	13.8	15.3	16.9	18.4	20	21.6	23.1	24.7	26.3	27.8	29.4	30.9	32.5	34.1	35.6	37.2	38.8	40.3	41.9	43.4	45	46.6	48.1	49.7	51.3	52.8
300	12.5	14.1	15.6	17.2	18.8	20.3	21.9	23.4	25	26.6	28.1	29.7	31.3	32.8	34.4	35.9	37.5	39.1	40.6	42.2	43.8	45.3	46.9	48.4	50	51.6	53.1
305	12.8	14.4	15.9	17.5	19.1	20.6	22.2	23.8	25.3	26.9	28.4	30	31.6	33.1	34.7	36.3	37.8	39.4	40.9	42.5	44.1	45.6	47.2	48.8	50.3	51.9	53.4
310	13.1	14.7	16.3	17.8	19.4	20.9	22.5	24.1	25.6	27.2	28.8	30.3	31.9	33.4	35	36.6	38.1	39.7	41.3	42.8	44.4	45.9	47.5	49.1	50.6	52.2	53.8
315	13.4	15	16.6	18.1	19.7	21.3	22.8	24.4	25.9	27.5	29.1	30.6	32.2	33.8	35.3	36.9	38.4	40	41.6	43.1	44.7	46.3	47.8	49.4	50.9	52.5	54.1
320	13.8	15.3	16.9	18.4	20	21.6	23.1	24.7	26.3	27.8	29.4	30.9	32.5	34.1	35.6	37.2	38.8	40.3	41.9	43.4	45	46.6	48.1	49.7	51.3	52.8	54.4
325	14.1	15.6	17.2	18.8	20.3	21.9	23.4	25	26.6	28.1	29.7	31.3	32.8	34.4	35.9	37.5	39.1	40.6	42.2	43.8	45.3	46.9	48.4	50	51.6	53.1	54.7
330	14.4	15.9	17.5	19.1	20.6	22.2	23.8	25.3	26.9	28.4	30	31.6	33.1	34.7	36.3	37.8	39.4	40.9	42.5	44.1	45.6	47.2	48.8	50.3	51.9	53.4	55
335	14.7	16.3	17.8	19.4	20.9	22.5	24.1	25.6	27.2	28.8	30.3	31.9	33.4	35	36.6	38.1	39.7	41.3	42.8	44.4	45.9	47.5	49.1	50.6	52.2	53.8	55.3
340	15	16.6	18.1	19.7	21.3	22.8	24.4	25.9	27.5	29.1	30.6	32.2	33.8	35.3	36.9	38.4	40	41.6	43.1	44.7	46.3	47.8	49.4	50.9	52.5	54.1	55.6
345	15.3	16.9	18.4	20	21.6	23.1	24.7	26.3	27.8	29.4	30.9	32.5	34.1	35.6	37.2	38.8	40.3	41.9	43.4	45	46.6	48.1	49.7	51.3	52.8	54.4	55.9
350	15.6	17.2	18.8	20.3	21.9	23.4	25	26.6	28.1	29.7	31.3	32.8	34.4	35.9	37.5	39.1	40.6	42.2	43.8	45.3	46.9	48.4	50	51.6	53.1	54.7	56.3
355	15.9	17.5	19.1	20.6	22.2	23.8	25.3	26.9	28.4	30	31.6	33.1	34.7	36.3	37.8	39.4	40.9	42.5	44.1	45.6	47.2	48.8	50.3	51.9	53.4	55	56.6
360	16.3	17.8	19.4	20.9	22.5	24.1	25.6	27.2	28.8	30.3	31.9	33.4	35	36.6	38.1	39.7	41.3	42.8	44.4	45.9	47.5	49.1	50.6	52.2	53.8	55.3	56.9
365	16.6	18.1	19.7	21.3	22.8	24.4	25.9	27.5	29.1	30.6	32.2	33.8	35.3	36.9	38.4	40	41.6	43.1	44.7	46.3	47.8	49.4	50.9	52.5	54.1	55.6	57.2
368	16.8	18.3	19.9	21.4	23	24.6	26.2	27.7	29.3	30.8	32.4	33.9	35.5	37.1	38.6	40.2	41.8	43.3	44.9	46.4	48	49.6	51.1	52.7	54.3	55.8	57.4
ANSI 1969	100	105	110	115	120	125	130	135	140	145	150	155	160	165	170	175	180	185	190	195	200	205	210	215	220	225	230

Better Ear (sum 500, 1,000, 2,000, 3,000 Hz)

Values are based on the following formula:

$$\frac{5 \times \%\ \text{impairment of better ear} + \%\ \text{impairment of poorer ear}}{6} = \text{binaural hearing impairment, (\%)}$$

The axes are the sum of hearing levels at 500, 1,000, 2,000 and 3,000 Hz. The sum for the worse ear is read at the side; the sum for the better ear is read at the bottom. At the intersection of the column for the worse ear and the column for the better ear is the hearing handicap.

235	240	245	250	255	260	265	270	275	280	285	290	295	300	305	310	315	320	325	330	335	340	345	350	355	360	365	368
50.6																											
50.9	52.5																										
51.3	52.8	54.4																									
51.6	53.1	54.7	56.3																								
51.9	53.4	55	56.6	58.1																							
52.2	53.8	55.3	56.9	58.4	60																						
52.5	54.1	55.6	57.2	58.8	60.3	61.9																					
52.8	54.4	55.9	57.5	59.1	60.6	62.2	63.8																				
53.1	54.7	56.3	57.8	59.4	60.9	62.5	64.1	65.6																			
53.4	55	56.6	58.1	59.7	61.3	62.8	64.4	65.9	67.5																		
53.8	55.3	56.9	58.4	60	61.6	63.1	64.7	66.3	67.8	69.4																	
54.1	55.6	57.2	58.8	60.3	61.9	63.4	65	66.6	68.1	69.7	71.3																
54.4	55.9	57.5	59.1	60.6	62.2	63.8	65.3	66.9	68.4	70	71.6	73.1															
54.7	56.3	57.8	59.4	60.9	62.5	64.1	65.6	67.2	68.8	70.3	71.9	73.4	75														
55	56.6	58.1	59.7	61.3	62.8	64.4	65.9	67.5	69.1	70.6	72.2	73.8	75.3	76.9													
55.3	56.9	58.4	60	61.6	63.1	64.7	66.3	67.8	69.4	70.9	72.5	74.1	75.6	77.2	78.8												
55.6	57.2	58.8	60.3	61.9	63.4	65	66.6	68.1	69.7	71.3	72.8	74.4	75.9	77.5	79.1	80.6											
55.9	57.5	59.1	60.6	62.2	63.8	65.3	66.9	68.4	70	71.6	73.1	74.7	76.3	77.8	79.4	80.9	82.5										
56.3	57.8	59.4	60.9	62.5	64.1	65.6	67.2	68.8	70.3	71.9	73.4	75	76.6	78.1	79.7	81.3	82.8	84.4									
56.6	58.1	59.7	61.3	62.8	64.4	65.9	67.5	69.1	70.6	72.2	73.8	75.3	76.9	78.4	80	81.6	83.1	84.7	86.3								
56.9	58.4	60	61.6	63.1	64.7	66.3	67.8	69.4	70.9	72.5	74.1	75.6	77.2	78.8	80.3	81.9	83.4	85	86.6	88.1							
57.2	58.8	60.3	61.9	63.4	65	66.6	68.1	69.7	71.3	72.8	74.4	75.9	77.5	79.1	80.6	82.2	83.8	85.3	86.9	88.4	90						
57.5	59.1	60.6	62.2	63.8	65.3	66.9	68.4	70	71.6	73.1	74.7	76.3	77.8	79.4	80.9	82.5	84.1	85.6	87.2	88.8	90.3	91.9					
57.8	59.4	60.9	62.5	64.1	65.6	67.2	68.8	70.3	71.9	73.4	75	76.6	78.1	79.7	81.3	82.8	84.4	85.9	87.5	89.1	90.6	92.2	93.8				
58.1	59.7	61.3	62.8	64.4	65.9	67.5	69.1	70.6	72.2	73.8	75.3	76.9	78.4	80	81.6	83.1	84.7	86.3	87.8	89.4	90.9	92.5	94.1	95.6			
58.4	60	61.6	63.1	64.7	66.3	67.8	69.4	70.9	72.5	74.1	75.6	77.2	78.8	80.3	81.9	83.4	85	86.6	88.1	89.7	91.3	92.8	94.4	95.9	97.5		
58.8	60.3	61.9	63.4	65	66.6	68.1	69.7	71.3	72.8	74.4	75.9	77.5	79.1	80.6	82.2	83.8	85.3	86.9	88.4	90	91.6	93.1	94.7	96.3	97.6	99.4	
58.9	60.5	62.1	63.6	65.2	66.8	68.3	69.9	71.4	73	74.6	76.1	77.7	79.3	80.8	82.4	83.9	85.5	87.1	88.6	90.2	91.8	93.3	94.9	96.4	98	99.6	100

Table 4. The Relationship of Binaural Hearing Impairment To Impairment of the Whole Person

% Binaural Hearing Impairment	% Impairment of the Whole Person	% Binaural Hearing Impairment	% Impairment of the Whole Person
0 - 1.7	0	50.0- 53.1	18
1.8- 4.2	1	54.2- 55.7	19
4.3- 7.4	2	55.8- 58.8	20
7.5- 9.9	3	58.9- 61.4	21
10.0-13.1	4	61.5- 64.5	22
13.2-15.9	5	64.6- 67.1	23
16.0-18.8	6	67.2- 70.0	24
18.9-21.4	7	70.1- 72.8	25
21.5-24.5	8	72.9- 75.9	26
24.6-27.1	9	76.0- 78.5	27
27.2-30.0	10	78.6- 81.7	28
30.1-32.8	11	81.8- 84.2	29
32.9-35.9	12	84.3- 87.4	30
36.0-38.5	13	87.5- 89.9	31
38.6-41.7	14	90.0- 93.1	32
41.8-44.2	15	93.2- 95.7	33
44.3-47.4	16	95.8- 98.8	34
47.5-49.9	17	98.9-100.0	35

Permanent impairment may result from any disorder causing disorientation in space or vertigo. Three regulatory systems, ocular (visual), kinesthetic (proprioceptive), and vestibular, are related to the vestibulo-ocular reflex. The evaluation of impairments of equilibrium may include consideration of one or more of these mechanisms.

This section is primarily concerned with permanent impairment resulting from defects of the vestibular (labyrinthine) mechanism and its central connections. The defects are evidenced by loss of equilibrium produced by: (1) loss of vestibular function; OR (2) disturbances of vestibular function.

Complete loss of vestibular function: This loss may be unilateral or bilateral. When the loss is unilateral, adequate central nervous system compensation may or may not occur. With total bilateral loss of vestibular function, equilibrium is totally dependent on the kinesthetic and visual systems, which are usually unable to compensate fully for movement or ambulation. Depending upon the extent of adjustment, the percentage of permanent impairment of the whole person may range from 0% to 95%.

Disturbances of vestibular function: These disorders are evidenced by vertigo (vestibular dysequilibrium) as defined above. In this chapter, light-headedness and abnormalities of gait not associated with vertigo are not considered.

Vertigo may be accompanied by varying degrees of nausea, vomiting, headache, immobility, ataxia, and nystagmus. Movement may increase the vertigo and these ancillary signs and symptoms. Peripheral vestibular (labyrinthine) disorders are often associated with hearing loss and tinnitus. While some vestibular disorders result in temporary impairment, others may be permanent. Evaluation of vestibular impairment should be performed when the condition is stable and maximum adjustment has been achieved.

For evaluating those patients with permanent disturbances of the vestibular mechanism, the following classification has been developed. The various classes provide a means by which a physician can correlate the patient's residual capacity for the usual activities of daily living and the extent of permanent impairment as a whole person. Use of this classification presupposes that the physician has established a firm diagnosis based on a carefully obtained history, thorough examination, and the use of appropriate objective tests, supplemented by sound clinical judgment. In that vestibular disorders cause a dynamic set of signs and symptoms, subject to peripheral changes and central nervous system compensatory mechanisms, final conclusions should be based on the patient's condition after it is medically stable.

Class 1—Impairment of the Whole Person, 0%:
A patient belongs in Class 1 when (a) signs of vestibular dysequilibrium are present without supporting objective findings; *and* (b) the usual activities of daily living can be performed without assistance.

Class 2—Impairment of the Whole Person, 5-10%:
A patient belongs in Class 2 when (a) signs of vestibular dysequilibrium are present with supporting objective findings; *and* (b) the usual activities of daily living are performed without assistance, except for complex activities such as bike riding or certain activities related to the patient's work, such as walking on girders or scaffolds.

Class 3—Impairment of the Whole Person, 15-30%:
A patient belongs in Class 3 when (a) signs of vestibular dysequilibrium are present with supportive objective findings; *and* (b) the patient's usual activities of daily living cannot be performed without assistance, except such simple activities as self care, some household duties, walking on the street, and riding in a motor vehicle operated by another person.

Class 4—Impairment of the Whole Person, 35-60%:
A patient belongs in Class 4 when (a) signs of vestibular dysequilibrium are present with supportive objective findings; *and* (b) usual activities of daily living cannot be performed without assistance, except self care.

Class 5—Impairment of the Whole Person, 65-95%:
A patient belongs in Class 5 when (a) signs of vestibular dysequilibrium are present with supportive objective findings; *and* (b) the usual activities of daily living cannot be performed without assistance, except self care not requiring ambulation; *and* (c) confinement to the home or premises is necessary.

9.2 The Face

The face and its structural components serve multiple functions in humans. The portal for deglutition is the mouth and lips. Disturbances in function can result in drooling or inability to contain food or liquid while eating. The lips and mouth also serve in vocal articulation, adding intelligibility to speech. The nose and mouth are the portal of entry for respiration. Impairment can be a result of neurologic disorders, such as partial or complete paralysis of the lips; scar formation and contracture of the lips; or loss of tissue.

The skin of the face has varied functions, such as body covering, resistance to trauma, sensory perception, and regulation of temperature and body fluids. Specific protective functions exist, such as coverage of the eye and its contents by the eyelid.

The face has a unique role in communication. No other part of the body serves as specific a function for personal identity and for expression of thought and emotion. Facial expressions are an integral part of normal living posture. A degree of normalcy is expected for effective verbal and nonverbal communication. Facial anatomy contributes to identity, expression, and normal functioning, and to the appearance of the forehead and cheeks; eyes, eyelids, and brows; lips and mouth; nose; and chin and neck.

In evaluating permanent impairment from a disorder of the face, functional capacity as well as structural integrity are considered. Impairment in this section is limited to abnormality in structural integrity only. (For loss of function, refer to sections regarding specific anatomical areas.) Loss of structural integrity can result from cutaneous disfigurement, such as that due to abnormal pigmentation or scars, or from loss of supporting structures, such as soft tissue, bone, or cartilage of the facial skeleton.

Class 1—Impairment of the Whole Person, 0-5%:
A patient belongs in Class 1 when the facial abnormality is limited to a disorder of the cutaneous structures, such as visible scars and abnormal pigmentation. (See Chapter 13.)

Class 2—Impairment of the Whole Person, 5-10%:
A patient belongs in Class 2 when there is loss of supporting structure of part of the face, with or without cutaneous disorder. Depressed cheek, nasal, or frontal bones constitute a Class 2 impairment.

Class 3—Impairment of the Whole Person, 10-15%:
A patient belongs in Class 3 when there is absence of a normal anatomical area of the face. Loss of an eye (see Chapter 8) or loss of part of the nose with the resulting cosmetic deformity, constitute a Class 3 impairment.

Class 4—Impairment of the Whole Person, 15-35%:
A patient belongs in Class 4 when facial disfigurement is so severe that it precludes social acceptance. Massive distortion of normal facial anatomy constitutes a Class 4 impairment. (See Chapter 14.)

Facial Disfigurement

The face is such a prominent feature of a person that it plays a critical role in his physical, psychological and emotional makeup. Facial disfigurement can affect all these components and can result in social and vocational handicap.

Disfigurement of the face can result from many causes, particularly burns, accidental injury, surgery, and infections. Effects upon individuals can vary tremendously. However, we recommend that "total disfigurement of the face" after treatment has been completed be deemed 15% to 35% impairment of the whole person. For assessment of impairment for associated behavioral changes, the reader is referred to Chapter 14.

Facial disfigurement can be considered total if it is severe and grossly deforming of face and features; also, it must involve at least the entire area between the brow line and the upper lip on both sides. Severe disfigurement above the brow line should be deemed, at a maximum, 1% impairment of the whole person. If it is severe below the upper lip, it may be deemed 8% impairment of the whole person. Specific prominent facial disfigurements should be deemed to have the following maximum values as impairments of the whole person:

Disfigurement	% Impairment of the Whole Person
Unilateral Total Facial Paralysis	5
Bilateral Total Facial Paralysis	8
Loss or Deformity of Outer Ear	2
Loss of the Entire Nose	25
Nasal Distortions in Physical Appearance	5

On the basis of the above guidelines, reasonable impairment values can be placed on other facial disfigurements.

9.3 The Nose, Throat, and Related Structures

For the purposes of this chapter, the nose, throat, and related structures include:

1. The nasal region: This consists of the external nose, the nasal cavity, and the nasopharynx.

2. The oral region: This consists of the mouth, teeth, tongue, hard and soft palate, region of the palatine tonsil, and oropharynx.

3. The neck and chest region: This consists of the hypopharynx, larynx, trachea, esophagus, and the bronchi.

The functions of these structures, and the order in which they will be discussed, are: (1) respiration; (2) mastication and deglutition; (3) olfaction and taste; and (4) speech. Permanent impairment may result from a deviation from normal in any of the above functions, and, because of their close relationship, more than one structure may be involved.

9.3a Respiration

Respiration, as used in this chapter, may be defined as the act or function of breathing, that is, the act by which air is inspired and expired from the lungs.

The respiratory mechanism includes the lungs and the air passages; the latter includes the nares, nasal cavities, mouth, pharynx, larynx, trachea, and bronchi.

The scope of this chapter limits discussion of permanent impairment to that produced by defects of the air passages. The reader is referred to Chapter 5 for a discussion of impairment of the lower airways and lung parenchyma.

The most commonly encountered defect of the air passages is obstruction, which may be partial (stenosis) or complete (occlusion). Obstructions and other air passage defects are evidenced primarily by dyspnea or so-called "unusual breathlessness." The "sleep apnea syndrome" may be related to functional upper airway obstruction.

Dyspnea is a cardinal factor that contributes to a patient's diminished capacity for the activities of daily living and to permanent impairment. This subjective complaint, indicating awareness of respiratory distress, is usually noticed first, and is most severe, during exercise. When dyspnea occurs at rest, respiratory dysfunction is probably severe. Dyspnea may or may not be accompanied by other pertinent signs or symptoms.

Patients with air passage defects may be evaluated in accordance with the classification in Table 5. Permanent impairment from obstructive sleep apnea should be evaluated using the criteria in Chapter 4.

9.3b Mastication and Deglutition

The act of eating includes mastication and deglutition. Numerous conditions of nongastrointestinal origin, singly or in combination, interfere with these functions. The imposition of dietary restrictions on the patient is usually the result. Such restrictions are, therefore, the most objective criteria by which to evaluate the permanent impairment of these patients. These criteria are:

Restriction	% Impairment of the Whole Person
1. The diet is limited to semi-solid or soft foods	5-10
2. The diet is limited to liquid foods	20-30
3. Ingestion of food requires tube feeding or gastrostomy	40-60

9.3c Olfaction and Taste

Only rarely does complete loss of the closely related senses of olfaction and taste seriously affect an individual's performance of the usual activities of daily living. The rare case almost invariably involves occupational considerations that are outside the scope of a physician's responsibility in the evaluation of permanent impairment.

For this reason, a single value of 3% impairment of the whole person is suggested for use in cases involving complete bilateral loss of either sense due to peripheral lesions. This value is to be combined with any other permanent impairment value pertinent to the case, using the Combined Values Chart.

Detection by the patient of any odor or taste, even though he or she cannot name it, precludes a finding of permanent impairment.

9.3d Speech

In this chapter, speech means the capacity to produce vocal signals that can be heard, understood, and sustained over a useful period of time. Speech ought to allow effective communication in the activities of daily living.

Table 5. Classes of Air Passage Defects

Class 1 0-10% impairment of the Whole Person.	Class 2 15-30% impairment of the Whole Person.†	Class 3 35-50% impairment of the Whole Person.	Class 4 Greater than 50% impairment of the Whole Person.
A recognized air passage defect exists.	A recognized air passage defect exists.	A recognized air passage defect exists.	A recognized air passage defect exists.
Dyspnea does *not* occur at rest.	Dyspnea does *not* occur at rest.	Dyspnea does *not* occur at rest.	Dyspnea occurs at rest, although patient is not necessarily bedridden.
Dyspnea is *not* produced by walking or climbing stairs freely, performance of other usual activities of daily living, stress, prolonged exertion, hurrying, hill-climbing, recreation* requiring intensive effort or similar activity.	Dyspnea is *not* produced by walking freely on the level, climbing at least one flight of ordinary stairs or the performance of other usual activities of daily living. Dyspnea IS produced by stress, prolonged exertion, hurrying, hill-climbing, recreation except sedentary forms, or similar activity.	Dyspnea IS produced by walking more than one or two blocks on the level or climbing one flight of ordinary stairs even with periods of rest; performance of other usual activities of daily living, stress, hurrying, hill-climbing, recreation or similar activity.	Dyspnea is aggravated by the performance of any of the usual activities of daily living beyond personal cleansing, dressing, grooming or its equivalent.
Examination reveals *one* or more of the following: partial obstruction of oropharynx, laryngopharynx, larynx, upper trachea (to 4th ring), lower trachea, bronchi, or complete obstruction of the nose (bilateral), or nasopharynx.	Examination reveals *one* or more of the following: partial obstruction of oropharynx, laryngopharynx, larynx, upper trachea (to 4th ring), lower trachea, bronchi, or complete obstruction of the nose (bilateral), or nasopharynx.	Examination reveals *one* or more of the following: partial obstruction of oropharynx, laryngopharynx, larynx, upper trachea (to 4th ring), lower trachea or bronchi.	Examination reveals *one* or more of the following: partial obstruction of oropharynx, laryngopharynx, larynx, upper trachea (to 4th ring), lower trachea or bronchi.

*Prophylactic restriction of activity such as strenuous competitive sport does not exclude patient from Class 1.

†Patients with successful permanent tracheostomy or stoma should be rated at 25% impairment of the whole person.

The causes and characteristics of abnormal speech are not considered. Consideration is given only to the degree of impairment relating to the individual's efficiency in using speech to make himself or herself understood in daily living. It is assumed that this evaluation pertains specifically to the production of voice and articulate speech, and not to the language content or structure of the patient's communication. Based on these assumptions, the primary problem is estimation of proficiency in using oral language, or measurement of the utility of speech as defined above. Esophageal speech is also included.

At this time there is no single, acceptable, proven test that will measure objectively the degrees of impairment from the many varieties of speech disorders. Therefore, it is recommended that speech impairment be evaluated clinically as to audibility, intelligibility, and functional efficiency.

Audibility: This is based on the patient's ability to speak at a level sufficient to be heard.

Intelligibility: This is based on the ability to articulate and to link the phonetic units of speech with sufficient accuracy to be understood.

Functional Efficiency: This is based on the ability to produce a serviceably fast rate of speech output, and to sustain this output over a useful period of time.

Other definable attributes of speech, such as acceptable voice quality, pitch, and melodic variation, are not evaluated except indirectly as they affect one of the three primary capacities of speech.

A classification chart, oral reading paragraph, and examining procedures for use in estimating speech impairment are described below.

Classification Chart

Judgments as to the amount of impairment should be made with reference to the classes, percentages, and examples provided in the classification chart (Table 6). The fifteen categories of the chart suggest activities or situations with different levels of impairment. Data gathered from direct observation of the patient or from interviews should be compared with these categories, and values should be assigned considering the specific impairments that are present.

Oral Reading Paragraph

The paragraph of 100 words entitled, "The Smith House," composed of 10 sentences, provides a uniform means of comparing a speech sample of the patient with the performance of normal speakers. The phonetic elements of the paragraph are selected particularly for their relevance to intelligibility of speech.

"The Smith House"

Larry and Ruth Smith have been married nearly 14 years. They have a small place near Long Lake. Both of

Table 6. Speech Classification Chart

	Audibility		Intelligibility		Functional Efficiency
Class 1 0-10% speech impairment	Can produce speech of intensity sufficient for *most* of the needs of everyday speech communication, although this sometimes may require effort and occasionally may be beyond the patient's capacity.	**Class 1** 0-10% speech impairment	Can perform *most* of the articulatory acts necessary for everyday speech communication, although listeners occasionally ask the patient to repeat and the patient may find it difficult or even impossible to produce a few phonetic units.	**Class 1** 0-10% speech impairment	Can meet *most* of the demands of articulation and phonation for everyday speech communication with adequate speed and ease, although occasionally the patient may hesitate or speak slowly.
Class 2 15-35% speech impairment	Can produce speech of intensity sufficient for *many* of the needs of everyday speech communication; is usually heard under average conditions; however, may have difficulty in automobiles, buses, trains, stations, restaurants, etc.	**Class 2** 15-35% speech impairment	Can perform *many* of the necessary articulatory acts for everyday speech communication. Can speak name, address, etc., and be understood by a stranger, but may have numerous inaccuracies; sometimes appears to have difficulty articulating.	**Class 2** 15-35% speech impairment	Can meet *many* of the demands of articulation and phonation for everyday speech communication with adequate speed and ease, but sometimes gives impression of difficulty, and speech may sometimes be discontinuous, interrupted, hesitant or slow.
Class 3 40-60% speech impairment	Can produce speech of intensity sufficient for *some* of the needs of everyday speech communication, such as close conversation; however, has considerable difficulty in such noisy places as listed above; the voice tires rapidly and tends to become inaudible after a few seconds.	**Class 3** 40-60% speech impairment	Can perform *some* of the necessary articulatory acts for everyday speech communication; can usually converse with family and friends, however, strangers may find it difficult to understand the patient; may often be asked to repeat.	**Class 3** 40-60% speech impairment	Can meet *some* of the demands of articulation and phonation for everyday speech communication with adequate speed and ease, but often can only sustain consecutive speech for brief periods, may give the impression of being rapidly fatigued.
Class 4 65-85% speech impairment	Can produce speech of intensity sufficient for a *few* of the needs of everyday speech communication; can barely be heard by a close listener or over the telephone, perhaps may be able to whisper audibly, but has no voice.	**Class 4** 65-85% speech impairment	Can perform a *few* of the necessary articulatory acts for everyday speech communication; can produce some phonetic units; may have approximations for a few words such as names of own family; however, unintelligible out of context.	**Class 4** 65-85% speech impairment	Can meet a *few* of the demands of articulation and phonation for everyday speech communication with adequate speed and ease, such as single words; or short phrases, but cannot maintain uninterrupted speech flow; speech is labored, rate is impractically slow.
Class 5 90-100% speech impairment	Can produce speech of intensity sufficient for *none* of the needs of everyday speech communication.	**Class 5** 90-100% speech impairment	Can perform *none* of the articulatory acts necessary for everyday speech communication.	**Class 5** 90-100% speech impairment	Can meet *none* of the demands of articulation and phonation for everyday speech communication with adequate speed and ease.

them think there's nothing like the country for health. Their two boys would rather live there than any other place. Larry likes to keep some saddle horses close to the house. These make it easy to keep his sons amused. If they wish, the boys can go fishing along the shore. When it rains, they usually want to watch television. Ruth has a cherry tree on each side of the kitchen door. In June they enjoy the juice and jelly.

Examining Procedures

General Orientation:

The examining physician should have normal hearing as defined in the earlier section on Hearing.

The setting of the examination should be a reasonably quiet office that approximates the noise level conditions of everyday living. The examiner should base judgments of impairment on two kinds of evidence: (1) direct observation of the patient's speech in the office, for example, during conversation, during the interview, and while reading and counting aloud; and

(2) reports pertaining to the patient's performances in situations of everyday living. The reports or the evidence should be supplied by observers who know the patient well. The standard of evaluation is the concept of a normal speaker's performance in average situations of everyday living. It is assumed in this context that an average speaker usually can perform as follows:

(1) Talk in a loud voice when the occasion demands it; (2) sustain phonation for at least 10 seconds in one breath; (3) complete at least a 10-word sentence in one breath; (4) form all of the phonetic units of American speech, and join them together intelligibly; and (5) maintain a rate of at least 75 to 100 words per minute, and sustain a flow of speech for a reasonable length of time.

Specific Instructions:

1. Place the patient approximately 8 ft from the examiner.

2. Interview the patient. This will permit observation of the patient's speech in ordinary conversation while obtaining information pertinent to his history.

Table 7. Speech Impairment as Related to Impairment of the Whole Person

% Speech Impairment	% Impairment of the Whole Person	% Speech Impairment	% Impairment of the Whole Person
0	0	50	18
5	2	55	19
10	4	60	21
15	5	65	23
20	7	70	24
25	9	75	26
30	10	80	28
35	12	85	30
40	14	90	32
45	16	95	33
		100	35

Note: Impairment of the *whole person* contributed by *speech impairment* may be rounded to the nearest 5% *only* when it is the *sole* impairment involved.

3. Listen to the patient's speech as the patient reads aloud the short paragraph, "The Smith House." For this exercise, seat the patient with the back towards the physician, maintaining a separation of 8 ft. Instruct the patient as follows: "You are to read this passage so that I can hear you plainly. Be sure to speak so that I can understand you."

4. If additional reading procedures are required, simple prose paragraphs from a magazine may be used. A nonreader may be requested to give name, address, the days of the week, the months of the year, etc. Additional evidence regarding the patient's rate of speech and ability to sustain it may be obtained by noting the time required to count to 100 by ones. Completion of the latter task in 60 to 75 seconds is accepted as normal.

5. Record judgment of the patient's speech capacity with regard to each of the three columns of the classification chart.

6. The degree of impairment of the speech function is equivalent to the greatest percentage of impairment recorded in any one of the three columns of the classification chart.

For example, speech capacity of a patient is judged to be:

Audibility	Intelligibility	Functional Efficiency
Class 1-10%	Class 3-50%	Class 2-30%

Then speech impairment is 50%, which on consulting Table 7 is seen to be 18% impairment of the whole person.

References

1. Guide for the evaluation of hearing handicap. *JAMA* 1979; 241:2055-2059.

2. Noble WG: *Assessment of Hearing Loss and Handicap in Adults*. New York, Academic Press, 1978.

3. ANSI Standard S3.6-1969, *Specifications for Audiometers*. American National Standards Institute, 1410 Broadway, New York, NY 10018.

4. Doty RL: A review of olfactory dysfunctions in man. *Am J Otolaryngol* 1979;1:57-59.

5. Bartoshuk LM: The psychophysics of taste. *Am J Clin Nutr* 1978; 31:1068-1077.

Chapter 10

The Digestive System

10.0 Introduction

The digestive system comprises the alimentary canal and its appendages, including the liver, biliary tract, and pancreas. The oral cavity and pharynx are considered elsewhere in the *Guides*.

The purpose of this chapter is to provide criteria for the evaluation of permanent impairment of the digestive system according to a person's ability to perform activities of daily living. A clinically established or objectively determined deviation from normal in the transport and assimilation of ingested food, the metabolism of nutrition, or the excretion of waste products may result in permanent impairment of varying degrees.

Before using the information in this chapter, the reader is urged to review Chapters 1 and 2, which provide a general discussion of the purpose of the *Guides* and of the situations in which they are useful; and which discuss techniques for the evaluation of the subject and for preparation of a report. The report should include the information found in the following outline, which is developed more fully in Chapter 2.

A. Medical Evaluation
1. Narrative history of medical conditions
2. Results of the most recent clinical evaluation
3. Assessment of current clinical status and statement of future plans
4. Diagnoses and clinical impressions
5. Expected date of full or partial recovery

B. Analysis of Findings
1. Impact of medical condition(s) on life activities
2. Explanation for concluding that the medical condition(s) has or has not become static or well-stabilized
3. Explanation for concluding that the individual is or is not likely to suffer from sudden or subtle incapacitation
4. Explanation for concluding that the individual is or is not likely to suffer injury or further impairment by engaging in life activities or by attempting to meet personal, social, and occupational demands
5. Explanation for concluding that accommodations and/or restrictions are or are not warranted

C. Comparison of Results of Analysis with Impairment Criteria
1. Description of clinical findings, and how these findings relate to specific criteria in the chapter
2. Explanation of each percent of impairment rating
3. Summary list of all impairment ratings
4. Overall rating of impairment of the whole person

10.1 Desirable Weight

For the purposes of determining impairment due to disorders of the upper digestive tract, "desirable" weight may be defined as follows:

1. If the examiner is able to determine by history or from previous medical records a weight before onset of the

Table 1. Desirable Weights in English and Metric by Sex, Height and Body Build
[Indoor Clothing Weighing 5 lb. (2.3 kg) for Men and 3 lb. (1.4 kg) for Women; and Shoes with 1 in. (2.5 cm) Heels]*

Men				**Women**			
Height in (cm)	**Weight** lb (kg) Small Frame	Medium Frame	Large Frame	**Height** in (cm)	**Weight** lb (kg) Small Frame	Medium Frame	Large Frame
62 (157)	128-134 (58.0-60.7)	131-141 (59.2-63.9)	138-150 (62.5-67.8)	58 (147)	102-111 (46.2-50.2)	109-121 (49.3-54.7)	118-131 (53.3-59.3)
63 (160)	130-136 (59.0-61.7)	133-143 (60.3-64.9)	140-153 (63.5-69.4)	59 (150)	103-113 (46.7-51.3)	111-123 (50.3-55.9)	120-134 (54.4-60.9)
64 (163)	132-138 (60.0-62.7)	135-145 (61.3-66.0)	142-156 (64.5-71.1)	60 (152)	104-115 (47.1-52.1)	113-126 (51.1-57.0)	122-137 (55.2-61.9)
65 (165)	134-140 (60.8-63.5)	137-148 (62.1-67.0)	144-160 (65.3-72.5)	61 (155)	106-118 (48.1-53.6)	115-129 (52.2-58.6)	125-140 (56.8-63.6)
66 (168)	136-142 (61.8-64.6)	139-151 (63.2-68.7)	146-164 (66.4-74.7)	62 (157)	108-121 (48.8-54.6)	118-132 (53.2-59.6)	128-143 (57.8-64.6)
67 (170)	138-145 (62.5-65.7)	142-154 (64.3-69.8)	149-168 (67.5-76.1)	63 (160)	111-124 (50.3-56.2)	121-135 (54.9-61.2)	131-147 (59.4-66.7)
68 (173)	140-148 (63.6-67.3)	145-157 (65.9-71.4)	152-172 (69.1-78.2)	64 (163)	114-127 (51.9-57.8)	124-138 (56.4-62.8)	134-151 (61.0-68.8)
69 (175)	142-151 (64.3-68.3)	148-160 (66.9-72.4)	155-176 (70.1-79.6)	65 (165)	117-130 (53.0-58.9)	127-141 (57.5-63.9)	137-155 (62.0-70.2)
70 (178)	144-154 (65.4-70.0)	151-163 (68.6-74.0)	158-180 (71.8-81.8)	66 (168)	120-133 (54.6-60.5)	130-144 (59.2-65.5)	140-159 (63.7-72.4)
71 (180)	146-157 (66.1-71.0)	154-166 (69.7-75.1)	161-184 (72.8-83.3)	67 (170)	123-136 (55.7-61.6)	133-147 (60.2-66.6)	143-163 (64.8-73.8)
72 (183)	149-160 (67.7-72.7)	157-170 (71.3-77.2)	164-188 (74.5-85.4)	68 (173)	126-139 (57.3-63.2)	136-150 (61.8-68.2)	146-167 (66.4-75.9)
73 (185)	152-164 (68.7-74.1)	160-174 (72.4-78.6)	168-192 (75.9-86.8)	69 (175)	129-142 (58.3-64.2)	139-153 (62.8-69.2)	149-170 (67.4-76.9)
74 (188)	155-168 (70.3-76.2)	164-178 (74.4-80.7)	172-197 (78.0-89.4)	70 (178)	132-145 (60.0-65.9)	142-156 (64.5-70.9)	152-173 (69.0-78.6)
75 (190)	158-172 (71.4-77.6)	167-182 (75.4-82.2)	176-202 (79.4-91.2)	71 (180)	135-148 (61.0-66.9)	145-159 (65.6-71.9)	155-176 (70.1-79.6)
76 (193)	162-176 (73.5-79.8)	171-187 (77.6-84.8)	181-207 (82.1-93.9)	72 (183)	138-151 (62.6-68.4)	148-162 (67.0-73.4)	158-179 (71.6-81.2)

*Source: 1979 Body Build Study, Society of Actuaries and Association of Life Insurance Medical Directors of America, 1980.
Copyright © 1983, The Metropolitan Life Insurance Company. Courtesy Statistical Bulletin, Metropolitan Life Insurance Company.

patient's digestive illness that he or she considers "usual," the examiner should use that weight as the "desirable" weight from which any deviations are measured.

2. If the examiner is not able to determine by history or from previous medical records a pre-illness "usual" weight, the examiner should refer to a table of "desirable" weights, and should determine deviations from the lower end of the range of the "desirable" weights for the patient's sex, height, and body build. Table 1, which is based on the 1979 Body Build Study by the Society of Actuaries and Association of Life Insurance Medical Directors of America, is recommended.

For an obese patient, the pre-illness weight may not be as physiologically "desirable" as the present weight; thus, the examiner should use judgment in assessing the relative importance of weight loss in determining the impairment rating.

In most cases, the examiner should use the definition shown under Number 1 above. The definition and reference in Number 2 will be helpful if Number 1 cannot be used.

10.2 Esophagus

Symptoms and signs of impairment include dysphagia, pyrosis or "heartburn," retrosternal pain, regurgitation, bleeding, and weight loss. One should be mindful that occasional, minor dyspepsia, "gas," and belching are within the experience of all normal persons.

Objective procedures useful in establishing esophageal impairment include, but are not limited to: (1) fluoroscopy and radiography with contrast materials; (2) peroral endoscopy; (3) cytology and/or biopsy; and (4) manometry.

Criteria for evaluating permanent impairment of esophageal function are those listed in Table 2.

Example of Class 1 Impairment of the Whole Person: A 44-year-old man complained of dysphagia six months ago after the ingestion of a broiled lobster. Now, symptoms referrable to esophageal disease cannot be elicited. Weight of 150 lb (68.1 kg) is within desirable limits for the man's height of 5 ft 10 in (1.78 meters).

Physical examination reveals a healthy-appearing man. The vital signs and the physical examination are normal. A chest radiograph and electrocardiogram are normal. Radiographic study of the upper gastrointestinal tract reveals a small sliding hiatal hernia.

Diagnosis: Hiatal hernia.

Impairment: 0% impairment of the whole person.

Comment: The symptoms are indicative of esophageal motor disorder and a hiatal hernia is present, but these have not interfered with normal nutrition, nor have they impaired the person's ability to perform the usual activities of daily living.

Example of Class 2 Impairment of the Whole Person:
A 59-year-old woman complains of having had almost daily substernal pain and dysphagia for five years. She feels better when she limits her diet to soft foods. Her symptoms are more severe when she becomes upset about the status of her invalid husband.

Physical examination reveals a woman 5 ft 7 in (1.70 meters) tall, of medium frame, appearing older than her stated age. Her blood pressure is 145/90 mm Hg. She weighs 118 lb (53.6 kg), which is less than 10% below her usual weight of 128 lb (58.0 kg). Chest radiograph and ECG are normal. Radiographic studies of the upper gastrointestinal tract reveal a corkscrew configuration or "curling," of the esophagus that is suggestive of diffuse spasm. This diagnosis is confirmed by esophageal motility studies.

Diagnosis: Diffuse spasm of the esophagus.

Impairment: 15% impairment of the whole person.

Comment: The patient's symptoms are persistent, and she is obliged to restrict her diet. Her weight is within 10% of the desirable level, and her daily activities have been impaired only slightly.

Example of Class 3 Impairment of the Whole Person:
A 49-year-old man complains of intermittent substernal pain, dysphagia, and nocturnal regurgitation of five years' duration. The dysphagia has been progressive. The man can swallow solid foods only by drinking large amounts of liquids. Before the onset of his illness, he weighed 180 lb (81.7 kg); now he weighs 155 lb (70.4 kg).

On physical examination, signs of weight loss are present. Height is 6 ft 2 in (1.88 meters). The vital signs are normal. Chest radiograph reveals widening of the mediastinum. An upper gastrointestinal tract study with x-rays reveals a markedly dilated and tortuous esophagus, which terminates in a filiform constrictive configuration. Dilation of the esophagus has been required about twice a year.

Diagnosis: Achalasia of the esophagus.

Impairment: 30% impairment of the whole person.

Comment: Symptoms have been persistent and progressive despite dietary limitation and esophageal dilation; weight loss has exceeded 10% of the desirable level. In this case, the impairment might be appreciably lessened if the patient could be persuaded to undergo surgical esophagomyotomy.

Example of Class 4 Impairment of the Whole Person:
The patient, a 58-year-old man, 5 ft 10 in (1.78 meters) in height, has almost complete esophageal obstruction. Five years ago he had a resection of the esophagogastric junction for cancer. Although there is no evidence of recurrence of the tumor, he has developed severe stenosing esophagitis. Surgical correction was attempted but was unsuccessful. At present, a gastrostomy tube is used for feeding. While the patient previously maintained a weight of 150 lb (68.1 kg), he now weighs 110 lb (49.9 kg). Dilation of the stricture is required about once a month to accommodate salivary secretions.

Diagnosis: Stenosing esophagitis.

Impairment: 55% impairment due to stenosing esophagitis and 10% impairment due to gastrostomy, which combine to 60% impairment of the whole person (see Combined Values Chart).

Comment: Symptoms and signs of disease have progressed despite exhaustive treatment, and further therapy can be only palliative. Weight loss has exceeded 20% of the desirable level. The prognosis is poor.

10.3 Stomach and Duodenum

Symptoms and signs of impairment include nausea, vomiting, pain, bleeding, obstruction, certain types of malassimilation, diarrhea, weight loss, and nutritional deficiencies that can include hematologic and neurologic manifestations.

Objective procedures useful in establishing impairment of the stomach and duodenum include, but are not limited to: (1) fluoroscopy and radiography employing contrast materials; (2) peroral endoscopy; (3) cytology and/or biopsy; (4) gastric secretory tests; (5) assimilation tests; and (6) stool examination.

Criteria for evaluating permanent impairment consequent to disease or injury of the stomach or duodenum are those listed in Table 2.

Example of Class 1 Impairment of the Whole Person:
A 28-year-old man complains of having had intermittent epigastric pain and burning over a five-year period. There is no history of nausea, vomiting, hematemesis, or melena. The man's height with shoes on is 5 ft 11 in (1.80 meters), and weight is 160 lb (72.6 kg). An upper gastrointestinal study reveals a deformed duodenal bulb without an ulcer crater or evidence of gastric retention.

Diagnosis: Duodenal ulcer, in remission.

Impairment: 5% impairment of the whole person.

Comment: Symptoms have been remittent, and the disease has been uncomplicated. Dietary restriction usually has not been necessary. Desirable weight and activities have been maintained.

Example of Class 2 Impairment of the Whole Person:

The patient, a 40-year-old man with a small frame body build, had intermittent ulcer symptoms over a period of 10 years. Bleeding occurred on three occasions. Blood replacement was necessary twice. The man was hospitalized about once a year for a period of one to two weeks. He consistently refused surgery. He had one episode of transient pyloric obstruction. At present, continual treatment is required. The patient's height with shoes on is 5 ft 8 in (1.73 meters), and weight, 130 lb (59.0 kg), which is 7% below desirable weight. Radiographs of the upper gastrointestinal tract reveal a marked cloverleaf deformity of the duodenum with an ulcer crater 3 mm in diameter.

Diagnosis: Active duodenal ulcer with history of complications.

Impairment: 15% impairment of the whole person.

Comment: The disease has been complicated, and symptoms have recurred despite medical therapy. There has been interference with the performance of daily activities. In this case, the patient has adamantly declined a surgical remedy, although this might appreciably lessen his impairment.

Example of Class 3 Impairment of the Whole Person:

A 50-year-old woman had a gastric resection for a duodenal ulcer two years ago. She now complains of episodes of light-headedness, sweating, and palpitation occurring 15 minutes after meals. The symptoms are partly relieved by diet and by lying down. Since the operation, her weight has decreased to approximately 15% below desirable weight.

Physical examination reveals a woman weighing 100 lb (45.4 kg) and standing 5 ft 3 in (1.60 meters) tall. A well-healed upper abdominal scar is present. The remainder of the physical examination is not remarkable. Upper gastrointestinal radiographs reveal evidence of a 70% gastric resection and a normally functioning gastrojejunostomy without evidence of ulceration.

Diagnosis: Postgastrectomy dumping syndrome.

Impairment: 30% impairment of the whole person.

Comment: The patient has symptoms impairing the performance of normal activities despite dietary restriction. She is unable to maintain weight within a 10% range of the desirable level.

Example of Class 4 Impairment of the Whole Person:

A 62-year-old man had a total gastric resection three years ago for carcinoma of the stomach. After the surgical procedure he complained of anorexia and developed progressive weight loss and signs of nutritional deficiency. Physical examination reveals a malnourished, elderly male. He is 5 ft 9 in (1.75 meters) tall and weighs 116 lb (52.7 kg). An upper abdominal scar is present, but no masses are palpable. The tongue is smooth and glistening. Slight pedal edema is present. Laboratory studies disclose anemia and hypoproteinemia. A satisfactory esophagojejunal anastomosis is demonstrated by radiography.

Diagnosis: Postoperative absence of the stomach with esophagojejunal anastomosis.

Impairment: 60% impairment due to gastric resection with esophagojejunal anastomosis, which is to be combined with an appropriate value for the anemia (see Chapter 7) to determine impairment of the whole person.

Comment: The patient's weight loss exceeds 20% of the desirable level, with signs of marked nutritional deficiency present. The patient clearly is unable to perform activities of normal daily living.

10.4 Small Intestine

Symptoms and signs of impairment include pain, diarrhea, steatorrhea, bleeding, obstruction, and weight loss, which often are associated with general debility and other extra-intestinal manifestations.

Objective procedures useful in establishing impairment of the small intestine include, but are not limited to: (1) fluoroscopy and radiography employing contrast materials; (2) peroral mucosal biopsy; and (3) measures of intestinal assimilation, for example, test for fecal fat excretion and urinary d-xylose excretion, C^{14} breath test, serum bile acid determination, and Schilling test.

Criteria for evaluating permanent impairment of small intestine function are those listed in Table 2.

Example of Class 1 Impairment of the Whole Person:

Ten years ago, a 45-year-old man who weighed 160 lb

Table 2. Classes of Impairment of the Upper Digestive Tract
(Esophagus, Stomach and Duodenum, Small Intestine, Pancreas)

Class 1 0-5% Impairment of the Whole Person	Class 2 10-20% Impairment of the Whole Person	Class 3 25-45% Impairment of the Whole Person	Class 4 50-75% Impairment of the Whole Person
Symptoms or signs of upper digestive tract disease are present or there is anatomic loss or alteration;	Symptoms and signs of organic upper digestive tract disease are present or there is anatomic loss or alteration;	Symptoms and signs of organic upper digestive tract disease are present or there is anatomic loss or alteration;	Symptoms and signs of organic upper digestive tract disease are present or there is anatomic loss or alteration;
and	**and**	**and**	**and**
Continuous treatment is not required;	Appropriate dietary restrictions and drugs are required for control of symptoms, signs and/or nutritional deficiency;	Appropriate dietary restrictions and drugs do not completely control symptoms, signs, and/or nutritional state;	Symptoms are not controlled by treatment;
and	**and**	**or**	**or**
Weight can be maintained at the desirable level;	Loss of weight below the "desirable weight"* does not exceed 10%.	There is 10-20% loss of weight below the "desirable weight"* which is ascribable to a disorder of the upper digestive tract.	There is greater than a 20% loss of weight below the "desirable weight"* which is ascribable to a disorder of the upper digestive tract.
or			
There are no sequelae after surgical procedures.			

*See Table 1.

(72.6 kg) required an operation because of recurrent and protracted abdominal pain, fever, and distention. Approximately 30 cm of the terminal ileum were resected; the histologic findings were consistent with regional enteritis. There has been no recurrence of the preoperative symptoms. The patient maintains a weight of 155 lb (70.3 kg) on an unrestricted diet and has two to three soft stools daily. Radiographs of the remaining small intestine are normal.

Diagnosis: Partial ileal resection for regional enteritis.

Impairment: 0% impairment of the whole person.

Comment: There has been no recurrence of symptoms that indicated disease of the small intestine 10 years ago. The patient maintains normal activity and requires no therapy.

Example of Class 2 Impairment of the Whole Person:
A 64-year-old woman, who is 5 ft 1 in (155 cm) tall, five years ago suffered diarrhea, weight loss, and vague abdominal pain; had a macrocytic anemia; and had small intestinal diverticula demonstrated by radiograph. Prior to her illness she weighed 120 lb (54.4 kg). All symptoms cleared on parenteral treatment with cyanocobalamin (vitamin B$_{12}$) and oral tetracycline. Two years ago, mild diarrhea recurred for three weeks and again subsided after oral therapy with tetracycline. Radiographs now reveal numerous jejunal diverticula. Nutri-

tion is normal, and her weight is maintained at 110 lb (49.9 kg). There are no symptoms on an unrestricted diet while the patient continues to take parenteral cyanocobalamin.

Diagnosis: Diverticulosis of the jejunum.

Impairment: 15% impairment due to diverticulosis of the jejunum, which is to be combined with an appropriate value for the anemia to determine impairment of the whole person.

Comment: This patient can perform the activities of daily living, but she is dependent on continuing therapy.

Example of Class 3 Impairment of the Whole Person:
This 38-year-old man, 5 ft 3 in (1.60 meters) tall, has diarrhea and loss of stamina, and had a 15% decrease in weight from 130 to 110 lb (59.0 to 49.9 kg) after a partial resection of the ileum involved with regional enteritis. Three to four bouts of partial intestinal obstruction each year have not required surgical intervention. Radiographs of the small intestine disclose changes consistent with regional enteritis. Impaired intestinal absorption is confirmed by appropriate tests. Dietary restriction, vitamin supplements, antidiarrheal agents, and on occasion corticosteroid therapy, have been required to help the patient maintain a reasonably satisfactory state of health.

Diagnosis: Recurrent regional enteritis with intestinal malabsorption and recurring partial intestinal obstruction after partial ileal resection.

Impairment: 40% impairment of the whole person.

Comment: The nutritional status of this patient has been impaired, and his weight deficit exceeds 10% of the desirable level, despite dietary and drug therapy.

Example of Class 4 Impairment of the Whole Person:
A 35-year-old woman developed volvulus, which required removal of a large portion of the jejunum and ileum one year ago. She now requires continuous dietary control with supplemental nutrition and use of drugs to diminish abdominal pains and diarrhea. Tetany and dehydration require frequent hospitalizations for fluid and electrolyte repletion. Stamina is diminished. Her weight remains 87 lb (39.5 kg), and it should be at least 127 lb (57.6 kg) for her height of 5 ft 5 in (1.65 meters) and medium build. Absorption of d-xylose and fat is impaired.

Diagnosis: Intestinal malabsorption secondary to extensive small-bowel resection for volvulus.

Impairment: 75% impairment of the whole person.

Comment: This patient's nutritional status has been markedly impaired by an irreversible defect of the small intestine. Her weight loss exceeds 20% of the desirable level, and her performance of daily activities is seriously impaired.

10.5 Colon, Rectum, and Anus

Symptoms and signs of impairment include pain, constipation, diarrhea, tenesmus, incontinence, bleeding, suppuration, appearance of fissures and fistulas, and varying degrees of fecal incontinence; systemic manifestations may include fever, weight loss, debility, and anemia.

Objective procedures useful in establishing impairment of the colon and rectum include, but are not limited to: (1) digital and endoscopic examination including anoscopy, proctoscopy, sigmoidoscopy, and colonoscopy; (2) fecal microscopy and culture; (3) biopsy; and (4) fluoroscopy and radiography with contrast materials.

Criteria for evaluating permanent impairment in function of the colon and rectum are those listed in Table 3.

Example of Class 1 Impairment of the Whole Person:
A 50-year-old woman has a protracted tendency to have mildly erratic bowel action with alternating constipation and diarrhea. Stools, while varying in consistency, contain no pathologic products. Proctosigmoidoscopy shows clear mucosa; barium enema examination outlines a normal colon with several diverticula in the sigmoid segment associated with circular muscle spasm.

Diagnosis: (1) Functional gastrointestinal disorder, that is, irritable bowel syndrome; and (2) diverticulosis coli.

Impairment: 0% impairment of the whole person.

Comment: The symptoms, while occasionally annoying, have not interfered with the patient's necessary activities; her treatment requires only minor dietary adjustment.

Example of Class 2 Impairment of the Whole Person:
A 28-year-old woman gives a 10-year history of recurring ulcerative colitis. During exacerbations, she has moderate diarrhea with abdominal discomfort and passes small amounts of blood. Sigmoidoscopy shows a granular, slightly friable bowel. Barium enema examination of the colon shows some loss of haustral markings in the descending and sigmoid colon. Fever and anemia are not present. Hospitalization has not been required. Her symptoms respond to a restricted diet, sedation, antispasmodics, constipating agents, and moderate limitation of activities.

Diagnosis: Mild ulcerative colitis, limited to descending colon, sigmoid and rectum.

Impairment: 15% impairment of the whole person.

Comment: The disease has been remittent, and the symptoms only occasionally have interfered with necessary activities; symptomatic and supportive therapy has adequately controlled the disease.

Example of Class 3 Impairment of the Whole Person:
A 35-year-old man has had Crohn's disease since the age of 19. He has been hospitalized on several occasions, requiring intensive therapy with transfusion of packed red blood cells because of anemia. His symptoms include intermittent abdominal cramps and diarrhea with occasional perianal suppuration. Examination discloses Crohn's disease affecting the terminal ileum, segments of the colon, and the perianal area. He declines elective proctocolectomy. He continues his sedentary occupation, but his weight is consistently 20% below the desirable level.

Table 3. Classes of Colonic and Rectal Impairment

Class 1 0-5% Impairment of the Whole Person	Class 2 10-20% Impairment of the Whole Person	Class 3 25-35% Impairment of the Whole Person	Class 4 40-60% Impairment of the Whole Person
Signs and symptoms of colonic or rectal disease are infrequent and of brief duration;	There is objective evidence of colonic or rectal disease or anatomic loss or alteration;	There is objective evidence of colonic or rectal disease or anatomic loss or alteration;	There is objective evidence of colonic or rectal disease or anatomic loss or alteration;
	and	**and**	**and**
and	There are mild gastrointestinal symptoms with occasional disturbances of bowel function, accompanied by moderate pain;	There are moderate to severe exacerbations with disturbance of bowel habit, accompanied by periodic or continual pain;	There are persistent disturbances of bowel function present at rest with severe persistent pain;
	and	**and**	**and**
Limitation of activities, special diet or medication is not required;	Minimal restriction of diet or mild symptomatic therapy may be necessary;	Restriction of activity, special diet and drugs are required during attacks;	Complete limitation of activity, continued restriction of diet, and medication do not entirely control the symptoms;
and	**and**	**and**	**and**
No systemic manifestations are present and weight and nutritional state can be maintained at a desirable level;	No impairment of nutrition results.	There are constitutional manifestations (fever, anemia, or weight loss).	There are constitutional manifestations (fever, weight loss, and/or anemia) present;
or			**or**
There are no sequelae after surgical procedures.			There is no prolonged remission.

Diagnosis: Crohn's enterocolitis.

Impairment: 35% impairment due to Crohn's disease, which is to be combined with an appropriate value for the anemia to determine the impairment of the whole person.

Comment: The disease, while remittent to varying degrees, interferes with the patient's pursuit of normal activities. He will require continuing treatment. His nutritional status is impaired.

Example of Class 4 Impairment of the Whole Person:
A 42-year-old woman has a 12-year history of chronic, recurring, ulcerative colitis that requires intensive therapy, limitation of activities, and numerous blood transfusions. As a result of malnutrition, infection, and transfusions, and as a further complication of her inflammatory bowel disease, the patient has developed jaundice and hepatomegaly. Extensive and severe involvement of the colon is demonstrated by sigmoidoscopic and radiographic studies. Fever and anemia persist. In the opinion of her physicians, surgery cannot be performed now because of her general debility and disease that involves several systems.

Diagnosis: Ulcerative colitis with associated liver disease.

Impairment: 60% impairment due to ulcerative colitis, which is to be combined with appropriate values for the liver disorder and anemia to determine impairment of the whole person.

Comment: The severe inflammatory bowel disease has been complicated by hepatobiliary disease. The patient's normal activities have been seriously impaired. It is possible that with intensive nutritional rehabilitation, a surgical remedy can be attempted, after which the impairment may be lessened.

10.6 Enterocutaneous Fistulas

Permanent enterocutaneous fistulas of the gastrointestinal tract, biliary tract, or pancreas, secondary to diseases of these structures, are evaluated as a part of the organ system primarily involved. Permanent, surgically created stomas usually are provided to compensate for anatomic losses and to allow either for ingress to or egress from the digestive tract.

If a patient has a permanent surgically created stoma, one of the values in the following table should be combined, using the Combined Values Chart, with a value based on criteria related to the involved organ.

Surgical Stoma	% Impairment of the Whole Person
Esophagostomy	10-15
Gastrostomy	10-15
Jejunostomy	15-20
Ileostomy	15-20
Colostomy	5-10

Criteria for evaluating permanent impairment of the anus are listed in Table 4.

Example of Class 1 Impairment of the Whole Person:
Five years ago a 45-year-old man had an acute pararectal abscess drained surgically. A fistula in ano resulted, with chronic drainage and recurrent bouts of acute infection. One year later a fistulectomy was performed. Since that time the man noted no recurrence of drainage or infection. Examination discloses a well-healed anal scar with distortion, but no weakness, of the anal sphincter.

Diagnosis: Healed fistula in ano.

Impairment: 0% impairment of the whole person.

Comment: The patient had documented anal disease that was appropriately treated and had a satisfactory resolution. His normal activities are not impaired.

Example of Class 2 Impairment of the Whole Person:
A 32-year-old woman has had Crohn's disease of the colon for 14 years, generally well controlled by medical therapy. However, during one exacerbation, a pararectal abscess developed that ruptured spontaneously and led to the development of a chronic fistula in ano. In addition, the patient experienced acute pain and bleeding at stool, and three years ago was found to have a chronic fissure in the posterior midline of the anal canal. Now, symptoms related to anal dysfunction occasionally recur, but generally they are well controlled by treatment. Surgery for the anal disorders is contraindicated in view of the patient's colonic disease.

Diagnosis: Chronic fistula in ano, chronic anal fissure, moderate intermittent impairment of anal function, associated with Crohn's disease of the colon.

Impairment: 10% impairment due to anal disorders, which is to be combined with an appropriate value for the colonic disorder to determine impairment of the whole person.

Comment: Anal function has been impaired but symptoms have been amenable to treatment when required. Her ability to perform normal activities has been only slightly impaired.

Example of Class 3 Impairment of the Whole Person:
Ten years ago a 56-year-old man developed a severe pararectal abscess that ruptured spontaneously. During the ensuing three years multiple recurrent infections occurred, with the opening of fistulous tracts in four other areas surrounding the anus. Surgical repair was undertaken in two stages, but this made necessary incision and excision of substantial portions of the sphincter. Recovery was complicated by severe wound infection. Since that time, the patient has had no recurrence of infection. However, he has had complete absence of fecal control. Although he practices daily rectal irrigations, he still soils himself almost daily. Examination discloses complete anatomic loss of sphincteric functions.

Diagnosis: Total anal incontinence secondary to anatomic loss of sphincter; complete loss of anal function.

Impairment: 25% impairment of the whole person.

Comment: The patient has uncontrollable fecal incontinence not amenable to further anorectal therapy.

10.7 Liver and Biliary Tract

Symptoms and signs of hepatobiliary impairment include pain, nausea, vomiting, anorexia, loss of strength and stamina, reduced resistance to infection, jaundice, and pruritus. Complications of advanced liver disease include ascites, anasarca, portal vein hypertension leading to esophageal varices and hemorrhage, and severe metabolic disturbances leading to hepatic encephalopathy and renal failure.

Objective procedures useful in establishing hepatobiliary impairment include, but are not limited to: (1) radiography employing contrast materials, including percutaneous and endoscopic cholangiography, and nuclide scintigraphy; (2) ultrasonography; (3) computerized tomography (CT scan); (4) angiography; (5) liver biopsy; and (6) selected laboratory tests to assess various functions of the liver and biliary ducts.

Criteria for evaluating permanent impairment of the liver and biliary tract are listed in Table 5.

Example of Class 1 Impairment of the Whole Person:
A 30-year-old man with a history of excessive alcohol consumption was hospitalized five years ago because of delirium tremens, fever, and jaundice. A liver biopsy revealed extensive fatty metamorphosis with steatonecrosis and minimal periportal fibrosis. Since being released from the hospital, he has drunk no alcoholic beverages, has felt well, and has exhibited excellent strength and appetite. Physical examination now shows a well-developed, muscular man without evidence of jaundice or ascites. The liver edge is firm and rounded and can be palpated 3 cm below the right costal margin. Liver function studies reveal: serum bilirubin 0.4 mg/100 ml; serum albumin 4.5 mg/100 ml; serum globulin 2.5 mg/100 ml; SGOT 35 units.

Table 4. Classes of Anal Impairment

Class 1 0-5% Impairment of the Whole Person	**Class 2** 10-15% Impairment of the Whole Person	**Class 3** 20-25% Impairment of the Whole Person
Signs of organic anal disease are present or there is anatomic loss or alteration;	Signs of organic anal disease are present or there is anatomic loss or alteration;	Signs of organic anal disease are present and there is anatomic loss or alteration;
or	**and**	**and**
There is mild incontinence involving gas and/or liquid stool;	Moderate but partial fecal incontinence is present requiring continual treatment;	Complete fecal incontinence is present;
or	**or**	**or**
Anal symptoms are mild, intermittent, and controlled by treatment.	Continual anal symptoms are present and incompletely controlled by treatment.	Signs of organic anal disease are present and severe anal symptoms unresponsive or not amenable to therapy are present.

Diagnosis: Slight hepatomegaly, probably due to fatty metamorphosis and portal fibrosis.

Impairment: 0% impairment of the whole person.

Comment: The pre-existing disease was documented, but recovery was satisfactory with only minimal evidence of residual liver impairment. The patient requires no treatment other than abstinence from alcohol, and he is able to engage in the activities of normal living.

Example of Class 2 Impairment of the Whole Person:
A 35-year-old man had acute viral hepatitis 10 years ago followed by a protracted convalescence. For the past six to seven years the disease has been quiescent, and the patient has had no jaundice, ascites, or gastrointestinal bleeding. His strength and nutritional state have been satisfactory except for limited stamina. Physical examination shows that he is well nourished and has good muscular development; several small spider angiomata are on the left shoulder; the liver is enlarged 4 cm below the right costal margin and has a firm, rounded edge; the spleen is palpable 1 cm below the left costal margin. Liver function studies reveal: serum bilirubin 2.1 mg/100 ml; serum albumin 4 gm/100 ml; serum globulin 4 gm/100 ml; SGOT 70 units. The serum hepatitis-B surface antigen and core antibody are positive. Liver biopsy shows chronic active hepatitis without cirrhosis.

Diagosis: Chronic active hepatitis B.

Impairment: 15% impairment of the whole person.

Comment: There is evidence of chronic active hepatitis and limited stamina, but the patient has been able to perform daily activities. Liver impairment is documented but of slight to moderate degree.

Example of Class 3 Impairment of the Whole Person:
A 48-year-old man had viral hepatitis at age 15, followed by recurrences of jaundice at ages 22 and 30. For the past six months he has had an intermittently poor appetite and an increase in fatigue. He has noted a slight yellowing of the skin. Physical examination shows that he appears to be chronically ill and minimally jaundiced. Several spider angiomata are seen on his neck and thorax. The liver and spleen are slightly enlarged. No ascites or edema are present. Laboratory studies reveal a normal blood count and urinalysis, serum bilirubin 2.8 mg/100 ml, serum albumin 3 gm/100 ml, serum globulin 4 gm/100 ml, and SGOT 180 units. Hepatitis B surface antigen and core antigen are absent from the serum. Examination of tissue obtained by needle biopsy shows chronic active hepatitis with extensive distortion of lobular architecture.

Diagnosis: Non-A, non-B chronic active hepatitis, and cirrhosis.

Impairment: 40% impairment of the whole person.

Comment: There is evidence of chronic, active, and probably progressive liver disease. The patient's ability to perform normal activities has been impaired.

Example of Class 4 Impairment of the Whole Person:
A 55-year-old woman has had repeated attacks of acute cholecystitis. She has experienced recurrent bouts of right upper quadrant pain, fever, jaundice, dark urine, nausea, vomiting, and severe pruritus. Laboratory studies are consistent with the presence of chronic biliary obstruction and permanent liver damage. Esophageal varices are demonstrated by radiography. Abdominal exploration discloses irreparable obstruction of the common bile duct. A liver biopsy reveals advanced biliary cirrhosis.

Diagnosis: Biliary cirrhosis, secondary to obstruction of common bile duct.

Impairment: 85% impairment of the whole person.

Table 5. Classes of Liver and Biliary Tract Impairment

Class 1 0-10% Impairment of the Whole Person	Class 2 15-25% Impairment of the Whole Person	Class 3 30-50% Impairment of the Whole Person	Class 4 Greater than 50% Impairment of the Whole Person
Liver Impairment			
There is objective evidence of persistent liver disease even though no symptoms of liver disease are present; and no history of ascites, jaundice, or bleeding esophageal varices within 3 years; **and** Nutrition and strength are good; **and** Biochemical studies indicate minimal disturbance in liver function; **or** Primary disorders of bilirubin metabolism are present.	There is objective evidence of chronic liver disease even though no symptoms of liver disease are present; and no history of ascites, jaundice, or bleeding esophageal varices within 3 years; **and** Nutrition and strength are good; **and** Biochemical studies indicate more severe liver damage than Class 1.	There is objective evidence of progressive chronic liver disease, or history of jaundice, ascites, or bleeding esophageal or gastric varices within the past year; **and** Nutrition and strength may be affected; **or** There is intermittent hepatic encephalopathy.	There is objective evidence of progressive chronic liver disease, or persistent ascites or persistent jaundice or bleeding esophageal or gastric varices, with central nervous system manifestations of hepatic insufficiency; **and** Nutritional state is poor.
Biliary Tract Impairment			
There is an occasional episode of biliary tract dysfunction.	There is recurrent biliary tract impairment irrespective of treatment.	There is irreparable obstruction of the bile tract with recurrent cholangitis.	There is persistent jaundice and progressive liver disease due to obstruction of the common bile duct.

Comment: The patient has sustained severe and irreparable impairment of the liver and biliary tract function. Her ability to perform normal activities has been seriously impaired.

10.8 Pancreas

Symptoms and signs of impairment of pancreatic function include pain, anorexia, nausea, vomiting, diarrhea, steatorrhea, jaundice, weight loss, muscle wasting, debility, and diabetes. Impairment from the endocrine function of the pancreas is discussed in Chapter 12.

Objective procedures useful in establishing impairment of pancreatic function include, but are not limited to: (1) radiography including plain or scout films of the abdomen, ultrasonography, CT scan, and endoscopic pancreatography; (2) determination of plasma glucose and glucose tolerance; (3) assay of pancreatic enzyme activity in blood, urine, and feces; (4) sweat electrolyte test; and (5) selected secretory tests such as the secretion test, and cytology.

Criteria for evaluating permanent impairment of pancreatic function are those listed in Table 2.

Example of Class 1 Impairment of the Whole Person: A 45-year-old woman has had epigastric pain associ-ated with an elevated serum amylase once or twice annually for the past three years. Despite a cholecystectomy for gallstones two years ago, the attacks continue to occur, usually after eating a large meal or drinking alcoholic beverages. A diet restricted in fat has corrected the patient's exogenous obesity but has not reduced her weight below a normal level. No clinical or laboratory evidence of pancreatic insufficiency is present.

Diagnosis: Recurrent pancreatitis.

Impairment: 5% impairment of the whole person.

Comment: The pre-existing disease was documented and treated appropriately. There is no present evidence of residual pancreatic impairment, and the patient is able to perform normal activities.

Example of Class 2 Impairment of the Whole Person: A 35-year-old, 6 ft 3 in (1.90 meters) man of medium build required partial pancreatectomy because of cyst formation and recurrent inflammation of the pancreas, after he was thrown against the steering wheel in an automobile crash. Despite treatment with pancreatic exocrine supplementation, he notes intermittent diarrhea and decreased stamina. He now weighs 164 lb (74.5 kg), while he previously had a weight of 180 lb (81.7 kg). Epigastric and back pain are sufficiently severe to require hospitalization once or twice a year. Steatorrhea is present.

Diagnosis: Chronic pancreatitis and exocrine insufficiency subsequent to trauma, with partial pancreatectomy.

Impairment: 20% impairment of the whole person.

Comment: Pancreatic exocrine function has been impaired, but the patient has been able to maintain a weight within 10% of his desirable weight. However, the patient's ability to perform normal activities has been somewhat impaired.

Example of Class 3 Impairment of the Whole Person:
Subsequent to a cholecystectomy and partial pancreatectomy, and despite dietary restriction and abstinence from alcohol, a woman who is 45 years old and 5 ft 8 in (1.73 meters) tall has had frequently recurring, severe, abdominal pain requiring medication for relief. Insulin is used daily for the control of diabetes mellitus. There has been a 15% reduction in weight below her desirable weight of 135 lb (61.3 kg) despite pancreatic exocrine supplementation.

Diagnosis: Chronic pancreatitis.

Impairment: 40% impairment due to chronic pancreatitis, which is to be combined with an appropriate value for the diabetes mellitus to determine the impairment of the whole person.

Comment: Both exocrine and endocrine functions of the pancreas have been impaired, and continuing treatment is required. The patient has been unable, despite treatment, to regain weight within 10% of the desirable level.

Example of Class 4 Impairment of the Whole Person:
A 47-year-old man first noted apathy, irritability, confusion, and "drunken behavior" six months ago. Total pancreatectomy and duodenectomy (Whipple procedure) subsequently were performed for an insulin-producing islet-cell tumor of the head of the pancreas. The patient now has a malabsorption syndrome with steatorrhea, partially controlled by pancreatic exocrine supplements. His diabetes is brittle and controlled only with difficulty by insulin.

Diagnosis: Pancreatic insufficiency subsequent to total pancreatectomy.

Impairment: 70% impairment due to pancreatic insufficiency, which is to be combined with an appropriate value for the diabetes mellitus to determine impairment of the whole person.

Comment: This patient's ability to perform normal activities has been seriously impaired by total loss of the pancreas, and his symptoms are controlled only partially by intensive therapy.

10.9 Hernias of the Abdominal Wall

Symptoms and signs of abdominal wall impairment include discomfort or pain at or near the site of herniation, typically intermittent and often associated with changes in posture or increased abdominal pressure; visible or palpable swelling or protrusion at the site of herniation, usually appearing and disappearing, depending on abdominal pressure; and more acute and intense pain of complication, notably incarceration and strangulation of the bowel. Incisional hernias can be unsightly; other symptoms, if any, tend to be related to the size of the hernia. Inguinal and femoral herniations are typically painful and entail a greater risk of grave complication. Most hernias of the abdominal wall are amenable to surgical correction.

Objective procedures useful in establishing impairment by hernias include, but are not limited to: 1) physical examination (most important), and 2) radiography, with or without the use of contrast agents.

Criteria for evaluating permanent impairment due to herniation of the abdominal wall are listed in Table 6.

Example of Class 1 Impairment of the Whole Person:
A 60-year-old woman required cholecystectomy three years ago for relief of calculous biliary tract disease. Her postoperative course was uneventful. The oblique, right upper quadrant wound healed but left a palpable defect in its medial extremity. There remains a slight, visible protrusion at this site when she rises from a supine position. She has no pain or discomfort in the region of the scar, which she perceives as unattractive.

Diagnosis: Uncomplicated incisional hernia.

Impairment: 0% impairment of the whole person.

Comment: The incisional hernia is asymptomatic and only mildly annoying to the patient. She is in no significant jeopardy of complication.

Example of Class 2 Impairment of the Whole Person:
For several years a 50-year-old man has been aware of a recurring protrusion in the right inguinal area when he exerts increased intra-abdominal pressure. The protru-

Table 6. Classes of Hernial Impairment

Class 1 0-5% Impairment of the Whole Person	Class 2 10-15% Impairment of the Whole Person	Class 3 20-30% Impairment of the Whole Person
Palpable defect in supporting structures of adominal wall; **and** Slight protrusion at site of defect with increased adominal pressure; readily reducible; **or** Occasional mild discomfort at site of defect, but not precluding normal activity.	Palpable defect in supporting structures of adominal wall; **and** Frequent or persistent protrusion at site of defect with increased abdominal pressure; still manually reducible; **or** Frequent discomfort, precluding heavy lifting, but not hampering normal activity.	Palpable defect in supporting structures of abdominal wall; **and** Persistent, irreducible, or irreparable protrusion at site of defect; **and** Limitation in normal activity.

sion has enlarged and entered the base of the scrotum but can be reduced painlessly. The patient has declined a recommended surgical repair, seemingly willing to accept the preclusion of heavy lifting. Otherwise, he maintains activities of daily living without discomfort.

Diagnosis: Reducible right indirect inguinal hernia.

Impairment: 10% impairment of the whole person.

Comment: The patient is functionally limited but chooses to live with his limitation. He has been made aware of the serious risk of an unrepaired inguinal hernia but nonetheless declines operation. His normally sedentary activities are not impaired.

Example of Class 3 Impairment of the Whole Person:
A 64-year-old man has had recurrent, bilateral inguinal hernias despite three previous attempts at repair: twice on the right and once on the left. The protrusions are partially reducible and give rise to only occasional discomfort. Fortunately, no complication has supervened. The patient is understandably reluctant to submit to further attempts at repair.

Diagnosis: Recurrent bilateral inguinal hernias, following unsuccessful herniorraphy.

Impairment: 30% impairment of the whole person.

Comment: Despite repeated surgical repair, the inguinal hernias have recurred bilaterally and are only partially reducible. The patient wears a supporting appliance. He is incapable of any lifting, and his activities of daily living are restricted.

References

1. Berk JE (ed): *Bockus' Gastroenterology.* Philadelphia, WB Saunders Co, 1985.

2. Sleisenger MH, Fordtran JS (eds): *Gastrointestinal Disease,* ed 3. Philadelphia, WB Saunders Co, 1983.

3. Schiff L, Schiff ER (eds): *Diseases of the Liver,* ed 6. Philadelphia, JB Lippincott, 1987.

4. Cecil R: *Cecil's Textbook of Medicine,* ed 17, Wyngaarden JB, Smith LH Jr (eds). Philadelphia, WB Saunders Co, 1985.

Chapter 11

The Urinary and Reproductive Systems

11.0 Introduction

This chapter provides criteria for evaluating the effects that permanent impairment of the urinary and/or reproductive systems has on the ability of an individual to perform the activities of daily living. The chapter discusses, in turn, (1) the upper urinary tract, and urinary diversions; (2) the bladder; (3) the urethra; (4) male reproductive organs; and (5) female reproductive organs.

Before using the information in this chapter, the reader is urged to review Chapters 1 and 2, which provide a general discussion of the purpose of the *Guides,* and of the situations in which they are useful; and which discuss techniques for the evaluation of the subject and for preparation of a report. The report should include the information found in the following outline, which is developed more fully in Chapter 2.

A. Medical Evaluation
1. Narrative history of medical conditions
2. Results of the most recent clinical evaluation
3. Assessment of current clinical status and statement of future plans
4. Diagnoses and clinical impressions
5. Expected date of full or partial recovery

B. Analysis of Findings
1. Impact of medical condition(s) on life activities
2. Explanation for concluding that the medical condition(s) has or has not become static or well-stabilized

3. Explanation for concluding that the individual is or is not likely to suffer from sudden or subtle incapacitation
4. Explanation for concluding that the individual is or is not likely to suffer injury or further impairment by engaging in life activities or by attempting to meet personal, social, and occupational demands
5. Explanation for concluding that accommodations and/or restrictions are or are not warranted

C. Comparison of Results of Analysis with Impairment Criteria
1. Description of clinical findings, and how these findings relate to specific criteria in the chapter
2. Explanation of each percent of impairment rating
3. Summary list of all impairment ratings
4. Overall rating of impairment of the whole person

11.1 Upper Urinary Tract

The parenchyma of the kidneys produces urine, which is conducted by the renal calyces, pelves, and ureters to the urinary bladder. The kidney is an important homeostatic regulatory organ. The manner in which renal and conduit abnormalities may affect the whole person can range from a clinically undetectable homeostatic change, to marked specific and generalized manifestations of deterioration of nephron reserve and urine transport.

Symptoms and signs of impairment of function of the upper urinary tract: These may include changes in micturition; edema; impairment of physical stamina; loss of weight and appetite; anemia; uremia; loin, abdominal, or costovertebral angle pain; chills and fever; hypertension and its complications; abnormalities in the appearance of the urine or its sediments; and biochemical changes in the blood. Renal disease may be revealed only on the basis of laboratory investigation.

Objective techniques useful in evaluating function of the upper urinary tract: Two clinically useful determinations of renal function, the renal clearance of endogenous creatinine and the 15-minute intravenous phenolsulfonphthalein (PSP) test, can ordinarily serve as guidelines for evaluating function of the upper urinary tract.

The glomerular filtration rate, which measures renal clearance of endogenous creatinine, gives a quantitative estimate of the total functioning nephron population. The reliability of clearance tests of renal function is improved by longer periods of urine collection; therefore, measurement of the 24-hour endogenous creatinine clearance should be used. The normal ranges of creatinine clearance are 130 to 200 liters/24 hr (90 to 139 ml/min) in men, and 115 to 180 liters/24 hr (80 to 125 ml/min) in women.

The 15-minute intravenous PSP test, although affected by stasis in conduit transport of urine, is a clinically useful determination of the general adequacy of renal tubular transport mechanisms. For the test to be valid, the patient must be adequately hydrated and precisely 1 cc of solution containing 6.0 mg of PSP must be injected intravenously, preferably by tuberculin syringe. The normal dye excretion is 25% or more in the urine within 15 minutes.

If there are any discrepancies in these two tests, that is, if the glomerular filtration rate is out of proportion to the PSP test, indicating tubular-glomerular imbalance, then it may be desirable to perform additional investigations, such as metabolic studies, serum and urine biochemical determinations, osmolalities, concentration and dilution tests, urinalyses, cultures, radiographic investigations, isotope renograms, and scans. Assessment of parenchymal disfigurement and/or conduit abnormality, which by virtue of clinical manifestations impair the function of the whole person, may require such diagnostic procedures as endoscopy with study of both or of individual kidneys, biopsy, arteriography, and uroradiography.

Criteria for Evaluating Impairment of the Upper Urinary Tract

In most instances of stable loss of upper urinary tract function, diminution in creatinine clearance is commensurate with depression of PSP excretion. If a discrepancy exists between these two tests, then additional diagnostic studies should be performed to determine which test is most representative of the loss of upper urinary tract function, and the results of that test should be used in determining the degree of impairment.

From a physiologic point of view, an individual with a solitary kidney may have no actual impairment of renal function; nevertheless, with that condition there exists an absence or loss of the normal safety factor that may be of potential significance in evaluating impairment, depending on the cause of the condition. The individual with a solitary kidney, regardless of cause, should be rated as having 10% impairment of the whole person because of a structural loss of an essential organ. This value is to be combined with any other permanent impairment, including any impairment in the remaining kidney, to determine the individual's impairment.

Deterioration of renal function requiring either peritoneal dialysis or hemodialysis would indicate severe impairment in the range of Class 4 Impairment, or 65% to 90% (see below). Successful renal transplantation may result in marked improvement of renal function, to the level of Class 2 Impairment, or 15% to 30%. However, transplant recipients require continuous observation and medication, which may add to their impairment. For this reason, and at the discretion of the evaluating physician, 0% to 5% may be added to the figure for impairment of renal function. Furthermore, impairment from complications of the disease or therapy, such as Cushingoid changes and osteoporosis, must be evaluated as they arise and combined with the renal impairment rating. Combining of ratings should be done as prescribed in the Combined Values Chart.

Class 1—Impairment of the Whole Person, 0-10%: A patient belongs in Class 1 when (a) diminution of upper urinary tract function is present, as evidenced by creatinine clearance of 75 to 90 liters/24 hr (52 to 62.5 ml/min) or PSP excretion of 15% to 20% in 15 minutes; *or* (b) intermittent symptoms and signs of upper urinary tract dysfunction are present that do not require continuous treatment or surveillance.

Example 1: When a 22-year-old man was 12 years of age, he developed backache, fever, hematuria, headache, and hypertension during an epidemic of [β]-hemolytic streptococcal tonsilitis. He was edematous and oliguric, and renal functions were depressed. The urine contained numerous red blood cells and red blood cell casts, and he passed 2.4 gm protein per 24 hours. The creatinine clearance was 72 liters/24 hr (50 ml/min).

After a severe illness with a long convalescence, the man improved and was well except for microscopic hematuria, which persisted for months but finally cleared. Six months after the illness, the creatinine clearance was 130 liters/24 hr (90 ml/min).

Current studies reveal a healthy man with no evidence of renal disease by biopsy and a creatinine clearance of 158 liters/24 hr (110 ml/min).

Diagnosis: Healthy man with kidneys that are completely recovered from poststreptococcal acute glomerulonephritis.

Impairment: 0% impairment of the whole person.

Example 2: A 40-year-old man had an acute episode of renal colic and later passed a small stone. He had two prior episodes of colic with spontaneous passage of stones. Urograms were interpreted as normal; no evidence of metabolic disease was present. Urine, creatinine clearance, and PSP determinations were within normal limits.

Diagnosis: Recurrent ureteral calculi.

Impairment: 5% impairment of the whole person.

Class 2—Impairment of the Whole Person, 15-30%:
A patient belongs in Class 2 when (a) dimunition of upper urinary tract function is present, as evidenced by creatinine clearance of 60 to 75 liters/24 hr (42 to 52 ml/min) or PSP excretion of 10% to 15% in 15 minutes; *or* (b) although creatinine clearance is greater than 75 liters/24 hr (52 ml/min), and PSP excretion is more than 15% in 15 minutes, symptoms and signs of upper urinary tract disease or dysfunction necessitate continuous surveillance and frequent treatment.

Example 1: A 45-year-old man with a history of nephritis as a child underwent an emergency appendectomy and drainage of an appendiceal abscess. Despite an adequate urinary output during the postoperative period, the serum creatinine rose to 2.8 mg/100 ml. Convalescence was prolonged; his anemia subsided gradually and physical stamina returned slowly.

Now, six months postoperatively, the patient feels well and is able to engage in most of his usual daily activities. The urine shows a trace of protein (0.75 gm/24 hr). Excretory urograms show no architectural abnormality, but the creatinine clearances range from 60 to 70 liters/24 hr (42 to 49 ml/min), and the PSP excretion ranges between 15% and 20% in 15 minutes.

Diagnosis: Asymptomatic persistent proteinuria as a result of childhood nephritis aggravated by surgery.

Impairment: 15% impairment of the whole person.

Example 2: A 50-year-old woman had a successful operation for parathyroid adenoma. However, she continues to have periodic attacks of pyelonephritis occasioned by residual calculi in both kidneys and she passes stones sporadically. The infrequent clinical attacks of pyelonephritis respond to antibiotics. The symptoms of her urinary tract infection are controlled by continuous medication. The creatinine clearance is stable at approximately 65 liters/24 hr (45 ml/min) and the PSP excretion at 10% in 15 minutes. The bilateral pyelocalyceal deformities and the size of the kidneys, as delineated by excretory urography, have not changed appreciably in a three-year period.

Diagnosis: Renal calculi and bilateral chronic pyelonephritis.

Impairment: 30% impairment due to upper urinary tract impairment, which is to be combined with an appropriate value for parathyroid impairment to determine the impairment of the whole person.

Example 3: A 52-year-old man had surgical reconstruction of his left lower ureter because of severe damage to its function from retroperitoneal fibrosis. Despite apparently normal architecture and function of the kidney on the side of the ureteral repair, vesicoureteral reflux can be demonstrated, and repeated attacks of pyelonephritis occur whenever antibacterial medication is discontinued. The creatinine clearance is 100 liters/24 hr (69 ml/min), and the PSP excretion is 25% in 15 minutes. Since the involved kidney is normal in appearance and shows no deterioration of function, no further surgical intervention is contemplated.

Diagnosis: Active, unilateral, chronic pyelonephritis, secondary to vesicoureteral reflux.

Impairment: 15% impairment of the whole person.

Example 4: A 28-year-old man with progressive chronic glomerulonephritis developed marked azotemia and oliguria requiring hemodialysis. Successful renal transplantation from his mother resulted in good renal function with creatinine clearance of 108 liters/24 hr. The patient is maintained on immuran and prednisone, requiring close observation for possible development of osteroporosis of the hip. The immunosuppression also increases the possibility of severe secondary infections.

Diagnosis: Functioning renal transplant.

Impairment: 25% impairment of the whole person due to renal disease and the need for continuous medication.

Comment: Should complications develop because of the therapy, the patient should be re-evaluated and the permanent impairment from the complications should be combined with the above impairment rating.

Class 3—Impairment of the Whole Person, 35-60%:

A patient belongs in Class 3 when (a) diminution of upper urinary tract function is present, as evidenced by creatinine clearance of 40 to 60 liters/24 hr (28 to 42 ml/min) or PSP excretion of 5% to 10% in 15 minutes; *or* (b) although creatinine clearance is 60 to 75 liters/24 hr (42 to 52 ml/min), and PSP excretion is 10% to 15% in 15 minutes, symptoms and signs of upper urinary tract disease or dysfunction are incompletely controlled by surgical or continuous medical treatment.

Example 1: A 52-year-old woman complained of chronic fatigue. On examination, she was found to have elevation of the serum creatinine and a moderate anemia. There was no clear-cut history of nephritis. A renal biopsy demonstrated diffuse proliferative glomerulonephritis. A high-dose excretory urogram delineated contracted kidneys with normal pyelocalyceal architecture. Results of urine culture were negative; creatinine clearance was 50 liters/24 hr (35 ml/min), and PSP excretion was 10% in 15 minutes.

Diagnosis: Chronic glomerulonephritis with contracted kidneys.

Impairment: 60% impairment due to upper urinary tract impairment, which is to be combined, using the Combined Values Chart, with an appropriate value for the anemia to determine the impairment of the whole person.

Example 2: A 48-year-old man has calculi in the minor calyces of both kidneys. He has a history of multiple endoscopic and open surgical procedures for stone removal. He has marked diminution in the size of one kidney and bilateral pyelographic architectural changes as a result of previous surgical procedures and recurrent pyelonephritis. Despite continuous antibacterial medication, the urine remains infected, and periodic episodes of chills, fever, and back pain occur. Creatinine clearance is 65 liters/24 hr (45 ml/min) and PSP excretion is 10% in 15 minutes.

Diagnosis: Renal calculi with bilateral recurrent pyelonephritis.

Impairment: 50% impairment of the whole person.

Example 3: A 48-year-old man was injured in an automobile crash and developed hematuria. Blood pressure was 150/90 mm Hg. Radiologic studies revealed that the left kidney was damaged. No other abnormalities were noted. The man was kept at bed rest in a hospital for a week and then discharged.

Six months later, the man began to complain of severe headaches. The blood pressure was found to be 240/160 mm Hg, and malignant hypertensive retinopathy was noted. Investigation revealed a creatinine clearance of 40 liters/24 hr (28 ml/min) and definite evidence of left renovascular hypertension. The left kidney was removed. Biopsies from the right kidney revealed malignant hypertensive changes. The histology of the left kidney revealed ischemia and juxtaglomerular hypertrophy.

Immediately after surgery, the patient's blood pressure fell to 170/110 mm Hg and, during the next six months, it leveled off at 155/95 mm Hg. The eyegrounds regressed to Grade II (Keith-Wagner classification), and creatinine clearance rose slowly to level off at 58 liters/24 hr (40 ml/min).

Diagnosis: Left nephrectomy for malignant hypertension due to post-traumatic renovascular ischemia of the left kidney; arteriolonephrosclerosis of the right kidney; and hypertensive vascular disease.

Impairment: 55% impairment due to arteriolonephrosclerosis and 10% impairment due to nephrectomy, which combine to 60% impairment of the urinary system; this should be combined with an appropriate value for the cardiovascular impairment to determine impairment of the whole person.

Class 4—Impairment of the Whole Person, 65-90%:

A patient belongs in Class 4 when (a) diminution of upper urinary tract function is present, as evidenced by creatinine clearance below 40 liters/24 hr (28 ml/min) or PSP excretion below 5% in 15 minutes; *or* (b) although creatinine clearance is 40 to 60 liters/24 hr (28 to 42 ml/min), and PSP excretion is 5% to 10% in 15 minutes, symptoms and signs of upper urinary tract disease or dysfunction persist, despite surgical or continuous medical treatment.

Example 1: A 44-year-old man with a family history of polycystic renal disease experienced sudden loin pain and noted gross hematuria. During two years preceding the acute episode, the man's serum creatinine rose from 8 mg/100 ml to 10 mg/100 ml, and he was maintained on a protein-restricted diet. Until the episode he was working regularly and was relatively asymptomatic.

Examination now discloses that the creatinine clearance is 35 liters/24 hr (24 ml/min), and the PSP excretion is less than 5% in 15 minutes. Endoscopy and retrograde urograms show bilateral deformities characteristic of polycystic kidneys.

Table 1. Classes of Upper Urinary Tract Impairment*

Class 1 0-10% Impairment of the Whole Person	Class 2 15-30% Impairment of the Whole Person	Class 3 35-60% Impairment of the Whole Person	Class 4 65-90% Impairment of the Whole Person
Diminution of upper urinary tract function is present as evidenced by creatinine clearance of 75 to 90 liters/24 hr (52 to 62.5 ml/min), or PSP excretion of 15% to 20% in 15 minutes.	Diminution of upper urinary tract function is present as evidenced by creatinine clearance of 60 to 75 liters/24 hr (42 to 52 ml/min), or PSP excretion of 10% to 15% in 15 minutes.	Diminution of upper urinary tract function is present as evidenced by creatinine clearance of 40 to 60 liters/24 hr (28 to 42 ml/min), or PSP excretion of 5% to 10% in 15 minutes.	Diminution of upper urinary tract function is present as evidenced by creatinine clearance below 40 liters/24 hr (28 ml/min), or PSP excretion below 5% in 15 minutes.
or	**or**	**or**	**or**
Intermittent symptoms and signs of upper urinary tract dysfunction are present that do not require continuous treatment or surveillance.	Although creatinine clearance is greater than 75 liters/24 hr (52 ml/min), or PSP excretion is more than 15% in 15 minutes, symptoms and signs of upper urinary tract disease or dysfunction necessitate continuous surveillance and frequent treatment.	Although creatinine clearance is 60 to 75 liters/24 hr (42 to 52 ml/min), or PSP excretion is 10% to 15% in 15 minutes, symptoms and signs of upper urinary tract disease or dysfunction are incompletely controlled by surgical or continuous medical treatment.	Although creatinine clearance is 40 to 60 liters/24 hr (28 to 42 ml/min), or PSP excretion is 5% to 10% in 15 minutes, symptoms and signs of upper urinary tract disease or dysfunction persists despite surgical or continuous medical treatment.

*Note: The individual with a solitary kidney, regardless of cause, should be rated as having 10% impairment of the whole person. This value is to be combined with any other permanent impairment (including any impairment in the remaining kidney) pertinent to the case under consideration. The normal ranges of creatinine clearance are: Males: 130 to 200 liters/24 hr (90 to 139 ml/min). Females: 115 to 180 liters/24 hr (80 to 125 ml/min). The normal PSP excretion is 25% or more in urine in 15 minutes.

Diagnosis: Bilateral polycystic renal disease; advanced renal insufficiency.

Impairment: 70% impairment of the whole person.

Example 2: A young woman became anuric following severe abruptio placentae. A percutaneous renal biopsy was performed. Diagnosis was renal cortical necrosis, and periodic courses of peritoneal dialyses were instituted. After 49 days of anuria and then oliguria, the urine output increased; on the 60th day the serum creatinine, which was 22 mg/100 ml, began to fall without peritoneal dialysis. Four months after the episode of anuria, the patient performs most of the activities of daily living despite severely compromised renal function. The creatinine clearance has leveled off at 11.5 liters/24 hr (8 ml/min).

Diagnosis: Renal cortical necrosis; severe chronic renal failure.

Impairment: 90% impairment of the whole person.

Example 3: A 56-year-old woman with chronic progressive glomerulonephritis is severely anemic, azotemic and oliguric and requires hemodialysis twice weekly. For one or two days after treatment she feels well and is able to perform household duties. On the days just prior to dialysis she is nauseated, lethargic, and edematous.

Diagnosis: Severe chronic renal failure.

Impairment: 90% impairment of the whole person.

This classification of upper urinary tract impairment is recapitulated in Table 1.

Urinary Diversion

Permanent, surgically-created forms of urinary diversion usually are provided to compensate for anatomic loss and to allow for egress of urine. They are evaluated as a part of, and in conjunction with, the assessment of the involved portion of the urinary tract.

Irrespective of how well these diversions function in the preservation of renal integrity and the disposition of urine, the following values for the diversions should be combined with those determined under the criteria previously given for the portion of the urinary tract involved:

Type of Diversion	% Impairment of the Whole Person
Uretero-Intestinal	10
Cutaneous Ureterostomy without Intubation	10
Nephrostomy or Intubated Ureterostomy	15

Example 1: A 56-year-old man with bilateral nephrostomies because of obliterative fibrotic ureteral disease had removal of renal calculi. An attempt to reconstitute normal conduit function through surgery

was unsuccessful. Urinary infection cannot be eradicated, and the patient complains mildly of hematuria when the nephrostomy tubes are changed and of occasional episodes of fever and flank pain. He continues to engage in most activities of daily living. The creatinine clearance is approximately 50 liters/24 hr (35 ml/min) and the PSP excretion is between 5% and 10% in 15 minutes.

Diagnosis: Pyeloureteral disease requiring bilateral nephrostomy diversion.

Impairment: 65% impairment due to pyeloureteral disease and 15% impairment due to bilateral nephrostomies, which combine to give 70% impairment of the whole person.

Example 2: A 52-year-old woman, seven years after anterior pelvic exenteration and uretero-ileostomy for carcinoma of the cervix, has no evidence of recurrent cancer. She has had calculi removed from both kidneys and she experiences periodic episodes of pyelonephritis even on continual medication. Radiographic changes suggesting pyelonephritis are present. The creatinine clearance is approximately 60 liters/24 hr (24 ml/min) and PSP excretion is about 10% in 15 minutes.

Diagnosis: Uretero-ileostomy urinary diversion and chronic bilateral pyelonephritis.

Impairment: 65% impairment due to bilateral pyelonephritis, 10% impairment due to uretero-ileostomy, and 55% impairment due to pelvic exenteration, that is, excision of bladder, lower ureters, uterus, cervix, vagina, fallopian tubes, and ovaries, which combine to 85% impairment of the whole person.

11.2 Bladder

The bladder is a voluntary controllable reservoir for urine that normally permits the patient to retain urine for several hours.

Symptoms and signs of impairment of function of the bladder: These may include urinary frequency, painful voiding (dysuria), urgency, incontinence, involuntary retention of urine, hematuria, pyuria, crystalluria, passage of urinary calculi, and a suprapubic mass.

Objective techniques useful in evaluating function of the bladder: These include, but are not limited to, cystoscopy, cystography, voiding cystourethrography, cystometry, uroflometry, urinalysis, and urine cultures.

Criteria for Evaluating Permanent Impairment of the Bladder

When evaluating permanent impairment of the bladder, the status of the upper urinary tract must also be considered. The appropriate impairment values for both should be combined using the Combined Values Chart in order to determine the extent of impairment of the whole person.

Class 1—Impairment of the Whole Person, 0-10%: A patient belongs in Class 1 when the patient has symptoms and signs of bladder disorder requiring intermittent treatment with normal function between episodes of malfunction.

Example: A 41-year-old woman was treated with radium 20 years ago for uterine fibroids. Recent episodes of urinary bleeding due to postradiation telangiectasia of the bladder required emergency hospitalization and vessel fulguration under anesthesia. The episodes occurred at intervals of from one to two weeks to six months. Between attacks, findings from blood and urine studies were normal. After each episode the patient was able to resume usual activities within seven days.

Diagnosis: Postradiation telangiectasia of the bladder.

Impairment: 10% impairment of the whole person.

Class 2—Impairment of the Whole Person, 15-20%: A patient belongs in Class 2 when (a) there are symptoms and/or signs of bladder disorder requiring continuous treatment; *or* (b) there is good bladder reflex activity, but no voluntary control.

Example 1: A 47-year-old man developed such progressive urinary frequency that he was voiding at intervals of every 10 to 15 minutes day and night. A diagnosis of interstitial cystitis was established, but the usual treatment, bladder dilation with various agents, was ineffective. The upper urinary tract was normal and uninfected. After a ureterosigmoidostomy the man was able to resume his usual activities.

Diagnosis: Contracted, fixed bladder requiring urinary diversion.

Impairment: 15% impairment due to contracted fixed bladder and 10% impairment due to ureterosigmoidostomy, which combine to 24% impairment of the whole person.

Note: The removal of the bladder for any reason and a resultant urinary diversion should be assigned a similar rating of impairment, that is, one of about 24%.

Example 2: A 42-year-old man with chronic renal infection resistant to antibiotic therapy developed a severe cystitis requiring him to empty his bladder at intervals of less than 30 minutes and making necessary his use of a urine collection device. His general physical condition was excellent; his urine contained numerous white blood cells and a few red blood cells.

The man refused urinary diversion through a surgical procedure. As a result, he cannot retain his urine long enough to permit him to perform many activities of daily living.

Diagnosis: Chronic cystitis.

Impairment: 20% impairment due to cystitis, which is to be combined with an appropriate value for the upper urinary tract disorder to determine the impairment of the whole person.

Class 3—Impairment of the Whole Person, 25-35%:
A patient belongs in Class 3 when the bladder has poor reflex activity, that is, there is intermittent dribbling, and no voluntary control.

Class 4—Impairment of the Whole Person, 40-60%:
A patient belongs in Class 4 when there is no reflex or voluntary control of the bladder, that is, there is continuous dribbling.

11.3 Urethra

In the female, the urethra is a urinary conduit containing a voluntary urethral sphincter. In the male, the urethra is a conduit for urine and seminal ejaculations that possesses a voluntary urethral sphincter and propulsive musculature.

Symptoms and signs of impairment of function of the urethra: These include dysuria, diminished urinary stream, urinary retention, incontinence, extraneous or ectopic openings, periurethral mass or masses, and diminished urethral caliber.

Objective techniques useful in evaluating function of the urethra: These include, but are not limited to, urethroscopy, urethrography, cystourethrography, endoscopy, urethrometry, and cystometrography.

Criteria for Evaluating Permanent Impairment of the Urethra

When evaluating permanent impairment of the urethra, one must also consider the status of the upper urinary tract and bladder. The values for all parts of the urinary system should be combined using the Combined Values Chart to determine the extent of impairment of the whole person.

Class 1—Impairment of the Whole Person, 0-5%:
A patient belongs in Class 1 when symptoms and signs of urethral disorder are present that require intermittent therapy for control.

Example: As a result of an injury, a 27-year-old man has a urethral stricture that requires dilation every few weeks. Between dilation he is free of symptoms, and he has difficulty only when the urethra gradually constricts, when he notices increasing difficulty in voiding. There is no upper urinary tract infection.

Diagnosis: Traumatic urethral stricture.

Impairment: 5% impairment of the whole person.

Class 2—Impairment of the Whole Person, 10-20%:
A patient belongs in Class 2 when there are symptoms and signs of a urethral disorder that cannot be effectively controlled by treatment.

Example 1: A 23-year-old man experienced considerable laceration of the ventral surface of the penis that created a surgically uncorrectable fistula. He was able to perform most of the activities of daily living, but could not void normally. He could ejaculate with sexual sensation, but the fistula was so situated that impregnation of his wife was impossible.

Diagnosis: Urethral fistula.

Impairment: 15% impairment due to urethral fistula and 10% impairment due to impaired sexual function, which combine to 24% impairment of the whole person.

Example 2: After an automobile crash, a 31-year-old man experienced a urethral stricture that necessitated weekly or biweekly urethral dilations. Because of the magnitude of the injury to the urethra, corrective surgery was ineffective. Repeated urinary tract infections secondary to urethral dilations continued to occur, and pyelonephritis developed. The man's creatinine clearance is 65 liters/24 hr (45 ml/min), and PSP excretion is 10% in 15 minutes.

Diagnosis: Traumatic urethral stricture with chronic pyelonephritis.

Impairment: 20% impairment due to urethral stricture and 25% impairment due to upper urinary tract damage, which combine to 40% impairment of the whole person.

Example 3: A 21-year-old factory worker was crushed between a lift and a wall. His bony pelvis was fractured, his urethra was totally severed at the apex of the prostate, and his perineum was severely lacerated. Immediate reconstructive urethral surgery was unsuccessful, and one year after the injury a ureterosigmoidostomy was necessary, which resulted in hydronephrosis of the right kidney and repeated urinary tract infections. Later, this diversion was converted to a conduit, and renal infection occurred only sporadically thereafter. The

At present, the worker is totally impotent. The pelvic fracture is healed and there is no evidence of musculoskeletal impairment, but because of occasional urinary tract infections the man periodically is unable to perform some activities of daily living. Creatinine clearance is 70 liters/24 hr (49 ml/min).

Diagnosis: Severed urethra, hydronephrosis with recurring urinary tract infections, and impotency.

Impairment: 20% impairment due to severed urethra, 30% impairment due to upper urinary tract impairment, 10% impairment due to uretero-ileostomy, and 30% impairment due to loss of sexual function, which combine to 65% impairment of the whole person.

11.4 Male Reproductive Organs

The male reproductive organs include the penis, scrotum, testes, epididymides, spermatic cords, prostate, and seminal vesicles. The values of impairment of the male reproductive organs are given in the following sections for men 40 to 65 years of age. These values may be increased by 50% of a given value for those below the age of 40 years, and decreased by 50% for those over the age of 65 years. For instance, a 50% increase of a 20% impairment equals a 30% impairment.

11.4a Penis

The penis has sexual functions of erection and ejaculation, and urinary functions. The latter are discussed in the section on urethra.

Symptoms and signs of impairment of function of the penis: These include abnormalities of erection and sensation, and partial or complete penile loss.

Criteria for Evaluating Permanent Impairment of the Penis

When evaluating impairment of the penis, it is necessary to consider impairment of both the sexual and the urinary functions. The degree of impairment of sexual function should be determined in accordance with the criteria that follow, and it should be combined with the appropriate value for an impairment of urinary function that is present to determine the impairment of the whole person.

Class 1—Impairment of the Whole Person, 5-10%: A patient belongs in Class 1 when sexual function is possible, but there are varying degrees of difficulty of erection, ejaculation, and/or sensation.

Example: A 32-year-old man suffered a compressive injury to the penile shaft. Healing occurred with partial cicatrization of the left mid corpus cavernosum. Bowstring curvature to the left occurs during erections. Sensation and ejaculation are normal, but pain results if intercourse is not very carefully consummated.

Diagnosis: Fibrosis of left mid corpus cavernosum, post-traumatic.

Impairment: 10% impairment of the whole person, which takes into consideration the patient's age.

Class 2—Impairment of the Whole Person, 10-15%: A patient belongs in Class 2 when sexual function is possible and there is sufficient erection, BUT ejaculation and sensation are absent.

Example: A 28-year-old man suffered a fractured pelvis with wide separation of the symphysis pubis, perivesical and periprostatic hematomas, and a tear of the prostatomembranous urethra. These injuries responded well to reparative surgery, and there was no subsequent urinary difficulty. Erection and intercourse are possible, but sexual sensation and ejaculation are absent.

Diagnosis: Post-traumatic urethral and genital insufficiency.

Impairment: 15% impairment of the whole person, which includes consideration for the patient's age.

Class 3—Impairment of the Whole Person, 20%: A patient belongs in Class 3 when no sexual function is possible.

Example: An 18-year-old boy suffered traumatic dislocation of the penis. Corporal repair and urethroplasty have preserved genital appearance and urethral function, but erection is not possible.

Diagnosis: Post-traumatic vascular and neurological penile insufficiency.

Impairment: 30% impairment of the whole person, which considers the patient's age.

11.4b Scrotum

The scrotum covers, protects, and provides a suitable environment for the testes.

Symptoms and signs of impairment of function of the scrotum: These include pain, enlargement, lack of testicular mobility, and inappropriate location of the testes.

Objective techniques useful in evaluating function of the scrotum: These include, but are not limited to, observation, palpation, and testicular examination.

Criteria for Evaluating Permanent Impairment of the Scrotum

Class 1—Impairment of the Whole Person, 0-5%: A patient belongs in Class 1 when there are symptoms and signs of scrotal loss or disease and there is no evidence of testicular malfunction, although there may be testicular malposition.

Example: A 38-year-old man had an injury resulting in loss of all scrotal skin. Split-thickness skin graft reconstructions gave a good cosmetic result. At present, there is no evidence of testicular malfunction, but testicular mobility is affected, and the patient experiences discomfort during exercise and in certain positions.

Diagnosis: Ablation of scrotal skin; split-thickness skin graft reconstruction of the scrotum.

Impairment: 5% impairment of the whole person, which includes due consideration of the patient's age.

Class 2—Impairment of the Whole Person, 10-15%: A patient belongs in Class 2 when (a) there are symptoms and signs of architectural alteration or disease such that the testes must be implanted in other than a scrotal position to preserve testicular function, and pain or discomfort is present with activity; OR (b) there is total loss of the scrotum.

Example: A 50-year-old man suffered extensive burns of the lower extremities, genitals, and abdomen. Skin grafting to the abdomen and lower extremities was satisfactory; however, it was necessary to transplant the testicles to the thighs to permit adequate skin coverage of the scrotal area.

Diagnosis: Burn ablation of the scrotum.

Impairment: 15% impairment of the whole person.

11.4c Testes, Epididymides, and Spermatic Cords

The testes produce spermatozoa, synthesize male steroid hormones, and provide the appearance and psychological badge of maleness. The epididymides and spermatic cords transport the spermatozoa.

Symptoms and signs of impairment of function of the testes, epididymides, and spermatic cords: These include local or referred pain; tenderness and change in size, contour, position, and texture; and abnormalities of testicular hormones and seminalfluid.

Objective techniques useful in evaluating function of the testes, epididymides, and spermatic cords: These include, but are not limited to, vasography; lymphangiography, spermatic arteriography and venography; biopsy; semen analysis; and studies of follicle-stimulating, ketosteroid, and hydroxysteroid hormones.

Criteria for Evaluating Permanent Impairment of Testes, Epididymides, and Spermatic Cords

Class 1—Impairment of the Whole Person, 0-5%: A patient belongs in Class 1 when (a) symptoms and signs of testicular, epididymal, and/or spermatic cord disease are present and there is anatomic alteration; *and* (b) continuous treatment is not required; *and* (c) there are no abnormalities of seminal or hormonal function; *or* (d) a solitary testis is present.

Example: A 36-year-old man has had repeated episodes of epididymo-orchitis due to recurrent prostatitis. He has symptoms of discomfort between attacks and clinical evidence of chronic epididymitis. He does not desire vas deferens ligation, because his seminal fluid is normal and he may desire additional children.

Diagnosis: Chronic epididymitis secondary to chronic prostatitis.

Impairment: 5% impairment due to epididymitis and 5% impairment due to prostatitis, taking into consideration the patient's age, which combine to give 10% impairment of the whole person.

Class 2—Impairment of the Whole Person, 10-15%: A patient belongs in Class 2 when (a) symptoms and signs of testicular, epididymal and/or spermatic cord disease are present and there is anatomic alteration; *and* (b) frequent or continuous treatment is required; *and* (c) there are detectable seminal or hormonal abnormalities.

Example: A 33-year-old man had evidence of interference with testicular blood supply after trauma, experiencing acute onset of swelling of the testes, hydrocele formation, and intense pain. One testis atrophied, and the other diminished in size. Procreative efforts, previously successful in producing offspring, were unavailing. At present, there are no systemic hormonal changes, but semen analysis reveals oligospermia.

Diagnosis: Testicular atrophy and oligospermia.

Impairment: 15% impairment of the whole person, which includes due consideration for the patient's age.

Class 3—Impairment of the Whole Person, 15-20%: A patient belongs in Class 3 when trauma or disease produces bilateral anatomical loss, or there is no detectable seminal or hormonal function of the testes, epididymides, or spermatic cords.

Example: A 17-year-old boy was injured by a farm machine, sustaining amputation of the scrotum and its contents.

Diagnosis: Traumatic gonadal ablation.

Impairment: 30% impairment due to gonadal ablation and 23% impairment due to scrotal loss, which include due consideration for the patient's young age, and 5% impairment due to lack of an endocrine gland; all values combine to give 49% impairment of the whole person.

11.4d Prostate and Seminal Vesicles

The prostate and seminal vesicles are involved with transport, nutritional modification, and maintenance of adequate environment for spermatozoa and semen. Impairment associated with urinary function is discussed in the section on urethra.

Symptoms and signs of impairment of function of the prostate and seminal vesicles: These may include local or referred pain; tenderness; changes in size and texture; disturbances in function of spermatic cords, epididymides and testes; oligospermia; hemospermia; and urinary abnormalities.

Objective techniques useful in evaluating function of the prostate and seminal vesicles: These include, but are not limited to, urography, endoscopy, ejaculatory duct catheterization, vasography, biopsy, and examination of prostatic excretions and of hormone excretion patterns.

Criteria for Evaluating Permanent Impairment of the Prostate and Seminal Vesicles

Class 1—Impairment of the Whole Person, 0-5%: A patient belongs in Class 1 when (a) there are symptoms and signs of prostatic and/or seminal vesicular dysfunction or disease; *and* (b) anatomic alteration is present; *and* (c) continuous treatment is not required.

Example: A 42-year-old man has had many episodes of acute prostatitis. He has episodes of mild perineal discomfort that occasionally require medication for pain.

Diagnosis: Chronic prostatitis with acute febrile episodes.

Impairment: 5% impairment of the whole person.

Class 2—Impairment of the Whole Person, 10-15%: A patient belongs in Class 2 when (a) frequent severe symptoms and signs of prostatic and/or seminal vesicular dysfunction or disease are present; *and* (b) anatomic alteration is present; *and* (c) continuous treatment is required.

Example: After drainage of a prostatic abscess, a 34-year-old man has continual symptoms and signs of prostatitis that he can tolerate only with the constant use of antibacterial medication.

Diagnosis: Recurrent acute and chronic prostatitis.

Impairment: 15% impairment of the whole person, which includes due consideration for the patient's age.

Class 3—Impairment of the Whole Person, 15-20%: A patient belongs in Class 3 when there has been ablation of the prostate and/or seminal vesicles.

11.5 Female Reproductive Organs

The female reproductive organs include the vulva, vagina, cervix, uterus, fallopian tubes, and ovaries. The degree of impairment of the female reproductive system is influenced by age, and especially by whether the woman is in the childbearing age group. The physiologic differences of premenopausal and postmenopausal women are considered in establishing the criteria in this chapter for evaluating the impairment of female reproductive organs.

11.5a Vulva-Vagina

The vulva has cutaneous, sexual, and urinary functions. The latter has been discussed in the section on the urethra. The vagina has a sexual function and serves as a birth passageway.

Symptoms and signs of impairment of function of the vulva-vagina: These include loss or altered sexual sensation; complete or partial absence; presence of vulvovaginitis, vulvitis, vaginitis, cicatrization, ulceration, stenosis, atrophy, hypertrophy, neoplasia, dysplasia, and/or spasm; difficulty with sexual intercourse, urination, and/or vaginal delivery; and secondary effects on underlying perineal structures.

Criteria for Evaluating Permanent Impairment of the Vulva-Vagina

Class 1—Impairment of the Whole Person, 0-10%:
A patient belongs in Class 1 when (a) symptoms and signs of disease or deformity of the vulva and/or vagina are present that do not require continuous treatment; *and* (b) sexual intercourse is possible; *and* (c) the vagina is adequate for childbirth during the premenopausal years.

Example: An obese 38-year-old married woman who has given vaginal birth to three living children experiences recurrent chronic dermatitis of the genitocrural area. At intervals, she requires treatment for intense pruritus and active dermatitis. Her discomfort is more marked during warm and humid weather. Laboratory cultures for fungal diseases are negative. The patient does not have diabetes. There is a remission of symptoms when her weight is controlled, when she avoids tight clothing, and when she observes careful hygienic measures. Sexual intercourse is possible if precautions are observed to avoid excessive vulvar irritation.

Diagnosis: Dermatitis of vulva, intertrigo.

Impairment: 0% impairment of the whole person.

Class 2—Impairment of the Whole Person, 15-25%:
A patient belongs in Class 2 when (a) symptoms and signs of disease or deformity of the vulva and/or vagina are present that require continuous treatment; *and* (b) sexual intercourse is possible with varying degrees of difficulty; *and* (c) during the premenopausal years, adequacy for vaginal delivery is limited.

Example: A 34-year-old married woman developed a rectovaginal fistula incidental to vaginal delivery of her second child. This was corrected surgically, but the woman developed severe vaginal stenosis. She required intermittent dilatation of the vagina under anesthesia and the continuous use of vaginal creams. These measures made sexual intercourse possible, but it was extremely painful and the patient lacked sexual sensation. A third pregnancy ended with cesarean section because vaginal delivery was deemed hazardous.

Diagnosis: Stenosis, vaginal, postoperative, severe.

Impairment: 20% impairment of the whole person, which includes due consideration for the patient's age.

Class 3—Impairment of the Whole Person, 30-35%:
A patient belongs in Class 3 when (a) symptoms and signs of disease or deformity of the vulva and/or vagina are present that are not controlled by treatment; *and* (b) sexual intercourse is not possible; *and* (c) during the premenopausal years, vaginal delivery is not possible.

Example: A para 2 30-year-old woman was injured in an automobile crash and suffered a severe traumatic laceration of the vagina, bladder, and rectum, leading to development of a vesicorecto-vaginal fistula. The vaginal depth was restricted to 2 cm, and a sinus tract 5 mm in diameter led to the cervix and provided escape for menstrual blood, feces, and urine. Sexual intercourse was impossible and pregnancy was deemed impossible. The recommended surgery was refused by the patient.

Diagnosis: Vesicorectovaginal fistula with partial absence of vagina.

Impairment: 35% impairment due to vaginal impairment, which includes consideration for the patient's age, and which is to be combined with appropriate values for the bladder and rectal impairments to determine the impairment of the whole person.

11.5b Cervix-Uterus

The cervix serves as a passageway for spermatozoa and menstrual blood, maintains closure of the uterus during pregnancy, and serves as a portion of the birth canal during vaginal delivery. The uterus is influenced during reproductive years by hormones that are elaborated by the ovaries. It serves as the organ of menstruation, a means of transportation of the spermatozoa, and the container of the products of fertilization. The uterus supplies the power for the first and third stages of labor and, in part, for the second stage.

Symptoms and signs of impairment of function of the cervix-uterus: These include abnormalities of menstruation, fertility, pregnancy, or labor; excessive size, stenosis, or atresia of the cervical canal; cervical incompetency during pregnancy; noncyclic hemorrhage; uterine displacement; dysplasia; and neoplasia.

Objective techniques useful in evaluating function of the cervix-uterus: These include, but are not limited to, cervical mucus studies; vaginal, cervical, and intra-uterine cytologic smears; biopsy; gas insufflation; probing and measuring with calibrated sounds; radiologic studies using radiopaque contrast media; blood and urine hormone studies; basal body temperature recordings; studies on sperm concentration, mobility, and viability; dilatation and curettage of the uterus; microscopic study of the endometrium; gynecography; culdoscopy; placental localization techniques; and intra-amniotic pressure studies.

Criteria for Evaluating Permanent Impairment of the Cervix-Uterus

Class 1—Impairment of the Whole Person, 0-10%:
A patient belongs in Class 1 when (a) symptoms and signs of disease or deformity of the cervix and/or uterus are present that do not require continuous treatment; *or* (b) cervical stenosis, if present, requires no treatment; *or* (c) there is anatomic loss of the cervix and/or uterus in the postmenopausal years.

Example 1: An obese 22-year-old married woman experienced menarche at age 14. Her menstrual cycles varied between 21 and 87 days until the age of 19, when they occurred between intervals of 26 to 40 days. Her menstrual periods averaged between two and three days, with no noncyclic bleeding. After medical treatment and good weight control, she reported her menstrual cycles became regular at 28 to 32-day intervals.

After 1½ years of marriage, during which no contraceptives were used, the woman became pregnant. During the second and third months of gestation, there was uterine bleeding that subsided with bed rest and medication. The pregnancy terminated spontaneously at 38 weeks with the delivery of a living infant weighing 2.6 kg (5 lb 12 oz). Menstrual periods after delivery averaged 32 days between cycles. Cytologic vaginal smears showed diminished hormone production. The uterus was small in size but normal in position and contour.

Diagnosis: Immature uterine development secondary to hormone deficiency.

Impairment: 0% impairment of the whole person.

Example 2: A 60-year-old married woman developed slight vaginal spotting of blood incidental to the lifting of heavy objects. Clinical examination disclosed no obvious pathologic lesion. The findings on cytologic, cervical, and vaginal smear studies were positive for malignant cells. On biopsy, carcinoma-in-situ was found. The cervix and uterine fundus were surgically removed.

Diagnosis: Carcinoma-in-situ of the cervix; absence of cervix and uterine fundus in a postmenopausal patient.

Impairment: 10% impairment of the whole person.

Class 2—Impairment of the Whole Person, 15-25%:
A patient belongs in Class 2 when (a) symptoms and signs of disease or deformity of the cervix and/or uterus are present that require continuous treatment; *or* (b) cervical stenosis, if present, requires periodic treatment.

Example: As the result of extensive cauterization of the cervix, a para 2 30-year-old woman developed partial stenosis of the cervix and incomplete retention of menstrual blood. Because of prolongation of menstruation and dysmenorrhea, cervical dilatation was necessary at two-month to four-month intervals. After two years, pregnancy occurred and resulted in the vaginal delivery of a healthy, full-term infant.

Diagnosis: Incomplete cervical stenosis.

Impairment: 15% impairment of the whole person.

Class 3—Impairment of the Whole Person, 30-35%:
A patient belongs in Class 3 when (a) symptoms and signs of disease or deformity of the cervix and/or uterus are present that are not controlled by treatment; *or* (b) cervical stenosis is complete; *or* (c) anatomic or complete functional loss of the cervix and/or uterus occurs in premenopausal years.

Example: As a result of a vaginal delivery, a 34-year-old woman suffered from severe prolapse of the uterus, which required surgical repair of the anterior and posterior vaginal walls, extensive amputation of the cervix, and posterior fixation of the uterus by plication of the broad ligaments. With careful management, three subsequent pregnancies were achieved, each of which ended in spontaneous abortion between 12 and 16 weeks' gestation, the result of premature dilation of the cervix. Objective evidence that there was almost no cervix indicated that a repair of the cervical incompetence was impossible.

Diagnosis: Partial absence of cervix; cervical incompetence.

Impairment: 30% impairment of the whole person.

11.5c Fallopian Tubes-Ovaries

The fallopian tubes transport ova and spermatozoa. The ovaries develop and release ova and elaborate female hormones.

Symptoms and signs of impairment of function of the fallopian tubes-ovaries: These include vaginal bleeding or discharge; stenosis of the tubes; abnormal morphology; pelvic mass; neoplasm; absent, infrequent, or abnormal ovulation; abnormal elaboration of hormones and menstrual dysfunction.

Objective techniques useful in evaluating function of the fallopian tubes-ovaries: These include, but are not limited to, air insufflation tests, cervical and vaginal cytologic smears, culdoscopy, pelvic roentgenography, hysterosalpingography, gynecography ovarian biopsy, blood and urine hormonal assays, and basal temperature studies.

Criteria for Evaluating Permanent Impairment of the Fallopian Tubes-Ovaries

Any associated endocrine impairment should be evaluated in accordance with criteria set forth in Chapter 12, The Endocrine System.

Class 1—Impairment of the Whole Person, 0-10%:
A patient belongs in Class 1 when (a) symptoms and signs of disease or deformity of the fallopian tubes and/or ovaries are present that do not require continuous treatment; *or* (b) only one fallopian tube and/or ovary is functioning in the premenopausal years; *or* (c) there is bilateral loss of function of the fallopian tubes and/or ovaries in the postmenopausal years.

Example: A 28-year-old married woman failed to become pregnant after six years of marriage, even though contraceptives were not used. Physical examination disclosed evidence of slight nodularity in the region of the fallopian tubes. Gas insufflation studies indicated partial stenosis of the tubes. Hysterosalpingography indicated tubal patency. After two years of treatment, the patient became pregnant and delivered a normal living infant.

Diagnosis: Partial stenosis of fallopian tubes.

Impairment: 5% impairment of the whole person.

Class 2—Impairment of the Whole Person, 15-25%:
A patient belongs in Class 2 when symptoms and signs of disease or deformity of the fallopian tubes and/or ovaries are present that require continuous treatment, but tubal patency persists and ovulation is possible.

Example: A 27-year-old para 2 woman developed generalized peritonitis following a rupture of the bowel incurred in an automobile crash. Because of the infection, she underwent a unilateral salpingo-oophorectomy. Subsequently, there was evidence of irregular and infrequent ovulation. Pelvic examination showed the presence of fibrous adhesions in the adnexal area. With treatment, ovulation and cyclic hormone elaboration occurred. A normal pregnancy ensued, resulting in the birth of a living infant. Continuous treatment was required to maintain a regular ovulatory cycle.

Diagnosis: Anovulatory menstruation; unilateral salpingo-oophorectomy.

Impairment: 15% impairment due to anovulatory menstruation and 10% impairment due to unilateral salpingo-oophorectomy, which combine to give 24% impairment of the whole person.

Class 3—Impairment of the Whole Person, 30-35%:
A patient belongs in Class 3 when (a) symptoms and signs of disease or deformity of the fallopian tubes and/or ovaries are present and there is total loss of tubal patency or total failure to produce ova in the premenopausal years; *or* (b) bilateral loss of the fallopian tubes and/or ovaries occurs in the premenopausal years.

Example: A 32-year-old mother of two children had severe pelvic infection. Diagnostic studies indicated total occlusion of the fallopian tubes at the level of the uterine cornu. A bilateral salpingectomy was performed.

Diagnosis: Bilateral salpingectomy.

Impairment: 30% impairment of the whole person.

References

1. Campbell MF: *Campbell's Urology,* ed 5, Walsh PC, Gittes RF, Perlmutter AD, Stamey TA (eds). Philadelphia, WB Saunders Co, 1986.

2. Glenn JF (ed): *Urologic Surgery,* ed 3. Philadelphia, JB Lippincott, 1983.

3. Danforth DN (ed): *Textbook of Obstetrics and Gynecology,* ed 5. Philadelphia, JB Lippincott, 1986.

Chapter 12

The Endocrine System

12.0 Introduction

The purpose of this chapter is to provide physicians with criteria they can use to evaluate permanent impairment of the endocrine system. The endocrine system is composed of the hypothalamic-pituitary complex, thyroid, parathyroids, adrenals, islet tissue of the pancreas, and gonads. The secretions of these ductless glands are hormones that regulate the activity of organs or tissues of the body. Examples of such regulation include control of growth, bone structure, sexual development and function, metabolism, and electrolyte balance. The various endocrine glands are usually interdependent, and a disorder of one gland may be reflected by dysfunction in one or more of the other endocrine glands which, in turn, may affect other body systems. This possibility should be considered when evaluating permanent impairment of the whole person.

Impairments involving the endocrine system usually result from altered hormonal secretion by one or more endocrine glands, or from the elaboration of hormonal substances by nonendocrine tissue. Dysfunction may be associated with morphologic changes in the endocrine gland or glands involved, such as atrophy, hypertrophy, hyperplasia, or neoplasia; or there may be no demonstrable morphologic changes.

The causes of abnormal secretion are not considered in this chapter; rather, the limitations that continued endocrine dysfunction places on the patient's efficiency in activities of daily living are considered.

Abnormal secretion of hormones usually can be corrected by treatment. When continuous treatment is necessary to maintain the patient, some degree of impairment may exist, even though the patient carries on most of the activities of daily living.

On the other hand, abnormal findings in other body systems may be associated with hypersecretion or hyposecretion of hormones, and some of these findings may persist indefinitely, even after therapy of the underlying hormonal dysfunction. Such impairment should be evaluated in accordance with criteria in the appropriate chapters, and, when appropriate, impairment ratings of other body systems should be combined with impairment ratings based on this chapter, using the Combined Values Chart to determine impairment of the whole person.

Neoplasms of the endocrine glands may produce nonhormonal permanent impairments manifested by pain or by effects involving other body systems. Such impairments should be evaluated with criteria set forth in the chapters concerning the respective body systems. It is recognized that, in addition to the abnormalities discussed in this chapter, others may occur that involve the endocrine system. If such abnormalities produce permanent impairment, the physician should attempt to assign a value based on the degree of the impairment and one that is consistent with established values.

The focus of this chapter is evaluation of physical impairment that may result from endocrine dysfunction. Since many of the endocrine abnormalities produce cosmetic and/or psychological abnormalities, the evaluator may wish to consider the criteria for impairment from mental and behavioral disorders that are discussed in Chapter 14. Similarly, many of the abnormalities require chronic replacement medications, perhaps for the lifetime of the individual. At the discretion of the evaluating physician, an added impairment of 0% to 5% may be allotted for this aspect of an endocrine disorder.

Before using the information in this chapter, the reader is urged to review Chapters 1 and 2, which provide a general discussion of the purpose of the *Guides*, and of the situations in which they are useful; and which discuss techniques for the evaluation of the subject and for preparation of a report. The report should include the information found in the following outline, which is developed more fully in Chapter 2.

A. Medical Evaluation
1. Narrative history of medical conditions
2. Results of the most recent clinical evaluation
3. Assessment of current clinical status and statement of future plans
4. Diagnoses and clinical impressions
5. Expected date of full or partial recovery

B. Analysis of Findings
1. Impact of medical condition(s) on life activities
2. Explanation for concluding that the medical condition(s) has or has not become static or well-stabilized
3. Explanation for concluding that the individual is or is not likely to suffer from sudden or subtle incapacitation
4. Explanation for concluding that the individual is or is not likely to suffer injury or further impairment by engaging in life activities or by attempting to meet personal, social, and occupational demands
5. Explanation for concluding that accommodations and/or restrictions are or are not warranted

C. Comparison of Results of Analysis with Impairment Criteria
1. Description of clinical findings, and how these findings relate to specific criteria in the chapter.
2. Explanation of each percent of impairment rating
3. Summary list of all impairment ratings
4. Overall rating of impairment of the whole person

12.1 Hypothalamic-Pituitary Axis

The intimate relationship between the hypothalamus and the pituitary requires that they be regarded as a unit. The hypothalamus produces chemical factors, such as releasing and inhibitory hormones, that influence anterior pituitary function, and factors that serve as hormones in their own right, such as antidiuretic hor-

mone (ADH) and oxytocin. The anterior lobe of the pituitary gland produces trophic hormones that control the activity of the thyroid gland (thyroid stimulating hormone, TSH), the adrenal gland (adrenocorticotropic hormone, ACTH), and the gonads (luteinizing hormone, LH, and follicle stimulating hormone, FSH).

Growth hormone is responsible for growth prior to epiphyseal closure and contributes to glucose homeostasis in the adult. Prolactin is necessary for lactation. The posterior lobe of the pituitary is an extension of hypothalamic neurons. ADH regulates the fluid balance of the body through its ability to influence the excretion of water. At present, there is no clearly understood function for oxytocin.

Permanent impairment due to altered function of the thyroid gland, adrenal glands and gonads will be discussed in subsequent sections of this chapter.

Symptoms and signs of impairment of the hypothalamic-pituitary axis: Hypothalamic and pituitary diseases can cause impairments through structural abnormalities or through alterations in hormone production. Structural changes resulting in visual field abnormalities, temporal lobe seizures, frontal lobe abnormalities, headaches, obstructive hydrocephalus, or nonendocrine hypothalamic dysfunction are considered in the section on the central nervous system in Chapter 4.

Hypersecretion of the anterior lobe may be evidenced by (a) prolactin hypersecretion due to a microadenoma or macroadenoma (prolactinoma), the most common cause; and (b) growth hormone hypersecretion due to pituitary adenoma. Prolactin excess per se results in hypogonadism, manifest in the female by oligomenorrhea, infertility, variable estrogen deficiency, and decreased libido, and in the male by decreased libido, impotence and/or infertility. Impairment from prolactin excess is equivalent to hypogonadotropic deficiency of the appropriate end organ, that is, secondary ovarian failure in the female and testicular failure in the male. Gonadal failure is discussed further in the reproductive section of this chapter.

Growth hormone hypersecretion results in gigantism prior to epiphyseal closure and in acromegaly in the adult. The manifestations of acromegaly include enlargement of the hands and feet, coarseness of facial features, and prognathism. Fatigue and increased perspiration are common symptoms. Acromegaly of long duration leads to morbidity from degenerative arthritis and to shortened life expectancy due to increased mortality from cardiovascular causes. Growth hormone excess may lead to glucose intolerance, or may precipitate or exacerbate diabetes mellitus.

Hyposecretion of the anterior lobe may cause isolated or multiple hormone deficiencies known as hypopituitarism. The deficiencies may be parital or complete. In childhood, hypopituitarism may be genetic, congenital, due to infiltrative disease, related to craniopharyngioma, due to a pituitary adenoma, or of unknown cause. In the adult years, pituitary tumors, infarction, particularly post partum, and surgical or radiotherapeutic interventions are the most common causes.

Hypopituitarism that begins in childhood leads to short stature, failure to enter puberty, and symptoms of thyroid and cortisol deficiency. In the adult, hypogonadism, manifested by impotence and amenorrhea, and thyroid hormone and cortisol deficiency appear. Post partum pituitary infarction results in an inability to lactate. Hypopituitarism in the diabetic results in decreasing insulin requirements. Pallor, fatigue, lethargy, weight loss, and weakness are also common symptoms.

Hyperfunction of the posterior lobe, which causes the syndrome of inappropriate antidiuretic hormone secretion (SIADH), may result from a variety of central nervous system disorders. However, it is rarely permanent. Inability of the kidneys to secrete a water load leads to hyponatremia if water intake is not restricted. Fatigue, lethargy progressing to confusion, coma, and seizures may result, depending upon the degree of hyponatremia.

Hypofunction of the posterior lobe results in ADH deficiency, causing diabetes insipidus. Hypofunction usually stems from disease involving the hypothalamus and/or pituitary stalk, and less commonly from disease of the pituitary gland itself. It may be hereditary, or it may be related to trauma, surgery, metastatic tumors, craniopharyngioma, histiocytosis X, or other conditions, or of unknown origin. If thirst is unimpaired, diabetes insipidus is predominantly an inconvenience, because of polyuria, polydipsia and nocturia. If thirst is impaired due to concomitant hypothalamic disease, then severe hypernatremia may result, leading to mental depression or even coma.

Objective techniques useful in evaluating function of the hypothalamic-pituitary axis: Structural abnormalities are evaluated by computerized tomography (CT scan), roentgenograms of the sella turcica, or polytomography. If a tumor is suspected, pneumoencephalography or metrizamide cisternography may be necessary to evaluate its extent. Angiography is required on occasion. Visual field examinations by perimetry complete the structural evaluation.

Hormonal function must be assessed, often by stimulation or suppression testing. In children, roentgenography for bone age to compare with physiologic and height age is useful.

Growth hormone deficiency is assessed by measuring the hormone in blood after stimulation testing with insulin, L-DOPA, arginine, or other agents. ACTH, and hence cortisol insufficiency, are assessed by stimulating testing with insulin or metyrapone. Baseline studies of cortisol function are of little utility.

The diagnosis of secondary hypothyroidism (pituitary and hypothalamic hypothyroidism) is made by demonstrating low concentrations of peripheral thyroid hormones without elevation of TSH. In this circumstance, roentgenograms of the skull and tests of pituitary function are needed to distinguish a hypothalamic from a pituitary origin. Secondary gonadal insufficiency, that is, hypogonadotropic hypogonadism or pituitary hypogonadism, requires the demonstration of end organ failure, with low testosterone in the male and low estrogen in the female, and low or normal levels of the gonadotropins LH and FSH.

ADH insufficiency requires the documentation of urine hypo-osmolality in the face of a stimulus to urine concentration, usually through water restriction. Subsequently, one must demonstrate an increase in urine osmolality in response to ADH administration. Prolactin deficiency is documented by low basal levels of the hormone and failure to rise after injection of thyrotropin-releasing hormone (TRH), chlorpromazine, or other stimulating agents.

Growth hormone excess is documented by failure to suppress growth hormone concentration after a glucose load. Prolactin excess is documented by measurement of elevated basal levels, and often by failure to rise after TRH injection. The SIADH is documented by hyponatremia with inappropriately elevated urine osmolality in the presence of normal cardiac, renal, adrenal, and thyroid function.

Criteria for evaluating permanent impairment of the hypothalamic-pituitary axis: The assessment of permanent impairment of the whole person from disorders of the hypothalamic-pituitary axis requires evaluation of (1) primary abnormalities related to growth hormone, prolactin, or ADH; (2) secondary abnormalities in other endocrine glands, such as thyroid, adrenal, and gonads, and; (3) structural and functional disorders of the central nervous system caused by anatomic abnormalities of the pituitary. Thus, the physician must evaluate each disorder separately, using guides in this chapter or in other chapters, such as those on the nervous system, visual system, and mental and behavioral disorders, combining the impairment ratings according to the Combined Values Chart.

Class 1—Impairment of the Whole Person, 0-10%:
A patient with hypothalamic-pituitary disease belongs in Class 1 when the disease can be controlled effectively with continuous treatment.

Example: A 19-year-old man developed severe thirst and increased frequency of urination after head trauma, from which he had otherwise fully recovered. His fluid intake and output ranged from 4 to 7 liters per day. Nocturia occurred 4 to 7 times, and thirst during the night was marked. His general health was excellent, except for fatigue related to interrupted sleep. On initial assessment, serum osmolality was 292 mOsm/kg and serum sodium concentration was 142 meq/L; urine osmolality was 120 mOsm/kg, and specific gravity was 1.003. There was no glycosuria. An attempt at water deprivation led to severe thirst with a serum osmolality of 302 mOsm/kg and urine osmolality of 150 mOsm/kg. After an initial ADH injection, urine osmolality rose to 450 mOsm/kg and urine volume diminished.

At first, management consisted of self-administered injections of pitressin tannate in oil every other day, which lowered the patient's urine output to 1200 ml/24 hours and prevented nocturia. More recently he has been maintained with good results on 0.1 ml twice daily of desamino-8-D arginine vasopressin (DDAVP), a long acting nasal spray. On this regimen he feels well and his urine output is well controlled. Symptoms recur if a dose of DDAVP is missed. No other endocrine disease has been found, and he is able to carry out the usual activities of daily living.

Diagnosis: Traumatic diabetes insipidus, controlled by treatment.

Impairment: 5% impairment of the whole person.

Class 2—Impairment of the Whole Person, 15-20%:
A patient with hypothalamic-pituitary disease belongs in Class 2 when the symptoms and signs are inadequately controlled by treatment.

Example: A 57-year-old man developed fatigue, hyperhidrosis, headaches, carpal tunnel syndrome, and enlargement of his hands, feet and nose. He also complained of pain in his knees and back and of decreased libido. He was found to have an enlarged sella turcia with suprasellar extension of a pituitary tumor, although there were no visual field abnormalities. His growth hormone level of 575 ng/ml was markedly elevated.

Despite an attempt at surgical excision and subsequent therapy with ionizing radiation, the man's growth hormone remained elevated at 100 ng/ml. He was unable to tolerate bromocriptine therapy. His testosterone level was low, but thyroid and adrenal function remained normal. His headaches were relieved, but symptoms of fatigue, excess perspiration, and joint discomfort continued. Libido improved with bimonthly injections of testosterone. The carpal tunnel syndrome required surgical therapy, which was successful.

Diagnosis: Acromegaly, moderately severe, inadequately controlled by therapy.

Impairment: 15% impairment due to acromegaly, and 5% impairment due to testosterone deficiency, which combine to 19% impairment of the whole person.

Class 3—Impairment of the Whole Person, 25-50%:
A patient with hypothalamic-pituitary disease belongs in Class 3 when severe symptoms and signs persist despite treatment.

Example: A 55-year-old man was seen initially at age 45 for an enlarged sella turcica. Evaluation revealed testosterone deficiency and no suprasellar extension of his tumor. The patient was not treated and was lost to follow-up. Later he was hospitalized with complaints of excruciating headache, visual loss, and impotence. On physical examination, his beard was markedly diminished, and a female escutcheon was noted. Testing of visual fields showed nearly complete loss of vision in the left eye and a temporal field defect in the right with some macular involvement. A skull roentgenogram revealed a massively enlarged sella turcica. A CT scan showed extensive suprasellar growth of the tumor with a suggestion of hemorrhage into the tumor.

The patient underwent emergency transsphenoidal pituitary decompression under coverage with glucocorticoids. Despite the decompressive procedure, vision in the left eye returned only to finger counting, and temporal field loss in the right eye continued. Preoperative prolactin concentration was 1000 ng/ml. Postoperative prolactin remained elevated at 660 ng/ml. In the postoperative period, a course of 4800 R to the sella turcica was given with ionizing radiation. Subsequent evaluation revealed elevated prolactin concentration of 280 ng/ml, low testosterone concentration, deficient cortisol response to hypoglycemia, and decreased thyroid function. Visual abnormalities were unchanged. The patient was unable to tolerate bromocriptine. Headaches were mild but persistent. Despite testosterone administration, the patient remained impotent.

Diagnosis: Prolactinoma (prolactin-secreting pituitary adenoma) with pituitary apoplexy, secondary panhypopituitarism, and partial blindness.

Impairment: 10% impairment due to pituitary dysfunction, 10% impairment due to secondary adrenal dysfunction, and 5% impairment due to secondary testosterone impairment, which combine to 23% impairment due to endocrine dysfunction; 33% impairment due to visual problems; and 10% impairment due to persistent headache. All of these combine to give 53% impairment of the whole person.

12.2 Thyroid

The thyroid gland, by its secretion of thyroid hormones, influences the metabolic rate of many organ systems throughout the body. Pathologic conditions causing impairments are hypersecretion and hyposecretion.

Symptoms and signs of impairment of function of the thyroid: *Hypersecretion* by the thyroid gland results in hyperthyroidism and may be manifested by nervousness, weight loss, heat intolerance, goiter, tachycardia, palpitation, diarrhea, tremor, and muscle weakness. Eye changes, such as exophthalmos, may be present.

Hyposecretion by the thyroid gland results in hypothyroidism and may be manifested by slowing of mental processes, lethargy, weakness, cold intolerance, dry skin, constipation, and myxedema. Late complications include myocardial insufficiency, effusions into body cavities, and coma. Hypothyroidism in infancy, including cretinism, may be associated with failure of skeletal and brain development and permanent mental retardation.

Objective techniques useful in evaluating function of the thyroid: Useful techniques include, but are not limited to, determination of (1) circulating thyroid hormones, total thyroxine (TT_4), free thyroxine (FT_4), triiodothyronine (T_3) and free triiodothyronine (FT_3); (2) circulating pituitary thyrotropin (TSH) level before and after stimulation with the hypothalamic thyrotropin-releasing hormone (TRH); (3) radioiodine uptake of the thyroid gland; and (4) the radiotriiodothyronine (T_3) resin or red blood cell uptake.

Criteria for evaluating permanent impairment of the thyroid: Hyperthyroidism is not considered to be a cause of permanent impairment, because the hypermetabolic state in practically all patients can be cor-

rected permanently by treatment. After remission of hyperthyroidism, there may be permanent impairment of the visual or cardiovascular systems, which should be evaluated using the chapters of this book for those systems.

Hypothyroidism in most instances can be satisfactorily controlled by the administration of thyroid medication. Occasionally, because of associated disease in other organ systems, full hormone replacement may not be possible.

Class 1—Impairment of the Whole Person, 0-10%: A patient belongs in Class 1 when (a) continuous thyroid therapy is required for correction of the thyroid insufficiency or for maintenance of normal thyroid anatomy; *and* (b) there is no objective physical or laboratory evidence of inadequate replacement therapy.

Example: A 45-year-old woman with symptoms of mild hypothyroidism had the diagnosis made by needle biopsy of lympho-epithelial goiter (Hashimoto's thyroiditis). She requires daily therapy with 0.20 mg of L-thyroxine to maintain a normal-sized thyroid, although her symptoms of hormone deficiency are relieved by a lower dose.

Diagnosis: Hashimoto's thyroiditis controlled by treatment.

Impairment: 5% impairment of the whole person.

Class 2—Impairment of the Whole Person, 15-20%: A patient belongs in Class 2 when (a) symptoms and signs of thyroid disease are present, or there is anatomic loss or alteration; *and* (b) continuous thyroid hormone replacement therapy is required for correction of the confirmed thyroid insufficiency; *but* (c) the presence of a disease process in another body system or systems permits only partial replacement of the thyroid hormone.

Example: A 65-year-old man has severe hypothyroidism with pronounced mental slowing, loss of memory, and apathy. He also has severe coronary artery disease with angina pectoris that can be precipitated by walking as little as 50 ft. TT_4 is 0.5 μg/100ml, and TSH is 100 μU/ml. Repeated trials and careful adjustment of doses of L-thyroxine disclose that a dose larger than 0.05 mg per day causes definite aggravation of his angina. Significant general debility from the hypothyroidism persists.

Diagnosis: Partially treated hypothyroidism.

Impairment: 20% impairment due to hypothyroidism, which is to be combined with an appropriate value for the cardiovascular impairment to determine the impairment of the whole person.

12.3 Parathyroids

The secretion of parathyroid hormone from the four parathyroid glands regulates the levels of serum calcium and phosphorus, which are essential to the proper functioning of the skeletal, digestive, renal, and nervous systems. The major abnormalities of the glands include hyperfunction, hypofunction, and carcinoma.

Symptoms and signs of impairment of function of the parathyroids: *Hypersecretion* of parathyroid hormone, or hyperparathyroidism, may be due to the hyperfunctioning of one gland, as with an adenoma, or of all four glands, as with hyperplasia, or due to a parathyroid carcinoma. Manifestations include lethargy, constipation, nausea, vomiting, and polyuria, and in extreme cases, bone pain, renal calculi, renal failure, and coma.

Hyposecretion of parathyroid hormone, or hypoparathyroidism, may be due to inadvertent removal of the parathyroid glands during thyroidectomy, or idiopathic, that is, due to unknown causes. Manifestations include chronic tetany, paresthesias, and seizures, and, particularly in idiopathic cases, cataracts, chronic moniliasis of the skin, alopecia, and hypofunction of other endocrine organs; the latter state may be associated with hypothyroidism, diabetes mellitus, or adrenal insufficiency.

Objective techniques useful in evaluating parathyroid function: Techniques of evaluating parathyroid gland function include determinations of serum calcium, phosphorus, albumin, creatinine, and parathyroid hormone levels, of calcium concentration in urine, and of urinary cyclic AMP response to intravenously administered parathyroid hormone. Intravenous pyelography and skeletal roentgenography may be useful.

Criteria for evaluating permanent impairment of the parathyroids: In most cases of hyperparathyroidism, surgical treatment results in correction of the primary abnormality, although secondary symptoms and signs may persist, such as renal calculi or renal failure, which should be evaluated according to criteria set forth in Chapter 11. If surgery fails, or if the patient

cannot undergo surgery, the patient may require long-term therapy, in which case the permanent impairment may be classified according to the following:

Severity of Hyperparathyroidism	% Impairment of the Whole Person
Symptoms and signs are easily controlled with medical therapy	0-10
There is persistent mild hypercalcemia, with mild nausea and polyuria	15-20
There is severe hypercalcemia, with nausea and lethargy	55-100

Hypoparathyroidism is a chronic condition of variable severity that requires long-term medical therapy in most cases. The degree of severity determines the degree of permanent impairment, according to the following:

Severity of Hypoparathyroidism	% Impairment of the Whole Person
Symptoms and signs easily controlled by medical therapy	0-5
Intermittent hypercalcemia and/or hypocalcemia, and more frequent symptoms in spite of careful medical attention	10-20

12.4 Adrenal Cortex

The adrenal cortex synthesizes and secretes adrenal cortical hormones. These hormones participate in the regulation of electrolyte and water metabolism and in the intermediate metabolism of carbohydrate, fat and protein. They also affect inflammatory response, cell membrane permeability, and antigen-antibody reactions, and play a role in the development and maintaining of secondary sexual characteristics.

Impairment of the whole person may result from hypersecretion or hyposecretion of the cortical hormones. Such an abnormality may be associated with dysfunction of another endocrine gland, for instance, the pituitary. If this occurs, impairment from the adrenal abnormality is evaluated together with the other dysfunction, using criteria set forth in the appropriate section of this chapter and the Combined Values Chart.

Symptoms and signs of impairment of function of the adrenal cortex: *Hypersecretion* of adrenal cortical hormones results from hyperplasia or from benign or malignant tumors of the adrenal cortex. The symptoms and signs of adrenal cortical disease may arise from hypersecretion of one or more of the following hormones: (1) glucocorticoid; (2) mineralocorticoids; (3) androgens; and (4) estrogens. In some instances, there may be hypersecretion of hormones in one category and hyposecretion of those in another.

Iatrogenic Cushing's syndrome secondary to nonphysiologic doses of glucocorticoids administered for systemic diseases such as bronchial asthma, systemic lupus erythematosis, or rheumatoid arthritis, is the most common syndrome of adrenal hormonal excess.

Among the diseases caused by hypersecretion of the adrenal cortical hormones are Cushing's syndrome, the adrenogenital syndrome, and primary aldosteronism. Hypersecretion of the adrenal cortex due to hyperplasia may be associated either with a tumor of the anterior pituitary gland or with a malignant tumor arising outside the endocrine system that causes ectopic ACTH secretion.

Hyposecretion of adrenal cortical hormones may be primary, resulting from surgical removal or destruction of the adrenals, as with Addison's disease, or secondary, resulting from decreased production of corticotropin. Therapy is guided by the number of hormonal deficiencies, which may be single, as in hypoaldosteronism, or multiple, as in adrenocortical destruction. One normal adrenal gland can compensate for loss of the other.

Objective techniques useful in evaluating function of the adrenal cortex include: (1) measurement of adrenal cortical hormones in the urine, such as, 17-ketosteroids, 17-hydroxycorticoids, free cortisol, and aldosterone and of hormones in the plasma such as cortisol and aldosterone; (2) measurement of ACTH, serum electrolytes, plasma glucose, and creatinine; (3) measurement of the effects of suppression and stimulation of adrenal cortical function; and (4) radiography of the adrenal glands, CT scan, arteriography, and venography of the skull, including polytomography of the sella turcica and of the spine.

Criteria for evaluating permanent impairment of the adrenal cortex: *Hypoadrenalism* is a lifelong condition that requires long-term replacement therapy with glucocorticoids and/or mineralocorticoids for proven hormonal deficiencies. Impairments should be classified according to the following scheme:

Severity of Hypoadrenalism	% Impairment of the Whole Person
Symptoms and signs controlled with medical therapy	0-10
Symptoms and signs controlled inadequately, usually during the course of acute illnesses	15-50
Severe symptoms of adrenal crisis during major illness, usually due to severe glucocortocoid deficiency and/or sodium depletion	55-100

Hyperadrenocorticism due to the chronic side effects of nonphysiologic doses of glucocorticoids (iatrogenic Cushing's syndrome) is related to dosage and duration of treatment and includes osteoporosis, hypertension, diabetes mellitus, and the effects involving catabolism that result in protein myopathy, striae, and easy bruising. Permanent impairment may range from 0% to 100%, depending on the severity and chronicity of the disease process for which the steroids are given. On the other hand, with diseases of the pituitary-adrenal axis, impairment may be classified as:

Severity of Hyperadrenocorticism	% Impairment of the Whole Person
Minimal, as with hyperadrenocorticism that is surgically correctable by removal of a pituitary or adrenal adenoma	0-10
Moderate, as with bilateral hyperplasia that is treated with medical therapy or adrenalectomy	15-50
Severe, as with aggressively metastasizing adrenal carcinoma	55-100

12.5 Adrenal Medulla

The adrenal medulla synthesizes and secretes primarily epinephrine, which functions in the regulation of blood pressure and cardiac output and, to some extent, affects the intermediate metabolism of the body.

The adrenal medulla is probably not essential to the maintenance of life or well-being. Hence, its absence does not constitute impairment of the whole person.

Hyperfunction of the adrenal medulla may stem from pheochromocytomas, or rarely, from hyperplasia of the chromaffin cells. Pheochromocytomas may arise at any site in the body that has sympathetic nervous tissue. The presence of a pheochromocytoma is usually associated with paroxysmal or sustained hypertension. Approximately 10% of pheochromocytomas are malignant. Pheochromocytomas may be multiple in an individual and may occur in families in association with medullary carcinoma of the thyroid and hyperplasia of the parathyroid, constituting the syndrome of multiple endocrine neoplasms, Type II.

Objective techniques useful in evaluating the function of the adrenal medulla include: (1) measurement of unmetabolized urinary catecholamines, including total catecholamines, epinephrine, and norepinephrine, and of their degradation products in urine, vanillylmandelic acid (VMA), and metanephrines; (2) measurement of the plasma catecholamines, epinephrine, norepinephrine, and dopamine; and (3) radiography of the adrenals, including arteriography, venography, and CT scan.

Criteria for evaluating permanent impairment of the adrenal medulla: Permanent impairment from pheochromocytoma may be classified using the following table:

Severity of Pheochromocytoma	% Impairment of the Whole Person
Minimal, as when the duration of hypertension has not led to cardiovascular disease and a benign tumor can be removed surgically	0-10
Moderate, as with inoperable malignant pheochromocytomas, if signs and symptoms of catecholamine excess can be controlled with blocking agents	15-50
Severe, as with widely metastatic malignant pheochromocytomas, in which symptoms of catecholamine excess cannot be controlled	55-100

12.6 Pancreas (Islets of Langerhans)

Insulin and glucagon are among the hormones secreted by the islets of Langerhans. Both hormones are required for the maintenance of normal metabolism of carbohydrate, lipid and protein. Impairment of the whole person may result from a deficiency or an excess of either hormone. Removal of normal pancreatic tissue during the resection of an islet cell neoplasm does not constitute endocrine impairment if, after the operation, carbohydrate tolerance is normal.

Symptoms and signs of impairment of function of the pancreatic islets: Abnormalities of islet cell function may be manifested by high plasma glucose levels, as in diabetes mellitus, or by low plasma glucose, as in hypoglycemia. Diabetes mellitus is classified into two main groups: insulin dependent (Type I) diabetes and noninsulin dependent (Type II) diabetes. People with insulin dependent diabetes mellitus, if untreated, will progress to stupor, coma, and death. This type of diabetes mellitus usually begins in the young, but it may occur at any age. People with noninsulin dependent diabetes generally are over 40 years old and overweight.

The main complications of diabetes mellitus and their associated impairments are: (1) retinopathy, causing visual impairment; (2) nephropathy, causing renal impairment; (3) arteriosclerosis, causing arteriosclerotic heart disease, and cerebrovascular and peripheral vascular disease; and (4) neuropathy.

Hypoglycemia occasionally causes impairment. Hypoglycemia may result from excessive insulin that is either produced endogenously or administered by injection. Hypoglycemia may be manifested by weakness, sweating, tachycardia, headache, muscular incoordination, blurred vision, loss of consciousness, and convulsions. Prolonged hypoglycemia or repeated severe attacks of hypoglycemia may lead to mental deterioration.

Objective techniques in evaluating impairment related to diabetes mellitus include, but are not limited to: (1) determination of fasting and postprandial plasma glucose levels; (2) determination of hemoglobin A_1c; (3) measurements of cholesterol and other lipids; (4) electrocardiogram; (5) ophthalmological examination; (6) tests of renal and bladder function; (7) Doppler testing of the peripheral circulation; (8) radiographs of chest, gastrointestinal tract, pelvis, or extremities, including arteriograms; and (9) neurological testing.

Criteria for evaluating permanent impairment related to diabetes mellitus are as follows:

Class 1—Impairment of the Whole Person, 0-5%: A patient with diabetes mellitus belongs in Class 1 if he or she has noninsulin dependent (Type II) diabetes mellitus that can be controlled by diet; the person may or may not have evidence of diabetic microangiopathy, as indicated by the presence of retinopathy and/or albuminuria greater than 30 mg/100 ml.

Example 1: Medical examinations disclosed 1+ glycosuria in a moderately obese 40-year-old man. Fasting plasma glucose was 160 mg/100 ml on two occasions. Retinal examination revealed no diabetic retinopathy and there was no albumin in the urine. After three months on a special diet, the man's weight was normal, and his fasting plasma glucose was 110 mg/100 ml.

Diagnosis: Noninsulin dependent (Type II) diabetes mellitus controlled by diet, without evidence of diabetic microangiopathy.

Impairment: 0% impairment of the whole person.

Example 2: An obese 45-year-old woman had elevated fasting plasma glucose, and physical examination disclosed retinal microaneurysms and dot and blot hemorrhages. There was no impairment of vision.

Diagnosis: Noninsulin dependent (Type II) diabetes mellitus with early diabetic retinopathy.

Impairment: 5% impairment of the whole person.

Class 2—Impairment of the Whole Person, 5-10%: A patient belongs in this classification when there is diagnosis of noninsulin dependent (Type II) diabetes mellitus; and when satisfactory control of the plasma glucose requires both a restricted diet and hypoglycemic medication, either an oral agent or insulin. Evidence of microangiopathy, as indicated by retinopathy or by albuminuria of greater than 30 mg/100 ml, may or may not be present.

Example 1: A 55-year-old man had the diagnosis of noninsulin dependent (Type II) diabetes mellitus without retinopathy or proteinuria. Although he lost weight on a prescribed diet, his plasma glucose could not be maintained within normal limits on diet alone. When he was on a restricted diet and an oral agent, his fasting serum glucose was 120 mg/100 ml.

Diagnosis: Noninsulin dependent (Type II) diabetes mellitus controlled by diet and oral agent.

Impairment: 5% impairment of the whole person.

Example 2: A 50-year-old man has had noninsulin dependent (Type II) diabetes mellitus for five years. At the onset of the disease, he had a fasting plasma glucose of 190 mg/100 ml when on a restricted diet and an oral hypoglycemic agent. Four years ago his right leg was amputated above the knee because of severe peripheral vascular disease that led to gangrene of the foot.

At present, the man adheres to a prescribed diet and takes 16 units of NPH insulin daily. On this regi-

men, his fasting plasma glucose is 125 to 140 mg/100 ml. He has no symptoms, nor does he spill sugar or acetone.

Diagnosis: Noninsulin dependent (Type II) diabetes mellitus with complications, requiring insulin to control hyperglycemia. Plasma glucose is satisfactorily controlled by diet and one daily injection of insulin.

Impairment: 10% impairment due to noninsulin dependent (Type II) diabetes mellitus, and 36% impairment due to amputation above the knee joint, which combine to give 42% impairment of the whole person.

Class 3—Impairment of the Whole Person, 15-20%: A patient belongs in this class when insulin dependent (Type I) diabetes mellitus is present with or without evidence of microangiopathy.

Example 1: A 33-year-old teacher has had insulin dependent (Type I) diabetes mellitus for five years. She originally presented with polyuria, polydipsia, and weight loss, and with a plasma glucose of 400 mg/100 ml and marked ketonuria. The condition is satisfactorily controlled with a prescribed diet and an injection of insulin before both breakfast and dinner. There is no evidence of microangiopathy.

Diagnosis: Insulin dependent (Type I) diabetes mellitus satisfactorily controlled by insulin and diet.

Impairment: 15% impairment of the whole person.

Example 2: A 40-year-old woman had onset of insulin dependent (Type I) diabetes mellitus 20 years ago, when she had polydipsia, polyuria, weight loss, and plasma glucose of 350 mg/100 ml. At present, the condition is satisfactorily controlled with diet and a daily injection of insulin. Physical examination discloses that background retinopathy is present.

Diagnosis: Insulin dependent (Type I) diabetes mellitus with diabetic microangiopathy and no visual impairment.

Impairment: 20% impairment of the whole person.

Example 3: A 45-year-old man has had insulin dependent (Type I) diabetes mellitus for 25 years. He has proliferative retinopathy, and he has an elevated creatinine level and a diminished creatinine clearance. His plasma glucose is controlled by a mixture of NPH and regular insulin given twice daily, 12 units before breakfast and 6 units before dinner. Ophthalmological examination reveals 70% impairment of vision of the right eye and 63% impairment of the left, which combine to give 65% impairment of the visual system.

Diagnosis: Insulin dependent (Type I) diabetes mellitus with complications; plasma glucose is satisfactorily controlled by diet and insulin.

Impairment: 20% impairment due to diabetes mellitus, and 65% impairment due to visual impairment, which should be combined with an appropriate value for the renal impairment to determine impairment of the whole person.

Class 4—Impairment of the Whole Person, 25-40%:
A patient belongs in Class 4 when the patient has the diagnosis of insulin dependent (Type I) diabetes mellitus, and when hyperglycemic and/or hypoglycemic episodes occur frequently in spite of conscientious efforts of both the patient and his or her physician.

Example 1: A 24-year-old male farmer has had labile insulin dependent (Type I) diabetes mellitus for 10 years. His physical activities vary greatly from day to day. Despite adherence to a prescribed diet that includes between-meal and bedtime snacks, and despite a carefully planned insulin program with both morning and evening injections, home plasma glucose tests vary greatly, and at times there are severe insulin reactions without warning. He is 10% underweight, but he shows no clinical or laboratory evidence of complications.

Diagnosis: Insulin dependent (Type I) diabetes mellitus, not adequately controlled by diet and insulin.

Impairment: 35% impairment of the whole person.

Example 2: A 35-year-old woman has had poorly controlled insulin dependent (Type I) diabetes mellitus for 15 years. Although fasting plasma glucose is often greater than 200 mg/100 ml, and the urine usually contains sugar, severe hypoglycemic reactions occur unpredictably several times a week. The patient is malnourished on a 3,000-calorie diet, which is combined with injections of 30 units of Lente insulin before breakfast and 10 units of Lente insulin before supper. She becomes fatigued easily, and she complains bitterly of burning pain in the feet and of difficulty in walking. Vibratory sensation and deep tendon reflexes are absent below the knees. Examination of the fundi reveals numerous microaneurysms, but there is no visual impairment.

Diagnosis: Insulin dependent (Type I) diabetes mellitus, with complications, not adequately controlled by diet and insulin.

Impairment: 40% impairment due to diabetes mellitus and 15% impairment due to peripheral neuritis, which combine to 49% impairment of the whole person.

Objective techniques useful in evaluating impairment related to hypoglycemia include, but are not limited to: (1) measurement of plasma glucose after overnight or longer periods of fasting; (2) measurement of plasma insulin after overnight fasting on several occasions; (3) roentgenograms of skull, chest, and abdomen; (4) tests of liver function; and (5) tests of adrenocortical and pituitary gland function.

Criteria for evaluating permanent impairment related to hypoglycemia are as follows:

Class I—Impairment of the Whole Person, 0%:
A patient has Class I impairment when surgical removal of an islet-cell adenoma results in complete remission of the symptoms and signs of hypoglycemia, and there are no postoperative sequelae.

Example: The wife of a 45-year-old man noted that with increasing frequency he had a bad temper upon arising that improved after breakfast. He did not use alcohol or tobacco. At 11:30 a.m. one morning, while at work, he suddenly became disturbed and lost consciousness. Upon emergency admission to a hospital, his plasma glucose level was 20 mg/100 ml. In spite of a high carbohydrate intake that included a large feeding at bedtime, he remained weak and irritable before breakfast, and his fasting plasma glucose never exceeded 35 mg/100 ml.

An abdominal examination and a chest radiograph disclosed no abnormalities, and pituitary, adrenal, and liver functions were normal. During an operation, a benign insulinoma 1.5 cm in diameter was excised from the head of the pancreas; the patient developed a pancreatic fistula that took three months to close. He was asymptomatic thereafter.

Diagnosis: Benign functioning islet-cell adenoma (insulinoma), with complete remission after an operation.

Impairment: 0% impairment of the whole person.

Class 2—Impairment of the Whole Person, 5-50%:
A patient with symptoms and signs of hypoglycemia has Class 2 impairment of the whole person ranging from 5% to 50%, depending on the degree of control obtained with diet and medications; and on how the condition affects activities of daily living.

Example: A 55-year-old man manifested alarming personality changes within a few weeks' time and had a seizure. A diagnosis of insulinoma was made. Laparotomy revealed an islet-cell adenocarcinoma, 5 cm in diameter, in the tail of the pancreas, with metastases in the liver. The spleen and main tumor mass were resected. The man experienced no impairment of hepatic function, and recovery from surgery was uneventful except for persistence of mild fasting hypoglycemia. This responded well to frequent feedings of a high-protein, high-carbohydrate diet and 40 mg of prednisone taken daily. Three months after returning to work, he still had occasional transient mental lapses, during one of which the plasma glucose level was 28 mg/100 ml. When the daily dosage of prednisone was raised to 60 mg, the symptomatic hypoglycemia improved, but manifestations of Cushing's syndrome became more prominent.

Diagnosis: Metastatic islet-cell adenocarcinoma, with incomplete control of symptoms.

Impairment: 50% impairment due to hypoglycemia and 10% impairment due to steroid-induced Cushing's syndrome, which combine to give 55% impairment of the whole person.

12.7 The Gonads

The gonads produce spermotozoa or ova and also produce the sex hormones, which affect physical and sexual development and behavior. The interstitial cells of the testes produce male hormones. The most significant hormones of the ovaries are estrogen from the follicles and progesterone from the corpora lutea. Changes in function of the gonads can be produced by tumors, trauma, infection, scarring, and surgical removal. Gonadal function may vary with changes in the pituitary-hypothalamus axis.

Symptoms and signs of impairment of function of the gonads: *Precocious puberty* in the male results in early, rapid growth and accelerated skeletal maturation. Occasionally a tendency toward this condition is familial. Precocious puberty in the female may be caused by an ovarian tumor, but usually a cause is not found; it can result in accelerated skeletal maturation. Some ovarian tumors may also cause masculinization. Certain ovarian conditions produce heavy and irregular menstrual periods.

Testicular hypofunction results in eunuchoidism or eunuchism. Symptoms are diminished sexual function, failure to develop or maintain secondary sexual characteristics, and, if there is onset before adolescence, growth of the body beyond the usual age because of delayed epiphyseal closure. There is usually lack of endurance and strength.

Ovarian hypofunction, with onset in preadolescence, may be characterized by primary amenorrhea, poor development of secondary sexual characteristics, and growth beyond the usual age due to delayed maturation of the skeleton. The menopause is a natural occurrence in older women, but it also can follow surgical removal of the ovaries. It may be accompanied by hot flashes, and by symptoms such as irritability, fatigue, and headaches. Osteoporosis and other changes may occur during later years.

Objective techniques useful in evaluating function of the gonads include, but are not limited to:
(1) measurements of plasma gonadotropins, testosterone, estrogen, and progesterone, and occasionally urinary 24-hour 17-ketosteroids; (2) radiographic determinations of bone age in children and adolescents; (3) evaluation of sella turcica size by radiography; (4) studies of sex chromatin and chromosomes; (5) testicular biopsy; (6) semen examination; (7) study of vaginal cytology; (8) culdoscopy or laparoscopy; (9) endometrial biopsy; and (10) ovarian biopsy.

Criteria for evaluating permanent impairment of the gonads: A patient with anatomic loss or alteration of the gonads that results in an absence, or abnormally high level, of gonadal hormones would have 0% to 5% impairment of the whole person. Impairment due to inability to reproduce, and other impairments associated with gonadal dysfunction, should be evaluated in accordance with the criteria set forth in Chapter 11.

Example 1: A 12-year-old girl complained of severe menorrhagia during the preceding six months. She had experienced vaginal bleeding since the age of nine years, at which time breast development began and pubic hair appeared. Also at that time, there was a spurt of growth, which slowed and then stopped during the 12th year. On physical examination her height was 4 ft 11 in (150 cm).

The girl's bone age was 17 years, and it seemed unlikely that she would grow taller. Urinary gonadotropin values were in the low normal range, while levels of urinary estrogens were elevated. The right ovary was enlarged to about five times its normal size. The ovary was removed surgically and found to contain a benign granulosa cell tumor. The left ovary was the size of an infant's and without visible follicles. A year after the operation, the patient had regular, normal menses.

Diagnosis: Precocious puberty caused by granulosa cell tumor of ovary.

Impairment: 0% impairment due to precocious puberty. The impairment of the whole person would be determined by the loss of one ovary. Note: Short stature is not considered a cause of impairment.

Example 2: A 31-year-old man complained of lack of sexual development and function, of a high-pitched voice, and of having no beard. He was tall, and had relatively long arms and legs. The penis was tiny and the scrotum and testes were small. The bone age was 18 years, the plasma testosterone was 70 ng/ml, and the plasma gonadotropins were low.

The man responded well to continuous treatment with testosterone. The penis became larger and there was adequate sexual functioning. The man had an increase in body and facial hair, and the voice became deeper. He continued to work as a railroad freight handler after the treatment.

Diagnosis: Hypogonadotropic hypogonadism.

Impairment: 5% impairment of the whole person.

12.8 Mammary Glands

The mammary glands make, store, and secrete milk. Absence of the mammary glands does not cause impairment of the whole person in males, but in females it will prevent nursing. In some endocrine disorders there may be galactorrhea in the female and gynecomastia in the male. Gynecomastia in the male may be accompanied by galactorrhea.

A female patient in the childbearing age with absence of the breasts, a patient with galactorrhea sufficient to require the use of absorbent pads, and a male patient with painful gynecomastia that interferes in the performance of daily activities, each would have 0% to 5% impairment of the whole person.

12.9 Metabolic Bone Disease

Metabolic bone disease, such as osteoporosis, vitamin D-resistant osteomalacia, and Paget's disease, may require continuous therapy. These conditions, unless accompanied by pain, skeletal deformity, or peripheral nerve involvement, should be rated at 0% impairment of the whole person. When continuous hormone and mineral therapy gives complete relief of symptoms, impairment of the whole person may be considered to be 3%. When continuous therapy is required to relieve pain, and the activities of daily living are restricted because of pain, the rating should be 5% to 15% impairment of the whole person. Any associated loss of motion should be evaluated in accordance with the criteria set forth in Chapter 3, which concerns the extremities and spine, and with those in Chapter 4, which concerns the nervous system.

Example: A 68-year-old woman has severe osteoporosis of the axial skeleton and, to a lesser extent, of the extremities. She has considerable local pain with motion of the spine, along with some generalized back ache and spasm related to partial collapse of T4 and T12. Pain persists in spite of prolonged therapy with anabolic agents, estrogens, vitamin D, and calcium.

Diagnosis: Postmenopausal osteoporosis with incomplete symptomatic control.

Impairment: 15% impairment of the whole person.

References

1. Williams RH: *Textbook of Endocrinology,* ed 7, Wilson JD, Foster DW (eds). Philadelphia, WB Saunders Co, 1985.

2. Felig P, Baxter J, Broadus A, Frohman L: *Endocrinology and Metabolism,* ed 2. New York, McGraw Hill, 1987.

3. Rifkin H, Raskin P (eds): *Diabetes Mellitus.* New York, American Diabetes Association, 1981.

4. Federman DD: Endocrinology, in Rubenstein E, Federman DD (eds): *Scientific American Medicine.* New York, Scientific American, Inc, 1987.

Chapter 13

The Skin

13.0 Introduction

This chapter provides criteria for evaluating the effect that permanent impairment of the skin and its appendages has on an individual's ability to perform or participate in the activities of daily living, including occupation.

The functions of the skin include: (1) providing a protective body covering; (2) participating in sensory perception, temperature regulation, fluid regulation, electrolyte balance, immunobiologic defenses, and resistance to trauma; and (3) regenerating the epidermis and its appendages.

The protective functions include, for example, barrier defenses against damage by chemical irritants and allergic sensitizers, invasion by micro-organisms, and injuries by ultraviolet light. Temperature regulation involves the proper function of the small blood vessels and sweat glands. The barrier defense against fluid loss is related to the intactness of the stratum corneum.

Immunobiologic defenses of the skin prevent and control infections by bacteria, viruses, or fungi. Alterations of skin sensory perception include pruritus, the decrease or loss of sensation, and hyperesthesia. Cutaneous and systemic disorders can alter one or more of these functions. An established deviation from normal in any of the functions may result in an anatomic or functional abnormality or loss and constitute a permanent impairment.

Permanent impairment of the skin is any anatomic or functional abnormality or loss, including an acquired immunologic capacity to react to antigens that persists after medical treatment and rehabilitation, and after a length of time sufficient to permit regeneration and other physiologic adjustments. The degree of permanent impairment of the skin may not be static. Therefore, findings should be subject to review and the patient's impairment should be re-evaluated at appropriate intervals.

Evaluation of impairment is usually possible through the exercise of sound clinical judgment based on a detailed medical history, a thorough physical examination, and the judicious use of diagnostic procedures. Laboratory aids include procedures such as patch, open, scratch, intracutaneous, and serologic tests for allergy; Wood's light examinations and cultures and scrapings for bacteria, fungi, and viruses; and biopsies.

Before using the information in this chapter, the reader is urged to review Chapters 1 and 2, which provide a general discussion of the purpose of the *Guides* and of the situations in which they are useful; and which discuss techniques for the evaluation of the subject and for preparation of a report. The report should include the information found in the following outline, which is developed more fully in Chapter 2.

A. Medical Evaluation
1. Narrative history of medical conditions
2. Results of the most recent clinical evaluation
3. Assessment of current clinical status and statement of future plans
4. Diagnoses and clinical impressions
5. Expected date of full or partial recovery

B. Analysis of Findings

1. Impact of medical condition(s) on life activities
2. Explanation for concluding that the medical condition(s) has or has not become static or well-stabilized
3. Explanation for concluding that the individual is or is not likely to suffer from sudden or subtle incapacitation
4. Explanation for concluding that the individual is or is not likely to suffer injury or further impairment by engaging in life activities or by attempting to meet personal, social, and occupational demands
5. Explanation for concluding that accommodations and/or restrictions are or are not warranted

C. Comparison of Results of Analysis with Impairment Criteria

1. Description of clinical findings, and how these findings relate to specific criteria in the chapter
2. Explanation of each percent of impairment rating
3. Summary list of all impairment ratings
4. Overall rating of impairment of the whole person

13.1 Methods of Evaluating Impairment

In the evaluation of permanent impairment resulting from a skin disorder, the actual functional loss is the prime consideration, although the extent of cosmetic or cutaneous involvement may also be important.

Impairments of other body systems, such as behavioral problems, restriction of motion or ankylosis of joints, and respiratory, cardiovascular, endocrine, and gastrointestinal disorders, may be associated with a skin impairment. When there is permanent impairment in more than one body system, the degree of impairment for each system should be evaluated separately and combined, using the Combined Values Chart, to determine the impairment of the whole person.

Manifestations of skin disorders may be influenced by physical and/or chemical agents that a patient may encounter. While the avoidance of these irritant agents, possibly through a change in occupation, might alleviate the manifestations of the skin disorder, the presence of a skin disorder should be recognized and evaluated in accordance with the criteria below.

13.2 Pruritus

Pruritus is frequently associated with cutaneous disorders. It is a subjective, unpleasant sensation that provokes the desire to scratch or rub. The sensation is closely related to pain, in that it is mediated by pain receptors and pain fibers when they are weakly stimulated. However, the itching sensation may be intolerable. Like pain, it may be defined as a unique complex made up of afferent stimuli interacting with the emotional or affective state of the individual and modified by that individual's past experience and present state of mind.

The sensation of pruritus has two elements, peripheral neural stimulation and central nervous system reaction, which are extremely variable in make-up and in time. The first element may vary from total absence of sensation to an awareness of stimuli as either usual or unusual sensations. The second element is also variable and is modified by the person's state of attentiveness, past experience, motivation at the moment, and stimuli such as exercise, sweating, and changes in temperature.

In evaluating pruritus associated with skin disorders, the physician should consider (1) how the pruritus interferes with the individual's performance of the activities of daily living, including occupation; and (2) to what extent the description of the pruritus is supported by objective skin findings, such as lichenification, excoriation, or hyperpigmentation. Subjective complaints of itching that cannot be substantiated objectively may require specialized referral.

13.3 Disfigurement

Disfigurement is an altered or abnormal appearance. This may be an alteration of color, shape, or structure, or a combination of these. Disfigurement may be a residual of injury or disease, or it may accompany a recurrent or ongoing disorder. Examples include giant pigmented nevi, nevus flammeus, cavernous hemangioma, and alterations in pigmentation.

With disfigurement there is usually no loss of body function and little or no effect on the activities of daily living. Disfigurement may produce either social rejection or impairment of self-image, with self-imposed isolation, life-style alteration or other behavioral changes. If, however, impairment due to disfigurement does exist, it is usually manifested by a change in behavior such as the individual's withdrawal from society. Then it should be evaluated in accordance with the criteria set forth in Chapter 14.

In some patients with altered pigmentation there may be loss of body function and interference in the activities of daily living, which should be evaluated in accordance with the criteria below.

The description of disfigurement is enhanced by good color photographs showing multiple views of the defect. The probable duration and permanency of the altered appearance should be stated.

The possibility of improvement in the altered appearance through medical or surgical therapy, and the extent to which the alteration can be concealed cosmetically, such as with hair pieces, wigs, or cosmetics, should be described in writing and should be depicted with photographs if possible.

13.4 Scars

Scars are cutaneous abnormalities that result from the healing of burned, traumatized, or diseased tissue, and they represent a special type of disfigurement. Scars should be described by giving their dimensions in centimeters and by describing their shape, color, anatomical location, and evidence of ulceration; their depression or elevation, which relates to whether they are atrophic or hypertrophic; their texture, which relates to whether they are soft and pliable or hard and indurated, thin or thick and smooth or rough; and their attachment, if any, to underlying bone, joints, muscles, or other tissues. Good color photography with multiple views of the defect enhances the description of scars.

The tendency of a scar to disfigure should be considered in evaluating whether impairment is permanent, or whether the scar can be changed, made less visible, or concealed. Function may be restored without improving appearance, and appearance may be improved without altering anatomical or physiological function. Assignment of a percentage of impairment because of behavioral changes related to a scar should be done according to the criteria set forth in Chapter 14.

If a scar involves the loss of sweat gland function, hair growth, nail growth, or pigment formation, the effect of such loss on performance of the activities of daily living should be evaluated. Furthermore, any loss of function due to sensory deficit, pain, or discomfort in the scar area should be evaluated according to the criteria in Chapter 4. Loss of function due to limited motion in the scar area should be evaluated according to criteria in Chapter 3, or if chest wall excursion is limited, in Chapter 5.

13.5 Patch Testing—Performance, Interpretation, and Relevance

Patch testing is not a substitute for an adequately detailed history. Nevertheless, when properly performed and interpreted, patch tests can make a significant contribution to the diagnosis and management of contact dermatoses.

The physician must be aware that patch testing can yield false positive and false negative results. Selecting the proper concentration of the suspected chemical, the proper vehicle, the proper site of application, and the proper type of patch are critical in assuring validity of the procedure. Making such selections and determining the relevance of the test results require considerable skill and experience.

A positive or negative patch test result should not be accepted at face value until the details of the testing procedures have been evaluated. While appropriate test concentrations and vehicles have been established for many common sensitizers, for most chemicals in existence there are no established vehicle and concentration standards. Further details about patch testing and its pitfalls are discussed in standard texts.

13.6 Criteria for Evaluating Permanent Impairment of the Skin

Class 1—Impairment of the Whole Person, 0–5%: A patient belongs in Class 1 when (a) signs or symptoms of skin disorder are present; *and* (b) with treatment, there is no limitation, or minimal limitation, in the performance of the activities of daily living, although exposure to certain physical or chemical agents might increase limitation temporarily.

Example 1: A 48-year-old white man has operated a unit manufacturing silver nitrate for 20 years. Five years ago he noted bluish discoloration of the inner canthi of his eyes, which progressed so that presently the sclerae, face, and arms are now decidedly bluish, and the unexposed skin shows a slightly bluish tint. There is also bluish pigmentation in the posterior nasal passages and around the turbinates and the fauces. Although he is aware of the condition, it does not bother him. His general health is good, and the remainder of the physical examination shows no abnormalities. The results of laboratory studies are within normal limits. Skin biopsy of the arm confirms the diagnosis of argyria.

Diagnosis: Argyria.

Impairment: 0% impairment of the whole person.

Comment: If impairment from cosmetic disfigurement also existed, it would be manifested by behavioral changes, which should be evaluated in accordance with the criteria set forth in Chapter 14.

Example 2: Three years ago a 62-year-old man developed a lichenoid purpuric dermatosis of the legs that was biopsied. He experienced no pruritus, and he received specific medication. Six months later an incomplete, annular, infiltrative lesion that caused no symptoms developed in the right antecubital fossa. A biopsy established the diagnosis of mycosis fungoides. Complete blood count and bone marrow and liver biopsies were normal. The lesion responded well to 300 rads of x-ray therapy.

Diagnosis: Mycosis fungoides.

Impairment: 0% impairment of the whole person due to mycosis fungoides.

Example 3: A 27-year-old male worker in a small paint manufacturing company developed acute contact dermatitis of the hands and arms. He related onset and exacerbations to preparation of batches of latex paint. Patch testing revealed a strong, allergic reaction to a 0.1% petrolatum mixture of a non-mercurial preservative, 2-n-4-isothiazolin-3-one, used by the company in its latex paints. The patient was unable to avoid latex paint completely, and his dermatitis continued. When he left the company to seek other employment, his dermatitis resolved completely.

Diagnosis: Allergic contact dermatitis due to a latex paint preservative.

Impairment: 0% impairment of the whole person.

Comment: The preservative to which the worker was allergic was manufactured for use only in latex paints. It is used widely in the paint manufacturing industry but not in other industries. The patient was restricted from employment in industries where he would come in contact with the offending chemical, but there was no limitation in the performance of activities of daily living. Although this worker has 0% impairment of the whole person, he may be disabled under some state workers' compensation statutes.

Example 4: A 52-year-old janitor had episodes of transient dermatitis of the hand from the detergents he used in wet work duties over the past 13 years. About 10 years ago, depigmentation developed on the sides of most fingers and over the dorsa of the hands and distal forearms. Recently other areas of depigmentation became apparent on the upper torso and thighs.

    The janitor used a germicidal disinfectant that contained para-tertiary butyl phenol (TBP). Patch tests revealed a 2+ reaction to TBP 1% in petrolatum but not to other common industrial allergens. A month later, the site of the positive patch test became depigmented. Ultraviolet light therapy in combination with oral 8-methoxypsoralen (PUVA therapy) failed to stimulate repigmentation over a one year period. Covering with cosmetics was unsatisfactory.

    The janitor also was required to perform outdoor maintenance work. Sunburn frequently occurred in the areas lacking pigmentation. Early actinic changes with wrinkling, bruising, and scaling of the skin were present.

Diagnosis: Occupational leukoderma due to a phenolic chemical, TBP.

Impairment: 5% impairment of the whole person.

Comment: This rating does not consider any impairment of the man's self-image or of social relationships that might develop, nor the effects that these might have on the worker's future occupational situation.

Class 2—Impairment of the Whole Person, 10-20%: A patient belongs in Class 2 when (a) signs and symptoms of skin disorder are present; *and* (b) intermittent treatment is required; *and* (c) there is limitation in the performance of some of the activities of daily living.

Example 1: An eczematous eruption developed beneath the wedding ring on the fourth finger of the left hand of a 28-year-old housewife shortly after the birth of her first child six years ago. The eruption gradually spread to involve areas on several fingers of both hands despite treatment and avoidance of all jewelry. The eruption persisted for several months, then subsided slowly. A severe flare-up of hand dermatitis occurred after the birth of her second child two years later. Presently chronic, low-grade dermatitis persists despite special precautions. Intermittent treatment is required to control the dermatitis. The patient has no previous history of eczema, hay fever, or asthma, and no family history of atopy. Her general health is good. Patch tests performed with various food, household, cosmetic, and diagnostic and therapeutic contactant tray materials were nonreactive.

Diagnosis: Chronic dermatitis of the hands, from undetermined multiple contact factors.

Impairment: 10% impairment of the whole person.

Comment: While the history of atopy is negative, the clinical events are highly suggestive of an atopic cutaneous reaction of recurrent nature. Allergic contact dermatitis was not demonstrated but the cutaneous reaction to low grade irritant agents seems clear.

Example 2: A 25-year-old man who has a family history of "eczema" and hay fever has had a recurrent pruritic eruption since the age of one month, when it was characterized by oozing lesions of the face, scalp, neck, and upper extremities. A diagnosis of infantile eczema was made shortly after the onset. He had periods of relatively complete remission, but even during these periods, lichenified patches in his antecubital, popliteal, and nuchal areas persisted. Exacerbations were severe at age 14, when he entered high school, and increased in frequency during college. In the past three years, he had two episodes requiring hospitalization. These were characterized by a pruritic, red papular eruption of the face, neck, upper trunk, and shoulders, followed by scaling and dryness.

When the eruptions flare, they respond to the frequent application of topical steroids, to oatmeal starch baths, oral antihistamines, and occasional courses of ataractics. When his acute eczematous eruption subsides, he benefits from the application of a nonmedicated emollient cream to the dry scaling areas. Extensive patch and scratch tests do not elicit significant positive reactions. His condition is made worse by cold weather, marked changes in environmental temperature, and stressful situations in his job or at home. No residual scarring occurs. Exacerbations may require confinement for as long as seven days, either at home or in the hospital, along with treatment by a physician.

Diagnosis: Atopic dermatitis.

Impairment: 15% impairment of the whole person.

Comment: Attacks of atopic dermatitis are precipitated by a variety of excitants often of a chemical nature. The need for frequent hospitalization and absence from work may require evaluation of the mental health status.

Example 3: A 45-year-old white man developed an eczematous eruption on his left arm and hand during spring, four years ago. The eruption was treated effectively by admitting him to the hospital and giving topical medications. After the man's discharge, the condition flared up, involving the right side of his face and neck and the left forearm to the bottom of his work shirt sleeve. The eruption responded incompletely to treatment but subsided in the fall. It returned the next spring and subsided in the winter, but during the next two years it persisted throughout the year. Further history was that the eruption on the exposed areas subsided to some degree when the man was off work but flared up within a day after his return, even on the night shift. He worked in the warehouse of a paperbox factory and handled only printed paper cartons. Illumination of the work area was exclusively by banks of fluorescent tubes contained in low-hanging fixtures.

Medical examination disclosed evidence of chronic dermatitis. There were no positive reactions from extensive patch tests with materials from the patient's work, home, or personal activities, or from those in the standard screening tray. The minimal erythema dose (MED) was significantly decreased. Photo patch tests with halogenated salicylanilides and fragrances were negative. However, within six hours after he was exposed to five minutes of light from an 8-watt fluorescent bulb, a severe erythema and edema developed in the exposed area. Five days later, this area was eczematous. Tests for urinary porphyrins were within normal limits.

Whenever the man was exposed to fluorescent light or sunlight, the eruption recurred. It was necessary for him to change jobs and to avoid all ultraviolet light exposure, including fluorescent lighting. He could be kept comfortable by intermittent use of topical corticosteroids and benzophenone sunscreen. Exacerbations that required treatment occurred periodically.

Diagnosis: Persistent photodermatitis, elicited and aggravated by ultraviolet light, including exposure to fluorescent light.

Impairment: 20% impairment of the whole person.

Comment: The presence of a light receptor being applied to the skin periodically or being contacted at work remains obscure, but the reactivity to light is well demonstrated. Clinically this case could represent a persistent light reactor.

Example 4: One year ago a 32-year-old black woman developed a 2 cm area of erythema and induration of the right malar eminence. One month later, similar spots appeared on the left side of her forehead, on the left cheek, at the right external auditory meatus, and at the interior aspect of the pinna of the left ear. At first the spots were erythematous and indurated, but then they became scaly and hyperpigmented, progressing to hypopigmentation with atrophic changes and some hair loss. Hyperpigmentation persisted at the margins of the lesions.

The patient limited her exposure to sunlight, and except for occasional mild pruritus, the lesions were asymptomatic. Various ointments and antimalarial medications were prescribed, but there was no improvement of the lesions. The patient became depressed about her appearance, and her friends reported that she avoided them and seemed withdrawn.

Diagnosis: Discoid lupus erythematosus.

Impairment: 15% impairment due to discoid lupus erythematosus, which is to be combined with an appropriate value for the behavioral disorder to determine the impairment of the whole person.

Example 5: A 30-year-old white man was employed in a rare metals refining plant. Inadvertently he was splashed with concentrated liquid zirconium chloride over the face, scalp, and neck. Immediately he was washed, and then he was taken to the hospital, where he remained for two days. Healing and epithelialization occurred without complications. He returned to work 22 days after the episode.

Examination one year after the incident discloses well demarcated areas of depigmentation on the right side of the face, extending from behind the right ear to the center of the face, and from the mid-temple area of the scalp to the chin. There are smaller areas of depigmentation on the left side of the neck and behind the right ear. Maximum dimensions of the depigmented areas on the right side of the face are 16 cm by 11 cm. There are narrow collars of hyperpigmentation around the depigmented areas.

Neurological examination indicates that all of the depigmented areas are hypersensitive to cold, heat, pinprick, and touch, and for some of these areas, low-temperature stimuli are mistakenly identified as "hot" and "burning." In contrast to the adjacent normal skin, the depigmented areas sunburn easily causing considerable discomfort. When the patient is operating a kiln in the plant or approaching a furnace, the affected side develops a stinging sensation. In the affected areas there is occasional muscle twitching.

The patient experiences considerable embarrassment when attempting to explain his disfigurement, and he avoids many kinds of social activities in which he previously participated. Examinations show that there has been no change during the last six months in the pigment loss, hyperesthesia, and intolerance to sunlight and warmth. Plastic surgery is not indicated.

Diagnosis: Chemical leukoderma after zirconium chloride burn.

Impairment: 20% impairment due to leukoderma, which is to be combined with an appropriate value for the behavioral problem to determine impairment of the whole person.

Example 6: A 40-year-old woman had purchased a sculptured nail kit consisting of liquid methylmethacrylate monomer and powdered methylmethacrylate polymer. When mixed and applied to the fingernails according to directions, the chemicals formed a paste, which hardened to clear plastic resembling artificial nails. Her nails were initially normal, but she eventually developed swelling and redness of the eponychial and paronychial areas with severe pain and paresthesia of all 10 fingers. The nails on all 10 fingers were lost. When the acute, inflammatory process subsided, she was patch tested and was positive to 5% methylmethacrylate monomer in olive oil.

The patient was followed for several years, during which time none of her fingernails regrew. The nail beds were exposed and keratinized, and the paronych-

ial areas continued to be swollen and tender. The paresthesia persisted although she had stopped using the sculptured nail kit. She complained of difficulty grasping, cold sensitivity, burning, tingling, and "pins and needles" sensation, especially when picking up small objects, such as coins and needles. She also had difficulty with other nonspecialized hand activities. The slightest trauma from ordinary daily activities aggravated the symptoms and increased the paresthesia in her fingers. She typically applied adhesive bandages over vaseline to her nails and wore gloves most of her waking hours. The patient was considerably anxious and depressed, requiring occasional psychiatric consultation.

Diagnosis: Chemical induced nail dystrophy and anonychia.

Impairment: 20% impairment due to chemically induced nail dystrophy, which is to be combined with appropriate values for the paresthesia (see Chapter 3), as well as for the behavioral disorder (see Chapter 14) to determine the impairment of the whole person.

Class 3—Impairment of the Whole Person, 25-50%: A patient belongs in Class 3 when (a) signs and symptoms of skin disorder are present; *and* (b) continuous treatment is required; *and* (c) there is limitation in the performance of many activities of daily living.

Example 1: Twenty-two months ago, a 50-year-old woman developed a persistently sore mouth. An examination revealed many eroded lesions of the tongue and oral mucous membranes. Subsequently the patient noted the appearance of vesicles, and then bullae, over the face, trunk, and extremities. In the hospital, the diagnosis of pemphigus vulgaris was made, this being substantiated by histologic, immunofluorescent, and cytologic procedures. Oral administration of steroids brought about a prompt remission of the disease.

A month after the hospital admission, the patient was discharged on steroid therapy. Bullae reappeared when withdrawal of the steroid was attempted, and therapy with azothiaprine was started. Oral erosions continued to appear, and therapy with cytoxan and then methotrexate also failed to control the disease. The patient experienced difficulty in eating and swallowing and was forced to puree her food. The debilitating effects of her disease also interfere with her speech and sleep.

Diagnosis: Pemphigus vulgaris.

Impairment: 25% impairment of the whole person.

Example 2: For the last six years, a 45-year-old man has had a persistent pruritic dermatitis involving both ankles, forearms, and hands, and occasionally the face and neck. These areas are excoriated and lichenified. He has had recurrent bouts of pyogenic infection, and on occasion regional nodes have become swollen and tender.

At the time of onset, the man's work as a nurseryman included general greenhouse activity such as planting, weeding, watering, fertilizing, and spraying with numerous pesticides and antifungal agents. Some of the chemicals were found to be primary irritants. Initially the man's dermatitis responded to topical therapy and to his avoiding irritants, but the condition would flare up after re-exposure. Eventually, avoiding incriminated agents and changing jobs was not followed by the subsiding of symptoms, which caused neurodermatitis, or the "itch-scratch" syndrome. Warm environments, sweating, and stress provoked episodes of severe itching. The man had no history of a prior dermatologic problem.

Three years ago, the patient began to have episodes of headache and memory loss, and to note periods of tenseness and apprehension accompanied by nausea and vomiting. He was treated intermittently for the mental disturbances, with little improvement of the neurodermatitis.

The patient has not engaged in nursery work for the past three years. He finds it difficult to tolerate other kinds of work, claiming they make his dermatitis worse. He is gainfully employed no more than six months during the year. At home he has been unable to perform household maintenance chores and to participate in social and recreational activities, and he has experienced difficulty sleeping.

Diagnosis: Persistent neurodermatitis secondary to occupational contact dermatitis.

Impairment: 30% impairment due to the skin disorder, which is to be combined with an appropriate value for the behavioral disorder (see Chapter 14) to determine the impairment of the whole person.

Example 3: A 28-year-old man has had acne vulgaris for the past 12 years. He has not responded to the conventional methods of treatment. During the last five years he has developed large cystic lesions and draining sinuses on his face, neck, and upper trunk. This has been accompanied by fever and aching joints. Scarring is severe. The large lesions on his back and chest have made it difficult for him to rest comfortably. In warm weather, clothing irritates his skin. He has had difficulty sleeping, participating in social and recreational activities, and obtaining employment. Sweating also aggravates the skin disorder considerably

Diagnosis: Acne vulgaris, acne conglobata; post-acne scar formation.

Impairment: 30% impairment of the whole person.

Example 4: A 22-year-old woman entered the hospital with fever, malaise, arthralgia, painful hands and feet and marked erythema, and edema of the face, the V of the neck, and the areas of the back not covered by her bathing suit. She also complained of abdominal pain and nausea. The acute episode was precipitated by a trip to the seashore, where she had sunbathed for several hours.

On physical examination, she had erythema, edema, and scaling of exposed body areas, generalized annular, atrophic plaques involving the trunk, palms, and soles. The liver was tender to palpation, and there was an apical systolic murmur. Funduscopic examination revealed perivascular hemorrhages and fluffy exudates. Laboratory tests showed hemolytic anemia, leukopenia, hypocomplementemia, hyperglobulinemia, albuminuria, hematuria, a positive lupus erythematosus cell test, and a high antinuclear antibody titer.

Steroid therapy was begun, and the patient responded well. However, the hematuria and albuminuria persisted, and she had to be maintained on steroids. She remained very tired most of the time, especially after slight exertion. Plaquenil therapy was begun for the severe cutaneous involvement with only a partial improvement of her palms and soles. She has considerable difficulty grasping, standing, and walking because of the severe skin disease.

Diagnosis: Systemic lupus erythematosus.

Impairment: 50% impairment due to lupus erythematosus, which is to be combined with appropriate values for impairments of the other involved systems, namely the hematopoietic, urinary, and visual systems, to determine the impairment of the whole person.

Class 4—Impairment of the Whole Person, 55-80%: A patient belongs in Class 4 when (a) signs and symptoms of skin disorder are present; *and* (b) continuous treatment is required, which may include periodic confinement at home or other domicile; *and* (c) there is limitation in the performance of many of the activities of daily living.

Example 1: A 55-year-old man, who had been employed for 30 years as a parts clerk at a construction company warehouse, injured his right leg severely in an automobile crash while at work. The injury was followed by a deep vein thrombophlebitis of the right leg that required six months of total and partial bed rest, both in a hospital and at home.

After recovery the man began to work at a chemical company. He wore an elastic stocking, but his right leg began to swell more and more each day. Four days after starting work, he spilled a can of caustic drain cleaner, causing second and third degree burns over 20% of the right lower leg. He was hospitalized for 12 weeks until the burn healed, leaving a scar but no thickening or contracture.

After four months, the man returned to work at the chemical company, but in spite of using elastic support stockings and diuretics, the edema in his leg became intolerable. He was unable to stay on his feet more than four hours at a time without significant swelling and discomfort. He began to develop stasis dermatitis with ulceration. Periodic treatment with Unna paste boots and occasional admissions to the hospital healed the ulcers only temporarily. After five years at the chemical company, he quit work and applied for workers' compensation benefits, alleging total disability.

At the time of evaluation the following were noted. Below the right knee there were marked pitting edema, post-inflammatory hyperpigmentation, scar formation, and ulceration. A large hypopigmented, atrophic, scaly scar, measuring 10 cm by 20 cm, on which there was no sensation of light touch, was found laterally, beginning 8 cm above the ankle and extending upward 20 cm. A stasis ulcer measuring 7 cm by 5 cm was noted over the right medial malleolus.

Diagnosis: Post-thrombophlebitis syndrome with stasis dermatitis and ulceration; scar formation secondary to chemical burn.

Impairment: 55% impairment of the whole person.

Comment: Future episodes of phlebitis, cellulitis and ulceration are to be expected. Diligent medical care will be required indefinitely.

In similar cases, a physician may be asked to apportion a percentage of the overall impairment between the two injuries. The reader is referred to the discussion of apportionment in Chapter 1.

Example 2: Raynaud's phenomenon was first observed in a 38-year-old man about five years ago. Four years ago, he noted difficulty in swallowing, and then he developed swelling and tightening of the skin of the fingers, which gradually and progressively worsened. Dressing and feeding became progressively more difficult.

Examination discloses that the patient has increased pigmentation with telangiectasia, primarily on the face, forearms, and dorsal surface of his hands.

He has a "pinched facies," and the skin over most of the body is hidebound. Chest excursion is limited. The fingers are held in flexion, and the patient has ulcerations on the distal phalanges of both index fingers. He is unable to extend his fingers because of stiffness, tightness, and pain.

The patient's weight is 20% below the desirable weight for height and age. Complete blood cell count is within normal limits, except for a sedimentation rate of 40 mm/hr. Urinalysis is normal, and the lupus erythematosus cell test and serologic test for syphilis are negative. An electrocardiogram and a chest roentgenogram are interpreted as normal. Roentgenographic examinations reveal a mild stenosis of the esophagus and disturbed peristaltic activity.

Diagnosis: Acrosclerotic scleroderma, mild stenosis of esophagus, and flexion deformity of fingers, with chronic ulcerations.

Impairment: 55% impairment due to scleroderma, which is to be combined with appropriate values for the stenosis of the esophagus and the flexion deformities to determine the impairment of the whole person.

Example 3: A 32-year-old white man was first admitted to the hospital because of a widespread pustular eruption associated with an acute conjuctivitis and severe arthritis of all joints of the hands, wrists, knees, ankles, and toes. He stated that he had been in good health until two months before this admission, when he developed an erythematous scaly eruption of the pretibial areas, which then spread to involve his upper extremities and hand. Shortly thereafter he developed pain, swelling, and erythema of the knees, and a urethral discharge. No organisms were grown in culture. The joints of the hands and feet were warm, red, and tender, with minimal swelling. A skin biopsy was compatible with exudative psoriasis. He was treated with topical therapy with no response, but he improved on systemic steroids and cytotoxic agents.

At the time of discharge, he was thought to have either Reiter's syndrome, keratoderma blennorhagica, or pustular psoriasis with psoriatic arthritis.

He was rehospitalized three months later with an acute and severe exacerbation of his skin eruption with severe pain, swelling, and deformity of all joints of his extremities. A skin biopsy again was diagnostic of exudative psoriasis. Radiographic examination of the hands and wrists demonstrated marked bony demineralization of the carpal bones and the proximal and distal heads of the metacarpal and all the phalanges. Joint space narrowing and periosteal reaction were present in the metacarpal bones of both hands. Flexion deformities were present in both hands. Five months later, after some improvement, he was discharged from the hospital. Presently, oral doses of steroids and cytotoxic agents are required for controlling the disease. He continues to have periodic flare-ups of his arthritis and psoriasis, which require hospitalization.

Diagnosis: Pustular psoriasis with psoriatic arthritis.

Impairment: 60% impairment due to psoriasis, which is to be combined with appropriate values for the limitations of joint motion to determine the impairment of the whole person.

Comment: The clinical features of Reiter's syndrome and pustular psoriasis may overlap. The presence of conjunctivitis and urethritis favors the former; small joint arthritis of the hands and feet favors psoriasis. The finding of HLA-B27 antigen in about 65% of cases of Reiter's syndrome, as well as in most patients with pustular psoriasis, indicates a further link between these conditions. Both may relapse and adversely affect the activities of daily living.

Example 4: A 56-year-old white man was admitted to the hospital because of a generalized pruritic eruption. His condition began 20 years ago with pruritic patches on his back and extremities. Despite topical therapy the eruption gradually became generalized, and many patches became infiltrated plaques. Recently nodular lesions have developed. Past treatment has included topical nitrogen mustard, PUVA, and electron beam therapy.

Physical examination revealed a generalized eruption consisting of erythematous scaly plaques, some of which were quite infiltrated. There were also many excoriations found on the trunk and extremities, and nodular tumors on his face and soles of his feet. Palpable axillary and inguinal lymph nodes were noted.

Laboratory tests showed normal values for fasting blood sugar, blood urea nitrogen, creatinine, uric acid, alkaline phosphatase, bilirubin, cholesterol, prothrombin time, sedimentation rate, and platelet counts. A skin biopsy confirmed a diagnosis of mycosis fungoides. There were no abnormalities found in bone marrow aspiration, and the results of serology rheumatoid factor, antinuclear factor, and ECG were negative. A biopsy specimen from an axillary lymph node showed mycosis fungoides infiltrating the node.

The chest radiograph showed some tortuosity of the thoracic aorta. The heart was normal in size and shape.

The patient was given a cytotoxic agent intravenously daily for five days with excellent results, followed by oral doses of the same cytotoxic agent. Moderate control of his eruption has been obtained with the cytotoxic agent and radiation therapy.

Diagnosis: Mycosis fungoides.

Impairment: 75% impairment of the whole person.

Comment: Late stage, widespread mycosis fungoides requires close medical surveillance. Morbidity is considerable, and the prognosis is poor. In most patients there is interference with some activities of daily living and they succumb within two to five years.

Example 5: A 35-year-old male technician inadvertently had exposures of about 12,000 rads to the hands and forearms while working on an x-ray machine. Within hours, an intense bluish-purple erythema appeared on the hands and wrists that was followed rapidly by the development of large, tense blisters filled with serous exudate. Treatment was symptomatic, and over the next few weeks the exposed areas became pigmented and atrophic, showing telangiectasia. Later, after only minor trauma, the exposed areas would develop large, tender ulcerations that would only partly heal.

During the next two years, the technician developed contractures that made it impossible for him to resume employment. He had to protect the affected skin from even minor injury, and he developed many limitations in his ability to care for himself. He became depressed and often thought of suicide. Excision of the ulcers and skin grafting were unsuccessful, the grafts quickly breaking down.

Diagnosis: Chronic radiation dermatitis with ulceration and scarring of both hands.

Impairment: 80% impairment due to radiation dermatitis, which is to be combined with appropriate values for the mental disorder to determine the impairment of the whole person.

Comment: The effects of such radiation exposure are life-long and progressive. Repeated skin ulceration will occur and adversely affect the activities of daily living and survival.

Class 5—Impairment of the Whole Person, 85-95%: A patient belongs in Class 5 when (a) signs and symptoms of skin disorder are present; *and* (b) continuous treatment is required, which necessitates confinement at home or other domicile; *and* (c) there is severe limitation in the performance of the activities of daily living.

Example 1: A 12-year-old girl has had photophobia for eight years. At the age of five years, she developed marked pigmentation of sun-exposed areas of the face, chest, arms, and legs. Since then, she has developed generalized freckling of the skin, several areas of

Table 1. Impairment Classification for Skin Disease

Class 1 0-5% Impairment of the Whole Person	Class 2 10-20% Impairment of the Whole Person	Class 3 25-50% Impairment of the Whole Person	Class 4 55-80% Impairment of the Whole Person	Class 5 85-95% Impairment of the Whole Person
A patient belongs in Class 1 when signs or symptoms of skin disorder are present	A patient belongs in Class 2 when signs and symptoms of skin disorder are present	A patient belongs in Class 3 when signs and symptoms of skin disorder are present	A patient belongs in Class 4 when signs and symptoms of skin disorder are present	A patient belongs in Class 5 when signs and symptoms of skin disorder are present
and	**and**	**and**	**and**	**and**
with treatment, there is no limitation, or minimal limitation, in the performance of the activities of daily living, although exposure to certain physical or chemical agents might increase limitation temporarily.	intermittent treatment is required **and** there is limitation in the performance of some of the activities of daily living.	continuous treatment is required **and** there is limitation in the performance of many activities of daily living.	continuous treatment is required which may include periodic confinement at home or other domicile **and** there is limitation in the performance of many of the activities of daily living.	continuous treatment is required, which necessitates confinement at home or other domicile **and** there is severe limitation in the performance of activities of daily living.

Signs or symptoms of skin disorders classified in Classes 1 and 2 may be intermittent and may not be present at the time of examination.

telangiectasia, and multiple basal and squamous cell epitheliomas. The condition is progressing in severity and the patient requires continuous observation and treatment. She has been confined to the home for the past year. Laboratory tests for blood and urine show normal values. Fecal and urinary porphyrin studies were negative.

Diagnosis: Xeroderma pigmentosum.

Impairment: 85% impairment of the whole person.

Comment: Xeroderma pigmentosum is a progressive disease with ultimate impairment approaching 100%. Development of metastatic carcinoma from squamous cell carcinomas or malignant melanoma can be expected, leading to early death.

Example 2: A 19-year-old boy developed bullous lesions shortly after birth; these have been present continuously since then, except for very minor and short remissions. Bullae appear after the slightest trauma and, at times, without apparent trauma, and heal with severe scarring. The boy's fingers now are tapered stumps. Bullae are present almost constantly in the mouth and pharynx, probably to the level of the esophagus. The boy requires continuous hospitalization. His weight is 40% below the desirable weight for his height. Roentgenography shows stricture of the esophagus.

Diagnosis: Epidermolysis bullosa dystrophica.

Impairment: 90% impairment due to epidermolysis bullosa dystrophica, which is to be combined with appropriate values for the stricture of the esophagus and the finger stumps to determine the impairment of the whole person.

Comment: This autosomal recessive disorder is one of the most impairing of all hereditary diseases, with impairment approaching 100%. Appropriate values for psychiatric complications should be combined with the physicial features of this disorder.

Example 3: A 25-year-old black man suffered burns on his body from a gasoline explosion three years prior to being seen by a dermatologist for impairment evaluation. He stated that he needed to soak 30 minutes a day with a teaspoon of alcohol and a teaspoon of Ivory soap in the water, after which he coated his body with Vaseline, but he still experienced a considerable amount of itching. He felt that he could not work with heavy equipment and be outdoors, because when he is out in the sun or in the heat he is not able to perspire and he becomes dizzy. However, he sweats extensively on his face. He has difficulty with writing, walking, and with nonspecialized hand activities because of scar formation. His ability to participate in group activities is greatly limited.

On physical examination approximately 85% of his body was involved in some dermatologic disease, including residual of burn scars; graft sites and donor sites; depigmentation in the axillae, palms, dorsum of the hands and ankles; partial destruction of the left ear; and thickened fingernails. The cheeks were mildly involved, but there was essentially no involvement of the neck and of a three-inch band around his waist. There was some hypertrophic scar formation involving approximately 20% of the individual skin.

Diagnosis: Residual skin damage with extensive scarring secondary to a gasoline explosion.

Impairment: 90% impairment of the whole person.

Comment: Approximately two years later, the patient was again seen by the dermatologist. He stated that his workers' compensation had been discontinued over a year ago. He also stated that the Social Security Administration had sent him to another physician for an evaluation of his problem, and that physician told him he could return to work. As a result, the Social Security Administration discontinued his payments, and he consulted an attorney.

Physical examination revealed no essential change in the skin except for minimal repigmentation in some areas. His subjective complaints were the same, and he still used Vaseline all over his body twice a day with soaking in the tub 30 minutes a day. The evaluation of the impairment of the whole person remained the same at 90%.

The criteria for evaluating permanent impairment due to skin disorders are recapitulated in Table 1.

References

1. Adams RM: *Occupational Skin Disease.* New York, Grune and Stratton, 1982.

2. *The Cosmetic Benefit Study.* Washington, DC, The Cosmetic, Toiletry and Fragrance Association, 1978.

3. Key MM: Confusing compensation cases. *Cutis 1967;* 3:965-969.

4. Maibach HJ, Gellin GA (eds): *Occupational and Industrial Dermatology.* Chicago, Yearbook Medical Publishers, 1982.

5. Fisher AA: Permanent loss of fingernails from sensitization and reaction to acrylics in a preparation designed to make artificial nails. *J Dermatol Surg Oncol 1980;* 6:70-71.

Chapter 14

Mental and Behavioral Disorders

14.0 Introduction

This chapter discusses impairments due to mental disorders and touches upon behavioral impairments which might complicate any condition. Fundamental principles of impairment and disability, as well as an overview of the assessment of the whole person, are provided in Chapters 1 and 2. The reader is referred to those sections for a discussion of these issues. This chapter incorporates some of those principles as they relate to impairments and functional limitations associated with mental disorders, and it presents guidelines for assessing impairment severity. Some of the material is taken from Social Security Administration regulations ("The Listings of Mental Impairments") developed by a workgroup of experts in disability due to mental impairments. The workgroup was cosponsored by the Social Security Administration and the American Psychiatric Association.

Three principles are central to assessing mental impairment:

1. Diagnosis is among the factors to be considered in assessing the severity and possible duration of the impairment, but it is by no means the sole criterion.

2. Motivation for improvement may be a key factor in the outcome of impairment.

3. A complete assessment requires a longitudinal history of the impairment, its treatment, and attempts at rehabilitation.

14.1 Diagnosis and Impairment

The Diagnostic and Statistical Manual of Mental Disorders (ed 3, revised in 1987), commonly known as DSM III R, is a widely accepted classification system for mental disorders. It is similar to another system, The International Classification of Diseases (ICD), also in widespread use. The criteria for mental disorders include a wide range of signs, symptoms, and impairments. Most mental disorders are characterized by one or more impairments. An individual may have a mental or behavioral impairment, however, without meeting the criteria for one of the mental disorders specified in the DSM III R or the ICD.

DSM III R calls for a multiaxial evaluation. Each of five axes refers to a different class of information. The first three constitute the official diagnostic evaluation, including the clinical syndromes and conditions that are the focus of treatment (Axis I), personality and developmental disorders (Axis II), and physical disorders and conditions that may be relevant to understanding and managing the care of the individual (Axis III). Axis IV (specifying and rating psychosocial stressors) and Axis V (rating adaptive functioning) may be particularly important for assessing severity of impairment.

Specific impairments: In judging the degree of mental impairment, it is important to recognize that there are various types of mental disorders, each of which, like a physical disorder, has its own natural history and unique characteristics. It is apparent that some major mental disorders are chronic. The term "remission" rather than "cure" is used to indicate improvement, and remission may be intermittent, long-term, or short-term, and may occur in stages rather than all at once. The degree of impairment may vary considerably among patients, and the severity of the impairment is not necessarily related to the diagnosis. Indeed, diagnosis alone is of limited relevance to the objective assessment of psychiatric impairment, because it does not permit sufficient insight into the nature of the impairment.

An episode of depression following a stressful life event, for instance, is often a short-term, self-limiting illness that may clear up when the stressful situation is relieved. Other affective disorders have their own patterns of recurrence and chronicity and often respond well to therapeutic interventions. Somatic and psychological treatment and adequate supervision are important in all affective disorders, because one outcome of partial, ineffective treatment may be suicide or attempted suicide. The schizophrenias are typically chronic disorders. Their onset can be insidious and recognized only in retrospect. Certain organic mental disorders, such as traumatic brain injury and lifelong mental retardation, are chronic. Treatment consists of minimizing the response to the pathology; for some patients, achieving only a degree of capability or habilitation may be a valid goal.

The types of mental dysfunctioning in various disorders are curiously similar, regardless of the specific diagnosis. Just as "fever" and "pain" are seen in different kinds of physical disorders, so "anxiety" and "hostility" may be observed in different kinds of mental disorders.

14.2 Evidence of Mental Impairments

The following recommendations on documentation are drawn from the "Listings of Mental Impairments" in regulations of the Social Security Administration.

The presence of a mental disorder should be documented primarily on the basis of reports from individual providers, such as psychiatrists and psychologists, and facilities such as hospitals and clinics. Adequate descriptions of functional limitations must be obtained from these or other sources which may include programs and facilities where the individual has been observed over a considerable period of time. Longitudinal data are particularly useful.

Information from both medical and nonmedical sources may be used to obtain detailed descriptions of the individual's activities of daily living; social func-

tioning; concentration, persistence, or pace; or ability to tolerate increased mental demands (stress). This information can be provided by programs such as community mental health centers, day care centers, sheltered workshops, etc. It can also be provided by others, including family members, who have knowledge of the individual's function. In some cases descriptions of activities of daily living or social functioning given by individuals or treating sources may be insufficiently detailed and/or may be in conflict with the clinical picture otherwise observed or described in the examinations or reports. It is necessary to resolve any inconsistencies or gaps that may exist in order to obtain a proper understanding of the individual's functional restrictions.

An individual's level of functioning may vary considerably over time. The level of functioning at a specific time may seem relatively adequate or, conversely, rather poor. Proper evaluation of the impairment must take any variations in level of functioning into account in arriving at a determination of severity of impairment over time. Thus, it is vital to obtain evidence from relevant sources over a sufficiently long period prior to the date of evaluation in order to establish the individual's severity of impairment. This evidence should include treatment notes, hospital discharge summaries, and work evaluation or rehabilitation progress notes if these are available.

Some individuals may have attempted to work or may actually have worked during the period of time pertinent to the determination of impairment. This may have been an independent attempt at work, or it may have been in conjunction with a community mental health or other sheltered program, which may have been of either short or long duration. Information concerning the individual's behavior during any attempt to work and the circumstances surrounding termination of the work effort are particularly useful in determining the individual's ability or inability to function in a work setting. Results of work evaluations and rehabilitation programs can be significant sources of relevant data in regard to vocational and related impairments.

The results of well-standardized psychological tests such as the Wechsler Adult Intelligence Scale (WAIS), the Minnesota Multiphasic Personality Inventory (MMPI), the Rorschach and the Thematic Apperception Test (TAT), may be useful in establishing the existence of a mental disorder. For example, the WAIS is useful in establishing mental retardation, and the MMPI, Rorschach, and TAT may provide data supporting several other diagnoses. Broad-based neuropsychological assessments using, for example, the Halstead-Reitan or the Luria-Nebraska batteries may be useful in determining brain function deficiencies, particularly in cases involving subtle findings such as may be seen in traumatic brain injury. In addition, the process of taking a standardized test requires concentration, persistence, and pace. Therefore, performance on such tests may provide useful data. Test results should, therefore, include both the objective data and a narrative description of clinical findings. Narrative reports of intellectual assessment should include a discussion of whether or not obtained IQ scores are considered valid and consistent with the individual's developmental history and degree of functional restriction.

14.3 Assessing Impairment Severity

The Social Security Administration's "Listings of Mental Impairments" suggest four areas for assessing the severity of mental impairments. Severity is assessed in terms of functional limitations on activities of daily living; social functioning; concentration, persistence and pace; and adaptive functioning in response to stressful circumstances. Independence, appropriateness, and effectiveness are all considered when assessing impairment severity. The four areas of functional limitation are discussed below:

1. **Activities of daily living** include activities such as self care and personal hygiene, communication, ambulation, attaining all normal living postures, travel, non-specialized hand activities, sexual function, sleep, and social and recreational activities (see Appendix A). In the context of the individual's overall situation, the quality of these activities is judged by their independence, appropriateness and effectiveness. It is necessary to define the extent to which the individual is capable of initiating and participating in activities independent of supervision or direction.

What is assessed is not simply the number of activities that are restricted but the overall degree of restriction or combination of restrictions. For example, a person who is able to cook and clean might still have marked restrictions of daily activities if he or she were too fearful to leave the home or neighborhood, hampering the ability to obtain treatment or even to shop.

2. **Social functioning** refers to an individual's capacity to interact appropriately and communicate effectively with other individuals. Social functioning includes the ability to get along with others, such as family members, friends, neighbors, grocery clerks, landlords, or bus drivers. Impaired social functioning may be demonstrated by a history of altercations, evictions, firings, fear of strangers, avoidance of interpersonal relation-

ships, social isolation, etc. Strength in social functioning may be documented by an individual's ability to initiate social contacts with others, communicate clearly with others, interact and actively participate in group activities, etc. Cooperative behaviors, consideration for others, awareness of others' feelings, and social maturity also need to be considered. Social functioning in work situations may involve interactions with the public, responding appropriately to persons in authority, such as supervisors, or cooperative behaviors involving coworkers.

Again, it is not the number of areas in which social functioning is impaired, but the overall degree of interference with a particular functional area or combination of such areas of functioning. For example, a person who is highly antagonistic, uncooperative, or hostile, but is tolerated by local storekeepers may nevertheless have marked restrictions in social functioning because that behavior is not acceptable in other social contexts, such as work.

3. **Concentration, persistence, and pace** refer to the ability to sustain focused attention sufficiently long to permit the timely completion of tasks commonly found in work settings. In activities of daily living, concentration may be reflected in terms of ability to complete tasks in everyday household routines. Deficiencies in concentration, persistence, and pace are best observed in work and work-like settings. Major impairment in this area can often be assessed through direct psychiatric examination and/or psychological testing, although mental status examination or psychological test data alone should not be used to accurately describe concentration and sustained ability to adequately perform work-like tasks. On mental status examinations, concentration is assessed by tasks such as having the individual subtract serial sevens from 100. In psychological tests of intelligence or memory, concentration is assessed through tasks requiring short-term memory or through tasks that must be completed within established time limits. In work evaluations, concentration, persistence, and pace are assessed through such tasks as filing index cards, locating telephone numbers, or disassembling and reassembling objects. Strengths and weaknesses in areas of concentration can be discussed in terms of frequency of errors, time it takes to complete the task, and extent to which assistance is required to complete the task. A person who appears to concentrate adequately on a mental status examination or in a psychological test situation may not do so in a more "real life" work-evaluation program.

4. Deterioration or decompensation in work or work-like settings refers to repeated failure to **adapt to stressful circumstances**, which cause the individual either to withdraw from that situation or to experience exacerba-

tion of signs and symptoms of his or her mental disorder (ie, decompensation) with an accompanying difficulty in maintaining activities of daily living, social relationships, and/or maintaining concentration, persistence, or pace (ie, deterioration that may include deterioration of adaptive behaviors). Stresses common to the work environment include decisions, attendance, schedules, completing tasks, interactions with supervisors, interactions with peers, etc.

14.4 Special Considerations

Particular problems are often involved in evaluating mental impairments in individuals who have long histories of repeated hospitalizations or prolonged outpatient care with supportive therapy and medication. Individuals with chronic psychotic disorders commonly have their lives structured in such a way as to minimize stress and reduce their signs and symptoms. Such individuals may be much more impaired for work than their signs and symptoms would indicate. The results of a single examination may not adequately describe these individuals' sustained ability to function. It is, therefore, vital to review pertinent information relative to the individual's condition, especially at times of increased stress.

Effects of structured settings: Particularly in cases involving chronic mental disorders, overt symptoms may be controlled or attenuated by psychosocial factors such as placement in a hospital, board and care facility, day treatment program, or other environment that provides similar structure. Highly structured and supportive settings may greatly reduce the mental demands placed on an individual. With lowered mental demands, overt signs and symptoms of the underlying mental disorder may be minimized. However, the individual's inability to function outside such a structured and/or supportive setting may not have changed. An evaluation of individuals whose symptoms are controlled or attenuated by psychosocial factors must consider the ability of the individual to function outside such highly structured settings.

Effects of medication: Attention must be given to the effect of medication on the individual's signs, symptoms, and ability to function. While psychotropic medications may control certain primary manifestations of a mental disorder, such as hallucinations, such treatment may or may not affect the functional limitations imposed by the mental disorder. In cases where overt symptoms are attenuated by psychotropic medications,

particular attention must be focused on the functional restrictions that may persist. These functional restrictions are also to be used as the measures of severity of impairment.

Neuroleptics, the medicines used in the treatment of some mental illnesses, may cause drowsiness, blunted affect, or other side effects involving other body systems. Such side effects must be considered in evaluating overall severity of impairment as well as the patient's functional capacity. A medication, necessary to control signs and symptoms such as hallucinations, may secondarily cause an "amotivational"-like syndrome.

Effects of rehabilitation: Of paramount importance to the evaluator is the degree of vocational limitation suffered by the individual, which may range from minimal to total. The severity of an impairment may vary with the course of the illness, and when an individual is ready for discharge, vocational skills may be intact, or the individual may have slight, moderate, or severe limitations that may or may not be reversible. The evaluator must judge the possible duration of any remaining impairment, whether remission may be fast or slow, whether it might be partial or total, and whether it is likely to remain stable or get worse. Upon such considerations will depend any clinical judgment about degree of impairment.

Rehabilitation is a sine qua non in treating most patients who have recovered or are recovering from the acute phase of mental disorder, especially a major mental disorder. Even if it is not possible to effect total "remission" or "cure," the outcome may be considered worthwhile if the individual has been able to move from one degree of impairment to one of a lesser degree.

For some persons, lack of motivation seems to be a major cause for continuing impairment. Yet, with proper rehabilitative measures many patients, including some patients with organic illnesses, achieve improvement of function. Determination of permanent impairment is often imprecise, and rarely is there certainty that it exists. The use of such a determination is pessimistic, providing an adverse prediction that may well be self-fulfilling. However, the tendency for physicians and others to minimize impairment of a psychiatric nature must also be considered. Patients may not be referred for potentially helpful rehabilitation.

An important aspect of rehabilitation is the recognition that an individual on certain types of medication may be able to sustain a satisfactory degree of functioning, whereas without medication, he or she might fail to do so. For instance, there may be only a slight problem in the thinking process while the patient is taking suitable medication, but a severe one if the patient is not taking medication. Another vital part of the rehabilitation effort is to educate family and potential employers about the importance of maintenance doses of the medication, as well as about the possibility that the patient may re-experience symptoms while taking or not taking medication.

Another consideration is that an employer needs reassurance that a worker on proper medication and in the proper job is a safe worker. An example is the control of epileptic seizures with medication. Education of the patient's family, employer, and fellow workers in such matters is vital and should be a part of the rehabilitation process.

Just as there are degrees of impairment, "total rehabilitation" may not be possible. To use an example from physical medicine, it is impossible for an amputated leg to be replaced, and the affected individual cannot hope to regain perfect, pre-injury ambulation. But a well-fitted prosthesis, accompanied by training in its use, can greatly improve ability to walk. If, in addition, the individual obtains suitable private or public transportation, he or she may well be totally restored to gainful employment, unless total ambulation is a requirement of the job. Even if it is, an employer could provide alternative tasks, or modify existing tasks so that they can be performed successfully by an amputee who makes skillful use of a suitable prosthesis.

Obviously, the analogy between the loss of a limb and the loss of capability resulting from a mental disorder has limitations. Nonetheless, it is important to recognize that residual impairment from a mental disorder may be just as real and severe as impairment resulting from a physical disorder or injury. The link between motivation and recovery may need strengthening in individuals impaired either by physical or mental illnesses, and this is a task for rehabilitation psychiatry. The provision by the employer of alternative tasks, or the modification of existing work conditions, may be an important part of restoration to vocational ability for a patient with mental illness, just as it is for one with a physical illness, or for one with an illness that combines elements of both.

Controversial impairment categories: Each of the various entitlement programs and systems of disability assessment may recognize some mental disorders and reject others as "legitimate" causes of mental impairment. There is controversy about the personality disorders (especially antisocial personality disorder) and about alcoholism and substance abuse and dependence. The adjustment disorders also present a dilemma to the evaluator. They are characterized by abnormal emotional responses to stressful life events that resolve in a short

period of time when the stressor is removed. Some experts do not consider these adjustments to life circumstances as "medical impairments."

Pain: The assessment of impairment due to the perception of pain, especially in circumstances in which the complaint exceeds what is expected based on physical findings, is complex and controversial. Although this issue is discussed elsewhere in the *Guides,* it is germane to mental and behavioral disorders. The perception of pain may be distorted by mental disorders. Pain may be an element in a somatic delusion in a patient with a major depression or a psychotic disorder. It may become the object of an obsessive preoccupation or a chief complaint in a conversion disorder. The latter has been called "psychogenic pain disorder" or "idiopathic pain disorder," but these terms are often used more loosely to describe any complaint of pain that is greater than the physician expects for the "normal" patient with the same physical findings. The more specific disorders with impairments in the perception of pain are somewhat easier to evaluate than cases in which the perception of pain is said to have a "psychogenic component." Such cases require specialized assessment, perhaps using a multidisciplinary, multispecialty approach.

Motivation: The assessment of motivation is problematic, in that motivation is often difficult to distinguish from mental impairment. When is an individual who is suffering from anhedonia and lack of energy, concentration, and initiative to be considered depressed, and when is such an individual "unmotivated?" This is a complicated clinical distinction. Ultimately it is a clinical judgment, aided by a careful investigation of the history of level of effort and accomplishment prior to the onset of an alleged impairment and a search for associated signs and symptoms of common mental disorders (such as psychosis and withdrawal in schizophrenia or sleep and appetite disturbance in major depression).

The issue of motivation cannot be ignored as a connecting link between impairment and disability. For some people, poor motivation is a major cause for continuing malfunction. The underlying character of the individual may be a major factor in whether or not he or she is likely to be motivated to benefit from rehabilitation. Personality characteristics usually remain unchanged throughout adult life. However, internal events, that is, psychological reactions, can influence the course of physical and mental illness. An individual who tends to be dependent may become more dependent as the course of the illness proceeds, and one who is inclined to act out impulses may develop a constant pattern of antisocial behavior. Indeed, the pathological development of an underlying character trait may become even more pronounced and more significant than the actual illness in deterring motivation for improved functioning. Thus, the degree of disability in the social and vocational context is not necessarily the same as the degree of impairment. The loss of function may be greater or less than the impairment might warrant, and the individual's performance may fall short of, or exceed, that usually associated with the impairment. Here the complex issue of "secondary gain" arises, involving not only the amount of compensation or financial benefit that may be awarded, but also the individual's lifestyle. The individual's motivation to recover and to be self-sufficient will either diminish or enhance the quality of life, in terms of social and vocational activities. Impairment may lead to an almost total or minimal disability depending on motivational factors. Often it is difficult for an evaluator to separate impairment and motivation. The evaluator may be able to see some clues in the clinical or family history, but these are likely to be only suggestive.

When considering the total background and underlying character and value system of the individual, it must be remembered that educational levels and financial resources of family members cannot be ignored. The evaluator should assess the usefulness of family influences, and if rehabilitation efforts are to be continued, the evaluator may recommend the inclusion of the family in the endeavor.

14.5 A Method of Evaluating Psychiatric Impairment

Although there is no available empirical evidence to support any method for assigning percentage of impairment of the whole person, the following approach to quantifying mental impairment is offered as a guide. Not everyone who has a mental or behavioral disorder is totally limited or totally impaired. Many individuals have specific limitations that do not preclude all of life's activities. On the other hand, there are individuals with less than chronic, unremitting impairments who are severely limited in some areas of function. These limiting impairments must be acknowledged as a significant concern. Some disability systems choose to recognize only rather complete disability (especially for work), while others recognize and compensate partial disability.

Medically determinable impairments in thinking, affect, intelligence, perception, judgment, and behavior are assessed by direct observation, formal mental status examination, and neuropsychological testing. Translating specific impairments directly and precisely into functional limitations, however, is complex and poorly

understood. For example, current research finds little relationship between psychiatric signs and symptoms (such as those found on a mental status examination) and the ability to perform competitive work. To bridge the gap between impairment and disability, the workgroup that advised the Social Security Administration on disability due to mental impairment identified the four areas of functional limitation discussed above. In a sense they are complex impairments of social functioning that may be directly related to work or other functional pursuits such as recreation, but there is no specific medical test for any one of the four categories of functional limitation. Observations made during the medical examination should be incorporated along with other relevant and important observations that go into an assessment of activities of daily living such as social functioning; concentration, persistence, and pace; and adaptive functioning.

Table 1 provides a guide for rating mental impairment in each of the four areas of functional limitation on a five-point ordinal scale, ranging from none to extreme. It might be useful to think of the following as "anchors" for each point on the scale. "None" means that there is no impairment noted in this area of function. "Mild" implies that any impairment that is discerned is compatible with most useful function. "Moderate" means that impairments that are found are compatible with some but not all useful function. "Marked" is a level of functional impairment that significantly impedes useful function. Taken alone, a marked impairment or limitation would not completely preclude function, but together with another marked limitation it may likely preclude useful function. "Extreme" means that the impairment or limitation is not compatible with useful function. For example, extreme limitation in activities of daily living implies complete dependency on another for personal care. In the area of social functioning extreme impairment implies that the individual engages in no meaningful social contact, such as a patient in a withdrawn, catatonic state. An extreme limitation in concentration, persistence, or pace means that the individual cannot attend to conversation or any productive task at all, such as might be seen in an acute confusional state or a complete loss of short-term memory. Extreme limitations in adaptive functioning are seen in individuals who cannot tolerate any change at all in routines or in their environment, such as those who cannot function, and decompensate or deteriorate whenever schedules of events change in an otherwise structured environment. Such individuals might have a psychotic episode whenever a meal is not served on time or might have a panic attack whenever they are left without companions in any environment.

In an otherwise ordinary individual one area of extreme impairment would be likely to preclude perfor-

Table 1. Impairment Due to Mental and Behavioral Disorders

Areas of Function	Class 1 No Impairment	Class 2 Mild Impairment	Class 3 Moderate Impairment	Class 4 Marked Impairment	Class 5 Extreme Impairment
Activities of Daily Living Social Functioning Concentration Adaptation	No impairments noted	Impairment levels compatible with most useful function	Impairment levels compatible with some but not all useful function	Impairment levels significantly impede useful function	Impairment levels preclude useful function

mance of any complex task, such as recreation or work. Two or more areas of marked limitation would also be likely to preclude performance of complex tasks without special support or assistance, such as provided in a sheltered environment. An individual who was impaired to a moderate degree in all four areas of function would be significantly limited in many, but not all, complex tasks. Mild and moderate limitations reduce overall performance but do not preclude performance.

Translating these guidelines for rating individual impairment on *ordinal* scales into a method for assigning percentage impairments, as if the ratings were made on precisely measured *interval* scales, is not recommended. For example, we cannot be certain that the difference in impairment between a rating of mild and moderate is the same as the difference between moderate and marked. Furthermore, a moderate impairment does not imply 50% limitation in useful function. Similarly, a rating of moderate impairment in all four areas of function does not imply a 50% impairment of the whole person. In reality, however, physicians often are required to make such judgments. It is important to remember that such judgments are based on clinical impression rather than on empirical evidence. In those circumstances in which it is essential to make a percentage rating, the ordinal scale might be of some help: one could assume that the extreme rating approaching 100% mental impairment is similar to a coma, which is the extreme impairment of central nervous system function and level of consciousness.

Eventually research may support the direct link between medical findings and percentage of mental impairment. Until that time the medical profession must refine its concepts of mental impairment, improve its ability to measure limitations, and continue to make clinical judgments.

Example: A 27-year-old single woman is referred for evaluation for mental impairment. She has a nine year history of chronic paranoid schizophrenia. She has not worked for longer than two months at a time since dropping out of business college at the age of 19 years. The young woman has lived at home, and was cared for and supported financially by her aging parents, who

recently moved to a retirement community. For the past three months she has been living in a cooperative apartment and has shown some ability to care for herself, although she needs to be reminded constantly to bathe, to take her medications, and to complete her household chores. She has little self-confidence and does not engage independently in any activities, including cooking, although when someone insists, she is capable of doing so. Once she initiates a task, she can complete it in a timely manner. She has no friends, never initiates a conversation, and when she is approached or prodded, she becomes terrified and occasionally abusive. The woman remains quite paranoid, concerned that everyone "knows my mind." Her attention span is limited to 25 to 30 minutes, however, and she frequently "blocks" in her speech and is unable to complete a thought. Although she has been hospitalized only twice, she frequently stops taking her neuroleptic medications, which are generally quite effective in controlling her delusions and hallucinations. Both times she was employed she became overwhelmed by the pressures of work deadlines, blamed her coworkers for slowing her down, stopped her medications, and required a return to intensive treatment. She handles some of the changes in her environment well but has considerable difficulty with the demands of time and with separation from her family.

Impairment: The evaluator concludes that her activities of daily living and social functioning are markedly impaired, and her ability to concentrate, maintain a reasonable pace, and adapt to change are, at best, moderately impaired. However, the evaluator feels that in more demanding social or vocational situations this woman would also be markedly impaired in concentration and adaptation. Therefore, he concludes that overall she is markedly impaired.

Reference

1. Social Security Administration: Federal Old-Age, Survivors and Disability Insurance: Listing of Impairments. Mental Disorders; Final Rule. Fed Reg 20 CFR Part 404 (Reg No 4) 50 (167), 35038-35070, 1985.

Appendix A

Glossary

Correct standardized usage of terminology related to the evaluation of medical impairment and disability is essential. Semantic distinctions between terms assume legal importance. This Glossary provides definitions of terms that are used in the *Guides,* and definitions of other terms related to impairment and disability evaluations that may be of interest to the reader, although they are not mentioned in the *Guides.* To assist the reader in distinguishing the evaluation of impairment from that of disability, this Glossary is in two sections: the first section contains terms related to impairment; the second section contains terms related to disability evaluation, workers' compensation, and employability.

Impairment

1. Activities of Daily Living

Activity	Example
Self care and personal hygiene	Urinating, defecating, brushing teeth, combing hair, bathing, dressing oneself, eating
Communication	Writing, typing, seeing, hearing, speaking
Normal living postures	Sitting, lying down, standing
Ambulation	Walking, climbing stairs
Travel	Driving, riding, flying

Activity	Example
Nonspecialized hand activities	Grasping, lifting, tactile discrimination
Sexual function	Having normal sexual function and participating in usual sexual activity
Sleep	Restful nocturnal sleep pattern
Social and recreational activities	Ability to participate in group activities

2. Apportionment: Apportionment is the determination of the degree to which each of various occupational or nonoccupational factors has contributed to a particular impairment. For each alleged factor, two criteria must be met:

(a) The alleged factor could have caused the impairment, which is a *medical* decision, and

(b) in the particular case, the factor did cause the impairment, which is a *nonmedical* determination.

3. Clinical Evaluation: The clinical evaluation is the collection of data by a physician for the purpose of determining the health status of an individual. The data include information obtained by history; clinical findings obtained from a physical examination; laboratory tests including radiographs, electrocardiograms, blood tests, and other special tests and diagnostic procedures; and measurements of anthropometric attributes and physiologic and psycho-physiologic functions.

4. Disfigurement: Disfigurement is an altered or abnormal appearance. It may be an alteration of color, shape, or structure, or a combination of these. Disfigurement may be a residual of an injury or disease, or it may accompany a recurrent or chronic disorder of function or disease. It may produce either social rejection or impairment of self-image, with self-imposed isolation, alteration of life style, or other changes in behavior.

5. Impairment: Impairment is the loss of, loss of use of, or derangement of any body part, system, or function.

Permanent impairment is impairment that has become static or well stabilized with or without medical treatment, or that is not likely to remit despite medical treatment of the impairing condition.

Evaluation or rating of impairment is an assessment of data collected during a clinical evaluation and the comparison of those data to the criteria contained in the *Guides.*

6. Intensity and Frequency: The intensity and the frequency of occurrence of symptoms or signs occasionally are useful in rating impairment. These can be graded as follows:

Intensity is:
(a) *minimal* when the symptoms or signs constitute an annoyance but cause no impairment in the performance of a particular activity;

(b) *slight* when the symptoms or signs can be tolerated but would cause some impairment in the performance of an activity that precipitates the symptoms or signs;

(c) *moderate* when the symptoms and signs would cause marked impairment in the performance of an activity that precipitates the symptoms or signs;

(d) *marked* when the symptoms or signs preclude any activity that precipitates the symptoms or signs.

Frequency is:
(a) *intermittent* when the symptoms or signs occur less than 25% of the time when awake;

(b) *occasional* when the symptoms or signs occur between 25% and 50% of the time when awake;

(c) *frequent* when the symptoms and signs occur between 50% and 75% of the time when awake;

(d) *constant* when symptoms and signs occur between 75% and 100% of the time when awake.

Disability, Workers' Compensation, and Employability

1. Aggravation and Causation: Aggravation and causation are related to the nonmedical determination that a factor that *can* cause a particular impairment in fact *did* cause the impairment (see Apportionment). In many benefit systems, causation and aggravation must be determined before entitlements are provided. In contrast to their involvement in traumatic injuries, the roles of occupational or environmental factors in causing or aggravating disorders of the various body systems often are not obvious to the lay person; thus evaluating their roles usually requires expert medical opinion. The expert's comments should include the identification of the specific environmental forces or agents and the dates and duration of their actions. An accurate chronicle of the clinical course of the disorder, with dates, times, and locations of environmental events, is helpful in the evaluation of causation and aggravation.

An aggravation, in order to have the legal impact of a causation, must be substantial and permanent, not merely speculative. Five types of aggravations are:

(a) an occupational disorder aggravated by a supervening nonoccupational disorder;

(b) an occupational disorder aggravated by a supervening other occupational condition arising out of and in the course of employment by the same employer;

(c) an occupational disorder aggravated by a supervening other industrial condition arising out of and in the course of employment by a different employer;

(d) an occupational disorder aggravated by a pre-existing nonoccupational condition;

(e) an occupational disorder aggravating a pre-existing nonoccupational condition.

2. Disability: Disability is the limiting loss or absence of the capacity of an individual to meet personal, social, or occupational demands, or to meet statutory or regulatory requirements.

Permanent disability occurs when the degree of capacity becomes static or well stabilized and is not likely to increase in spite of continuing medical or rehabilitative measures. Disability may be caused by medical impairment or by nonmedical factors.

Evaluation or rating of disability is a nonmedical assessment of the degree to which an individual does or does not have the capacity to meet personal, social, or occupational demands, or to meet statutory or regulatory requirements.

3. Employability: Employability is the capacity of an individual to meet the demands of a job and the conditions of employment.

4. Employability Determination: Employability determination is a management assessment of the individual's capacity to meet the demands of a job and the conditions of employment. The management carries out an assessment of performance capability to estimate the likelihood of performance failure and an assessment of the likelihood of future liability in case of human failure. If either likelihood is too great, then the individual will not be considered employable in a particular job.

5. Medical Determination Related to Employability: The medical determination of employability is a statement by a physician about the relationship of an individual's health to the demands of a specific job, such as the demands for performance, reliability, integrity, durability, and overall useful service life as defined by the employer. The physician must ensure that the medical evaluation is complete and detailed enough to obtain the clinical information needed to draw valid conclusions. The physician's tasks are: to identify impairments that could affect performance and to determine whether or not the impairments are permanent; and to identify impairments that could lead to sudden or gradual incapacitation, further impairment, transmission of a communicable disease, or other adverse conditions.

In estimating the risk factors, the physician should indicate whether or not the individual represents a greater risk to the employer than someone without the same medical condition, and indicate the limits of the physician's ability to predict the likelihood of an untoward occurrence.

6. Possibility and Probability: Possibility and probability are nonspecific terms without true statistical or legal meanings. They refer to the likelihood that an injury or illness was caused by a stipulated employment or other event. *Possibility* sometimes is used to imply a likelihood of less than 50%. *Probability* sometimes is used to imply a likelihood of greater than 50%.

Pain and Impairment

Introduction

Any discussion about the concept of impairment and disability arising primarily from pain will be controversial. Perhaps this reflects that understanding pain, especially chronic pain, lacks a measure of precision and confidence, which might be desirable. However, despite such reservations, it would be difficult to overstate the importance of this particular topic.

Chronic pain is endemic in our society. Paradoxically, however, the scope of knowledge concerning chronic pain has not been clearly identified or catalogued. The medical profession as a whole has been slow to identify chronic pain as a specific medical disorder. Consequently, there has been scant research resulting in too few available data. There are, however, several sobering facts concerning chronic pain:

• Sixty to 100 billion dollars are spent annually in the United States on chronic pain syndromes. This represents approximately ¼ of the annual health care budget.

• Five hundred and fifty million sick days are lost annually because of chronic pain syndromes among the full-time working population.

• Eighty million individuals suffer from chronic recurring headaches.

• Thirty million individuals are afflicted with chronic lower back problems.

Indeed, the medical, legal, social and economic consequences of chronic pain are devastating. The Research Briefing Panel on Pain and Pain Management of the National Academy of Sciences in 1985 reported that "the discomfort and suffering associated with [chronic pain] disturb the quality of life and can produce complex and profound alterations in behavior. As a consequence, pain is a major health problem."

In 1979 the federal government became interested in this problem when the National Institute of Neurological and Communicative Disorders and Stroke formed a panel on pain. The report of the panel to the National Advisory Neurological and Communicative Disorders and Stroke Council was published by the U.S. Department of Health, Education and Welfare on June 1, 1979 (NIH publication #81-1912). Stimulated by Congressional concerns over conflicting judicial and administrative findings concerning impairment from pain, a twenty-member Commission on the Evaluation of Pain was appointed by the Secretary of Health and Human Services under the authority of the Social Security Disability Benefits Reform Act of 1984. Comprising experts in the fields of medicine, law, insurance and disability administration, the Commission began deliberations in April 1985. In its report of June 1986 to the Secretary, the Commission noted that, under existing Social Security law, there must first be a finding of medically determined physical or mental impairment that could reasonably be expected to produce pain in order for an individual to be considered disabled. The

Commission then proceeded with a lengthy assessment of the various ramifications that are pertinent to the issue of impairment and disability pertaining to pain.

It has been said that pain is the bond that unites mankind. Indeed, life without pain is inconceivable and undesirable, since without such a warning system, an individual would sustain irrevocable harm. Despite the fact that all individuals experience pain, recognize pain, and respond to pain, there has been considerable difficulty in defining pain. Even more difficulty has been encountered in validating the presence of pain, which is a purely subjective phenomenon. Assessment of pain has been further complicated by its social and psychological ramifications. Pain itself cannot be observed; pain itself cannot be measured.

The International Association for the Study of Pain (IASP) defines pain as "an unpleasant sensory and emotional experience associated with actual or potential tissue damage and described in terms of such damage." The Commission on the Evalution of Pain defines pain as a "complex experience, embracing physical, mental, social, and behavioral processes which compromises the quality of life of many individuals." The Commission recognizes the two categories of pain, acute and chronic. The Commission also recognizes the existence of a chronic pain syndrome. Embodied in all of these definitions is the concept that pain is a subjective, unpleasant, physical and emotional experience associated with the perception of physical harm.

Basic Concepts

Inherent in the definition, and basic to any discussion, is the concept that pain is a complex, multifaceted phenomenon with physical, behavioral, social, and economic dimensions. Pain is a bio-psycho-social problem involving medical, legal, social, and environmental elements in our society.

Students of Algology (the study of human pain) tend to conceptualize pain as involving four interrelated phases: nociception, central pain, perception, and pain response.

Nociception

Tissue damage results in noxious stimuli giving rise to complex neuro-electrical and neuro-chemical mechanisms, which transmit pain impulses from the site of injury along the peripheral and central nervous system. This physical component of pain represents the primary sensory arc defined within neuro-anatomical and neuro-physiological parameters. Nociceptive pain is generally well understood by the medical profession and constitutes the majority of human experience with acute pain.

Central Pain

Sometimes referred to as deafferentation pain, this subset of pain results from excitation of the central nervous system in the absence of any specific noxious stimulus. Phantom limb pain and thalamic pain serve as examples.

Pain Perception

The conscious awareness of an unpleasant sensation defined as pain is most often described in terms of suffering. The value judgments an individual attaches to pain perception are unique and depend on multiple factors, such as genetic endowment, ethnic and cultural traits, education, value system, motivation, expectations, cognitive awareness, and many other considerations involving external and internal influences and conditioned stimuli.

Pain Response

The individual's unique reaction to perceived pain is dependent on the internal and external milieu of the individual. Internally it involves both the central nervous system and the autonomic nervous system. Externally, an individualized response is a conditioned behavioral reaction, which may be adaptive or maladaptive. It is important to recognize that pain behavior is the only facet of the pain complex that is apparent to the external milieu. Pain behavior becomes a "window" through which others may appreciate and evaluate the pain experience of an individual, an experience that otherwise is a purely subjective phenomenon. Hence, pain behavior represents an important link between the individual and his or her environment. In the instance of the chronic pain syndrome, it serves as the basis for a disability rating.

To the four phases of pain described above, a fifth dimension—secondary reactive pain, or acquired pain—might be added. Maladaptive pain behavior frequently includes prolonged periods of inactivity and immobilization. This, in turn, results in deconditioning, joint contractures, postural imbalances, musculoskeletal deterioration and neuromuscular "dystrophy." Such conditions, in turn, give rise to further generation of nociceptive stimuli, thereby creating perpetuation and augmentation of a biological feedback loop.

Categories of Pain

By convention pain has been categorized as "acute" and "chronic," which inadvertently implies a chronology that actually is of minor importance to the understanding of the various categories of pain.

Acute Pain

This alerting mechanism is an early warning signal that protects an individual from somatic tissue damage. Acute pain is generally of recent onset and of short duration. It seldom represents a major diagnostic or therapeutic problem. The physical injury giving rise to the noxious stimulus results in pain perception and pain behavior, which are usually commensurate with and appropriate to the underlying pathogenesis. Appropriate management includes establishing a correct diagnosis and providing palliative measures, such as analgesic medication and immobilization of the injured part. Pain abatement accompanies tissue healing. Impairment and/or disability rarely transcend the underlying pathology.

Acute Recurrent Pain

This subset of acute pain represents a somewhat more complex concept. It refers to episodic noxious sensations resulting from tissue damage in chronic disorders, such as arthritis, tic douloureux, and malignant neoplasms. The teleological significance, diagnostic evaluation, and medical management of acute recurrent pain remain basically the same as those of acute pain. Acute recurrent pain may be controlled effectively with traditional modalities of treatment, such as analgesic medication and immobilization. However, because of the chronicity of the underlying pathological process, the intensity and the duration of health care and the resulting impairment and/or disability are considerably greater in magnitude. Acute recurrent pain at times has been erroneously referred to as chronic pain, thereby giving rise to further confusion of the concept.

Chronic Pain

Chronic pain, frequently referred to as chronic intractable pain or chronic benign pain (referring to its nonmalignant etiology), represents the nidus of the chronic pain syndrome. In striking contrast to the intrinsically utilitarian value of acute pain, chronic pain represents a useless, malevolent, and destructive force. Not a symptom of an underlying acute somatic injury, it must be considered a pathological disorder in its own right. It is chronic, long lived and progressive. Pain perception is markedly enhanced. Pain behavior becomes maladaptive and counterproductive. Both pain perception and pain behavior are grossly disproportionate to any underlying noxious stimulus. Tissue damage, often trivial at its inception, generally has healed and no longer serves as an underlying generator of pain.

Chronic pain improperly diagnosed and inadequately treated results in deteriorating coping mechanisms and pacing skills. Under such circumstances, peristent chronic pain results in progressive limitations and functional capacity, which contribute to the evolution of the chronic pain syndrome. Within the framework of this definition, chronic pain may exist in the absence of chronic pain syndrome, but chronic pain syndrome always presumes the presence of chronic pain.

Truly, the chronic pain syndrome represents a bio-psycho-social phenomenon of maladaptive behavior with far reaching medical, social, and economic consequences. Early detection and prompt, effective intervention require a high index of suspicion. The presence of two or more of the following characteristics (the six "D"s) should be considered as establishing the diagnosis of a chronic pain syndrome.

Duration: By its very nature, chronic pain is of long duration, persisting and progressing long after tissue damage has healed. Whereas in the past, the term "chronic pain" has been applied to pain of greater than six months duration, it is now recognized that the chronic pain syndrome can be diagnosed as early as two to four weeks after its onset. Recent studies have suggested there may be underlying predisposing factors that could perhaps be isolated and identified, thus permitting prevention of the chronic pain syndrome through premorbid intervention.

Dramatization: Patients with chronic pain syndrome tend to use emotionally charged words to describe their pain, suffering, and handicap. Their physical presentation is replete with exaggerated histrionic deportment. They frequently provide a theatrical display of the signature of pain, including moaning, groaning, gasping, facial grimacing, posturing, pantomime, and other exaggerated mannerisms. All this reflects maladaptive conditioned behavior.

Drugs: Substance abuse in the form of prescription drugs and/or alcohol is a frequent stigma of the chronic pain syndrome. Chronic pain patients become dependent on their physicians, and consequently are known as excessive utilizers of health care. They are subjected to repetitive diagnostic studies, which generally are inconclusive and contradictory. They become the willing recipients of multiple drugs, which frequently interact in an adverse manner. They demand passive modalities of perpetual physical therapy, which, although pleasant for the moment, provide no lasting benefit. Finally, when all else fails, the chronic pain patients are subjected to well intended, but poorly conceived, sequential surgical procedures ("we have tried everything else"), which again provide no lasting benefit, but all too often result in further pain and disability. In the terminal phases, the chronic pain patients are often referred to psychiatrists ("it must be in your head") only to be told they they have no mental illness and would, in fact, be "all right" if it were not for their intrinsic pain.

Despair: The chronic pain syndrome results in major emotional upheavals. Patients frequently exhibit high scores on neuropsychological tests in the area of hypochondriasis and hysteria. Dysphoric manifestations include depression, apprehension, irritability, and hostility. Chronic pain patients become embittered, defensive, rigid, and paradoxical. Pacing and coping mechanisms are severely impaired. Low self-esteem and a lack of self-worth result in impaired self-reliance and in the externalization of the locus of control. Finally, despondency and despair pave the road to self-destructive behavior.

Disuse: Pain of musculoskeletal origin frequently results in prolonged and excessive immobilization. Self-imposed splinting, validated by medical admonitions to "be careful" and to "take it easy," result in progressive muscular dysfunction, postural imbalances, joint contractures and generalized deconditioning. Passive modalities of physical therapy further aggravate the problem, irrespective of the value of transient symptomatic pain relief. Prolonged disuse results in secondary acquired pain, which further aggravates and perpetuates the chronic pain cycle.

Dysfunction: Bereft of adequate pacing and coping skills, chronic pain patients begin to withdraw from the social fabric. They disengage from work activities. They retreat from recreational endeavors. They tend to alienate friends and family. They begin to descend a spiral staircase of increasing isolation, eventually restricting their activities to the bare essentials of daily living. Bereft of social contacts, shunned by loved ones, rebuffed by the health care system, isolated by society, and deprived of financial sustenance, the chronic pain patient becomes truly an invalid in the physical, emotional, social, and economic sense.

The presence of a chronic pain syndrome should be strongly suspected if a patient does not respond to appropriate medical care within a reasonable period of time, or if the patient's verbal or nonverbal pain behavior transcends the expected response to a given noxious stimulus. Patients suspected of having a chronic pain syndrome should be promptly referred for evaluation and treatment to physicians specializing in chronic pain medicine (algology).

A discussion of the universe of pain would be incomplete without brief mention of two other subcategories of pain.

Psychogenic Pain

Psychogenic pain, which is referred to as Somatoform Pain Disorder in the Diagnostic and Statistical Manual, Third Edition (Revised), is considered within the diagnostic and therapeutic scope of psychiatry. It differs from the chronic pain syndrome, which cannot be considered a mental disorder.

Malingering

Defined as the conscious and deliberate feigning of an illness or disability, malingering involves the fabrication of symptoms and complaints in order to achieve a specific goal. There is consensus among algologists that malingering is readily detected with appropriate medical and psychological tests. It is an infrequent occurrence among the population of chronic pain patients.

Acute pain and chronic pain are not mutually exclusive. Chronic pain may develop and coexist in an individual with acute pain, though it is more likely to occur in an individual with acute recurrent pain stemming from a chronic medical disorder. For example, a patient with a malignant neoplasm is quite likely to be afflicted with acute recurrent pain requiring effective pain management. In certain instances, pain perception and pain behavior will become disproportionate to the underlying somatic disorder and noxious stimuli. In such circumstances, chronic pain will become superimposed on the pre-existing acute recurrent pain and the patient no longer will be responsive to traditional methods of medical intervention. When coping mechanisms become impaired, maladaptive behavior reaches such proportions as to interfere with functional activity. The patient then can be considered as having the chronic pain syndrome.

In summary, chronic pain is not a purely physical problem; chronic pain is not purely a psychological problem; chronic pain is not a manifestation of fabrication or delusion. Chronic pain and the chronic pain syndrome are truly multidimensional bio-psycho-social phenomena.

Pain Management

It would be a disservice to leave this section without interjecting a note of optimism. Although chronic, progressive, consumptive, and destructive, chronic pain is not hopeless. It is treatable, but spontaneous improvement is rare. Early diagnosis and prompt intervention can restore an individual with the chronic pain syndrome to full functional capacity.

Many algologists tend to consider chronic pain as representing a failure of traditional health care. Indeed, it has been well documented that failure to establish an early diagnosis, continued emphasis on repetitive diagnostic studies, excessive and inappropriate use of medication, prolonged use of passive physical therapy modalities, prolonged immobilization and inactivation, and poorly conceived surgical intervention, all inevitably led to perpetuation and augmentation of the chronic pain syndrome.

Other nonmedical vectors also are operative. The Commission on the Evaluation of Pain noted that there are multiple variations on the theme of rewarding illness behavior and providing disincentives for recovery. Pain often provides the rationalization for quitting an unpleasant work situation. Pain may provide a legitimate attention-getting device when other efforts fail. Pain may provide unrealistic expectations for financial rewards through a legal or administrative system. Society has constructed an intricate subconscious feedback process, whereby suffering and pain behavior result in intangible rewards, whereas recovery and well behavior may seem to result in deprivation. In this context, the chronic pain syndrome results not only from activities of the medical profession, but also from activities of the legal profession and activities of the insurance industry.

Paradoxically, society, as well as the medical profession, view individuals with the chronic pain syndrome with frustration, suspicion, disdain, and anger. Such prejudicial presumptions create major barriers to prompt diagnosis and effective management. They serve to further isolate and alienate patients with a chronic pain syndrome.

Inasmuch as chronic pain and the chronic pain syndrome are multifactorial problems, appropriate evaluation and management requires a multidisciplinary and interdisciplinary effort of concerned health professionals. Comprehensive rehabilitation (physical, pharmaceutical, psychological, social, vocational), operant conditioning, and cognitive training represent the benchmarks of a chronic pain program. Treatment may be on an outpatient or inpatient basis, but should be structured and individualized.

The Commission on the Evaluation of Pain, noted that "chronic pain and chronic pain syndrome are inadequately understood," that there is a "need to assess the magnitude of the problem" and that there is a "need for input by specialists in pain behavior and pain management." The Commission recommends that 1) the scope and body of knowledge of chronic pain be recognized and defined; 2) adequate funding be provided for research and education in the field of algology; 3) physicians should be encouraged to seek specialty training in the field of pain medicine (algology); and 4) facilities for the comprehensive management of pain should be established and accredited.

Impairment

There has been little consensus and much confusion about the extent and nature of impairment that results solely from chronic pain and the chronic pain syndrome.

Physicians, medical organizations, third party payors, and regulatory and governmental agencies have held divergent and shifting viewpoints. The Commission recognized the problem, but after much deliberation, it was unable to set criteria that would clearly provide measures of impairment related to pain. Instead the Commission recommended further study of the problem. It noted that "chronic pain and its consequences are inadequately understood by patients, the health care system, the general public, and the Social Security Admininstration." It recognized the distinction between acute and chronic pain and noted that chronic pain patients have a multifaceted problem, which includes somatic pathology and behavioral responses. The Commission recognized that the chronic pain syndrome is a complex condition with physical, mental, and social components. It also noted that, despite numerous attempts, the development of methodologies for the objective measurement of pain were not available. Finally, it recognized the inadequacy of the data base concerning disability related primarily to pain. For these reasons, the Commission recommended that the problem be studied further in conjunction with the Institute of Medicine of the National Academy of Sciences. Several members of the Commission filed a minority report, which requested that there be no further delay in the recognition of chronic pain as a legitimate source of impairment within the Social Security Administration.

Perhaps further confusion is introduced into this discussion by the inconsistent usage of the terms "impairment" and "disability." The *Guides* provide the following definitions:

> *"Impairment is the loss of, loss of use of, or derangment of any body part, system or function."*

> *"Disability is the limiting, loss or absence of the capacity of an individual to meet personal, social, or occupational demands, or to meet statutory or regulatory requirements."*

"Impairment" is seen as an adverse alteration in the physical and/or mental health status of an individual resulting from anatomical, physiological, chemical, or psychiatric abnormalities. The focus is patient oriented. "Disability" is seen as an administrative finding that an individual is unable to engage in certain activities by reason of medical impairment and other nonmedical considerations. The focus is task oriented. Based upon such operational definitions, the following thoughts about pain are offered as guidelines:

Acute pain: Impairment and any resulting disability are primarily a function of the underlying pathological process, giving rise to physical tissue damage and nociceptive pain. In most instances, impairment and disability will be partial and temporary.

Acute recurrent pain: The considerations of impairment and any resulting disability are the same as in acute pain. However, given the chronic nature of the underlying pathological process, impairment and disability could well be total and permanent.

Chronic pain: It is in this area in which most of the divergence of opinion arises and in which there is considerable controversy. In the presence of the chronic pain syndrome, evaluation of impairment and any resulting disability should be deferred until the disorder has been appropriately evaluated and managed, and the condition can be considered static or stabilized.

Furthermore, distinguishing between impairment and disability becomes important:

Impairment: Since chronic pain by definition is primarily a perceptual, maladaptive behavioral problem; since pain per se cannot be validated objectively or quantitated, and since the underlying substrate of somatic pathology is minimal or nonexistent, it follows that little, if any, impairment exists in most instances of the chronic pain syndrome. However, consideration should be given in instances where there is a significant somatic substrate, either as the primary nociceptive generator or as the secondary acquired regenerator. Allowances should also be made for bonafide psychogenic factors resulting in alterations in mental health, although it should be recognized that psychogenic pain is not the same as chronic pain, but is a psychiatric disorder that should be treated by specialists in that field.

Disability: Since the chronic pain syndrome is a bio-psycho-social problem with major social, economic, and environmental ramifications, it would seem that disability may become a major issue. Chronic pain patients may, indeed, have major limitations of functional capacity over and above any possible impairment. Such disability must be defined by the individual's limitations of functional capacity in the sphere of activities of daily living, social interaction, recreational pursuits, and work endeavors. This will require nonmedical assessment, particularly when countervailing nonmedical influences, such as legal or occupational problems, motivate the patient to maximize the chronic pain syndrome.

In conclusion, using the definitions contained in these *Guides*, one might address the topic of pain as follows: Does chronic pain result in—

impairment—perhaps, but not often;
disability—probably, but to a variable degree;
handicap—almost certainly.

References

1. Osterweis M, Kleinman A, Mechanic D (eds): *Pain and Disability: Clinical, Behavioral and Public Policy Perspectives. Report of the Institute of Medicine Committee on Pain, Disability and Chronic Illness Behavior.* Washington, DC, National Academy Press, 1987.

2. *Report of the Commission on the Evaluation of Pain.* US Department of Health and Human Services, Social Security Administration Office of Disability. SSA Pub. No. 64-031. Washington, D C, March 1987.

3. Cousins MJ, Phillips GD (eds): *Acute Pain Management.* New York, Churchill Livingstone, 1986.

4. Barber J, Adrian C (eds): *Psychological Approaches to the Management of Pain.* New York, Brunner Mazel, 1982.

5. Aronoff GM (ed): *Evaluation and Treatment of Chronic Pain.* Baltimore, Urban and Schwarzenberg, 1985.

6. Gildenberg PL, DeVaul RA (eds): *The Chronic Pain Patient: Evaluation and Management.* Basel, Switzerland, S Karger AG, 1985.

Combined Values Chart

The values are derived from the formula $A + B(1-A)$ = combined value of A and B, where A and B are the decimal equivalents of the impairment ratings. In the chart all values are expressed as percents. To combine any two impairment values, locate the larger of the values on the side of the chart and read along that row until you come to the column indicated by the smaller value at the bottom of the chart. At the intersection of the row and the column is the combined value.

For example, to combine 35% and 20% read down the side of the chart until you come to the larger value, 35%. Then read across the 35% row until you come to the column indicated by 20% at the bottom of the chart. At the intersection of the row and column is the number 48. Therefore, 35% combined with 20% is 48%. Due to the construction of this chart, the larger impairment value must be identified at the side of the chart.

If three or more impairment values are to be combined, select any two and find their combined value as above. Then use that value and the third value to locate the combined value of all. This process can be repeated indefinitely, the final value in each instance being the combination of all the previous values. In each step of this process the larger impairment value must be identified at the side of the chart.

	1	2	3	4	5	6	7	8	9	10	11	12	13	14	15	16	17	18	19	20	21	22	23	24	25	26	27	28	29	30	31	32	33	34	35	36	37	38	39	40	41	42	43	44	45	46	47	48	49	50
1	2
2	3	4
3	4	5	6
4	5	6	7	8
5	6	7	8	9	10
6	7	8	9	10	11	12
7	8	9	10	11	12	13	14
8	9	10	11	12	13	14	14	15
9	10	11	12	13	14	14	15	16	17
10	11	12	13	14	15	15	16	17	18	19
11	12	13	14	15	15	16	17	18	19	20	21
12	13	14	15	16	16	17	18	19	20	21	22	23
13	14	15	16	16	17	18	19	20	21	22	23	23	24
14	15	16	17	17	18	19	20	21	22	23	23	24	25	26
15	16	17	18	18	19	20	21	22	23	24	24	25	26	27	28
16	17	18	19	19	20	21	22	23	24	24	25	26	27	28	29	29
17	18	19	19	20	21	22	23	24	24	25	26	27	28	29	29	30	31
18	19	20	20	21	22	23	24	25	25	26	27	28	29	29	30	31	32	33
19	20	21	21	22	23	24	25	25	26	27	28	29	30	30	31	32	33	34	34
20	21	22	22	23	24	25	26	26	27	28	29	30	30	31	32	33	34	34	35	36
21	22	23	23	24	25	26	27	27	28	29	30	30	31	32	33	34	34	35	36	37	38
22	23	24	24	25	26	27	27	28	29	30	31	31	32	33	34	34	35	36	37	38	38	39
23	24	25	25	26	27	28	28	29	30	31	31	32	33	34	35	35	36	37	38	38	39	40	41
24	25	26	26	27	28	29	29	30	31	32	32	33	34	35	35	36	37	38	38	39	40	41	41	42
25	26	27	27	28	29	30	30	31	32	33	33	34	35	36	36	37	38	39	39	40	41	42	42	43	44
26	27	27	28	29	30	30	31	32	33	33	34	35	36	36	37	38	39	39	40	41	42	42	43	44	45	45
27	28	28	29	30	31	31	32	33	34	34	35	36	36	37	38	39	39	40	41	42	42	43	44	45	45	46	47
28	29	29	30	31	32	32	33	34	34	35	36	37	37	38	39	40	40	41	42	42	43	44	45	45	46	47	47	48
29	30	30	31	32	33	33	34	35	35	36	37	38	38	39	40	40	41	42	42	43	44	45	45	46	47	47	48	49	50
30	31	31	32	33	34	34	35	36	36	37	38	38	39	40	41	41	42	43	43	44	45	45	46	47	48	48	49	50	50	51
31	32	32	33	34	34	35	36	37	37	38	39	39	40	41	41	42	43	43	44	45	45	46	47	48	48	49	50	50	51	52	52
32	33	33	34	35	35	36	37	37	38	39	39	40	41	42	42	43	44	44	45	46	46	47	48	48	49	50	50	51	52	52	53	54
33	34	34	35	36	36	37	38	38	39	40	40	41	42	42	43	44	44	45	46	46	47	48	48	49	50	50	51	52	52	53	54	54	55
34	35	35	36	37	37	38	39	39	40	41	41	42	43	43	44	45	45	46	47	47	48	49	49	50	51	51	52	52	53	54	54	55	56	56
35	36	36	37	38	38	39	40	40	41	42	42	43	43	44	45	45	46	47	47	48	49	49	50	51	51	52	53	53	54	55	55	56	56	57	58
36	37	37	38	39	39	40	40	41	42	42	43	44	44	45	46	46	47	48	48	49	49	50	51	51	52	53	53	54	55	55	56	56	57	58	58	59
37	38	38	39	40	40	41	41	42	43	43	44	45	45	46	46	47	48	48	49	50	50	51	51	52	53	53	54	55	55	56	57	57	58	58	59	60	60
38	39	39	40	40	41	42	42	43	44	44	45	45	46	47	47	48	49	49	50	50	51	52	52	53	54	54	55	55	56	57	57	58	58	59	60	60	61	62
39	40	40	41	41	42	43	43	44	44	45	46	46	47	48	48	49	49	50	51	51	52	52	53	54	54	55	55	56	57	57	58	59	59	60	60	61	62	62	63
40	41	41	42	42	43	44	44	45	45	46	47	47	48	48	49	50	50	51	51	52	53	53	54	54	55	56	56	57	57	58	59	59	60	60	61	62	62	63	63	64
41	42	42	43	43	44	45	45	46	46	47	47	48	49	49	50	50	51	52	52	53	53	54	55	55	56	56	57	58	58	59	59	60	60	61	62	62	63	63	64	65	65
42	43	43	44	44	45	45	46	47	47	48	48	49	50	50	51	51	52	52	53	54	54	55	55	56	57	57	58	58	59	59	60	61	61	62	62	63	63	64	65	65	66	66
43	44	44	45	45	46	46	47	48	48	49	49	50	50	51	52	52	53	53	54	54	55	56	56	57	57	58	58	59	60	60	61	61	62	62	63	64	64	65	65	66	66	67	68
44	45	45	46	46	47	47	48	48	49	50	50	51	51	52	52	53	54	54	55	55	56	56	57	57	58	59	59	60	60	61	61	62	62	63	64	64	65	65	66	66	67	68	68	69
45	46	46	47	47	48	48	49	49	50	51	51	52	52	53	53	54	54	55	55	56	57	57	58	58	59	59	60	60	61	62	62	63	63	64	64	65	65	66	66	67	68	68	69	69	70
46	47	47	48	48	49	49	50	50	51	51	52	52	53	54	54	55	55	56	56	57	57	58	58	59	60	60	61	61	62	62	63	63	64	64	65	65	66	67	67	68	68	69	69	70	70	71
47	48	48	49	49	50	50	51	51	52	52	53	53	54	54	55	55	56	57	57	58	58	59	59	60	60	61	61	62	62	63	63	64	64	65	66	66	67	67	68	68	69	69	70	70	71	71	72
48	49	49	50	50	51	51	52	52	53	53	54	54	55	55	56	56	57	57	58	58	59	59	60	60	61	62	62	63	63	64	64	65	65	66	66	67	67	68	68	69	69	70	70	71	71	72	72	73
49	50	50	51	51	52	52	53	53	54	54	55	55	56	56	57	57	58	58	59	59	60	60	61	61	62	62	63	63	64	64	65	65	66	66	67	67	68	68	69	69	70	70	71	71	72	72	73	73	74
50	51	51	52	52	53	53	54	54	55	55	56	56	57	57	58	58	59	59	60	60	61	61	62	62	63	63	64	64	65	65	66	66	67	67	68	68	69	69	70	70	71	71	72	72	73	73	74	74	75	75

Combined Values Chart (continued)

	1	2	3	4	5	6	7	8	9	10	11	12	13	14	15	16	17	18	19	20	21	22	23	24	25	26	27	28	29	30	31	32	33	34	35	36	37	38	39	40	41	42	43	44	45	46	47	48	49	50
51	51	52	52	53	53	54	54	55	55	56	56	57	57	58	58	59	59	60	60	61	61	62	62	63	63	64	64	65	65	66	66	67	67	68	68	69	69	70	70	71	71	72	72	73	73	74	74	75	75	76
52	52	53	53	54	54	55	55	56	56	57	57	58	58	59	59	60	60	61	61	62	62	63	63	64	64	64	65	65	66	66	67	67	68	68	69	69	70	70	71	71	72	72	73	73	74	74	75	75	76	76
53	53	54	54	55	55	56	56	57	57	58	58	59	59	60	60	61	61	61	62	62	63	63	64	64	65	65	66	66	67	67	68	68	69	69	69	70	70	71	71	72	72	73	73	74	74	75	75	76	76	77
54	54	55	55	56	56	57	57	58	58	59	59	59	60	60	61	61	62	62	63	63	64	64	65	65	66	66	66	67	67	68	68	69	69	70	70	71	71	71	72	72	73	73	74	74	75	75	76	76	77	77
55	55	56	56	57	57	58	58	59	59	60	60	60	61	61	62	62	63	63	64	64	64	65	65	66	66	67	67	68	68	69	69	69	70	70	71	71	72	72	73	73	73	74	74	75	75	76	76	77	77	78
56	56	57	57	58	58	59	59	60	60	60	61	61	62	62	63	63	63	64	64	65	65	66	66	67	67	67	68	68	69	69	70	70	71	71	71	72	72	73	73	74	74	74	75	75	76	76	77	77	78	78
57	57	58	58	59	59	60	60	60	61	61	62	62	63	63	63	64	64	65	65	66	66	66	67	67	68	68	69	69	69	70	70	71	71	72	72	72	73	73	74	74	75	75	75	76	76	77	77	78	78	79
58	58	59	59	60	60	61	61	61	62	62	63	63	63	64	64	65	65	66	66	66	67	67	68	68	68	69	69	70	70	71	71	71	72	72	73	73	74	74	74	75	75	76	76	76	77	77	78	78	79	79
59	59	60	60	61	61	61	62	62	63	63	64	64	64	65	65	66	66	66	67	67	68	68	68	69	69	70	70	70	71	71	72	72	73	73	73	74	74	75	75	75	76	76	77	77	77	78	78	79	79	80
60	60	61	61	62	62	62	63	63	64	64	64	65	65	66	66	66	67	67	68	68	68	69	69	70	70	70	71	71	72	72	72	73	73	74	74	74	75	75	76	76	76	77	77	78	78	78	79	79	80	80
61	61	62	62	63	63	63	64	64	65	65	65	66	66	66	67	67	68	68	68	69	69	70	70	70	71	71	72	72	72	73	73	73	74	74	75	75	75	76	76	77	77	77	78	78	79	79	79	80	80	81
62	62	63	63	64	64	64	65	65	65	66	66	67	67	67	68	68	68	69	69	70	70	70	71	71	72	72	72	73	73	73	74	74	75	75	75	76	76	76	77	77	78	78	78	79	79	79	80	80	81	81
63	63	64	64	64	65	65	66	66	66	67	67	67	68	68	69	69	69	70	70	70	71	71	72	72	72	73	73	73	74	74	74	75	75	76	76	76	77	77	77	78	78	79	79	79	80	80	80	81	81	82
64	64	65	65	65	66	66	67	67	67	68	68	68	69	69	69	70	70	70	71	71	72	72	72	73	73	73	74	74	74	75	75	76	76	76	77	77	77	78	78	78	79	79	79	80	80	81	81	81	82	82
65	65	66	66	66	67	67	67	68	68	69	69	69	70	70	70	71	71	71	72	72	72	73	73	73	74	74	74	75	75	76	76	76	77	77	77	78	78	78	79	79	79	80	80	80	81	81	81	82	82	83
66	66	67	67	67	68	68	68	69	69	69	70	70	70	71	71	71	72	72	72	73	73	73	74	74	75	75	75	76	76	76	77	77	77	78	78	78	79	79	79	80	80	80	81	81	81	82	82	82	83	83
67	67	68	68	68	69	69	69	70	70	70	71	71	71	72	72	72	73	73	73	74	74	74	75	75	75	76	76	76	77	77	77	78	78	78	79	79	79	80	80	80	81	81	81	82	82	82	83	83	83	84
68	68	69	69	69	70	70	70	71	71	71	72	72	72	72	73	73	73	74	74	74	75	75	75	76	76	76	77	77	77	78	78	78	79	79	79	80	80	80	80	81	81	81	82	82	82	83	83	83	84	84
69	69	70	70	70	71	71	71	71	72	72	72	73	73	73	74	74	74	75	75	75	76	76	76	76	77	77	77	78	78	78	79	79	79	80	80	80	80	81	81	81	82	82	82	83	83	83	84	84	84	85
70	70	71	71	71	72	72	72	72	73	73	73	74	74	74	75	75	75	75	76	76	76	77	77	77	78	78	78	78	79	79	79	80	80	80	81	81	81	81	82	82	82	83	83	83	84	84	84	84	85	85
71	71	72	72	72	72	73	73	73	74	74	74	74	75	75	75	76	76	76	77	77	77	77	78	78	78	79	79	79	79	80	80	80	81	81	81	81	82	82	82	83	83	83	83	84	84	84	85	85	85	86
72	72	73	73	73	73	74	74	74	75	75	75	75	76	76	76	76	77	77	77	78	78	78	78	79	79	79	80	80	80	80	81	81	81	82	82	82	82	83	83	83	83	84	84	84	85	85	85	85	86	86
73	73	74	74	74	74	75	75	75	75	76	76	76	77	77	77	77	78	78	78	78	79	79	79	79	80	80	80	81	81	81	81	82	82	82	82	83	83	83	84	84	84	84	85	85	85	85	86	86	86	87
74	74	75	75	75	75	76	76	76	76	77	77	77	77	78	78	78	78	79	79	79	79	80	80	80	81	81	81	81	82	82	82	82	83	83	83	83	84	84	84	84	85	85	85	85	86	86	86	86	87	87
75	75	76	76	76	76	77	77	77	77	78	78	78	78	79	79	79	79	80	80	80	80	81	81	81	81	82	82	82	82	83	83	83	83	84	84	84	84	85	85	85	85	86	86	86	86	87	87	87	87	88
76	76	76	77	77	77	77	78	78	78	78	79	79	79	79	80	80	80	80	81	81	81	81	82	82	82	82	82	83	83	83	83	84	84	84	84	85	85	85	85	86	86	86	86	87	87	87	87	88	88	88
77	77	77	78	78	78	78	79	79	79	79	80	80	80	80	80	81	81	81	81	82	82	82	82	83	83	83	83	83	84	84	84	84	85	85	85	85	86	86	86	86	86	87	87	87	87	88	88	88	88	89
78	78	78	79	79	79	79	80	80	80	80	80	81	81	81	81	82	82	82	82	82	83	83	83	83	84	84	84	84	84	85	85	85	85	85	86	86	86	86	87	87	87	87	87	88	88	88	88	89	89	89
79	79	79	80	80	80	80	80	81	81	81	81	82	82	82	82	82	83	83	83	83	83	84	84	84	84	84	85	85	85	85	86	86	86	86	86	87	87	87	87	87	88	88	88	88	88	89	89	89	89	90
80	80	80	81	81	81	81	81	82	82	82	82	82	83	83	83	83	83	84	84	84	84	84	85	85	85	85	85	86	86	86	86	86	87	87	87	87	87	88	88	88	88	88	89	89	89	89	89	90	90	90
81	81	81	82	82	82	82	82	83	83	83	83	83	83	84	84	84	84	84	85	85	85	85	85	86	86	86	86	86	87	87	87	87	87	87	88	88	88	88	88	89	89	89	89	89	90	90	90	90	90	91
82	82	82	83	83	83	83	83	83	84	84	84	84	84	85	85	85	85	85	85	86	86	86	86	86	87	87	87	87	87	87	88	88	88	88	88	88	89	89	89	89	89	90	90	90	90	90	90	91	91	91
83	83	83	84	84	84	84	84	84	85	85	85	85	85	85	86	86	86	86	86	86	87	87	87	87	87	87	88	88	88	88	88	88	89	89	89	89	89	89	90	90	90	90	90	90	91	91	91	91	91	92
84	84	84	84	85	85	85	85	85	85	86	86	86	86	86	86	87	87	87	87	87	87	88	88	88	88	88	88	88	89	89	89	89	89	89	90	90	90	90	90	90	91	91	91	91	91	91	92	92	92	92
85	85	85	85	86	86	86	86	86	86	87	87	87	87	87	87	87	88	88	88	88	88	88	88	89	89	89	89	89	89	90	90	90	90	90	90	90	91	91	91	91	91	91	91	92	92	92	92	92	92	93
86	86	86	86	87	87	87	87	87	87	87	88	88	88	88	88	88	88	89	89	89	89	89	89	89	90	90	90	90	90	90	90	90	91	91	91	91	91	91	91	92	92	92	92	92	92	92	93	93	93	93
87	87	87	87	88	88	88	88	88	88	88	88	89	89	89	89	89	89	89	89	90	90	90	90	90	90	90	91	91	91	91	91	91	91	91	92	92	92	92	92	92	92	92	93	93	93	93	93	93	93	94
88	88	88	88	88	89	89	89	89	89	89	89	89	90	90	90	90	90	90	90	90	91	91	91	91	91	91	91	91	91	92	92	92	92	92	92	92	92	93	93	93	93	93	93	93	93	94	94	94	94	94
89	89	89	89	89	90	90	90	90	90	90	90	90	90	91	91	91	91	91	91	91	91	91	92	92	92	92	92	92	92	92	92	93	93	93	93	93	93	93	93	93	94	94	94	94	94	94	94	94	94	95
90	90	90	90	90	91	91	91	91	91	91	91	91	91	91	92	92	92	92	92	92	92	92	92	92	93	93	93	93	93	93	93	93	93	93	94	94	94	94	94	94	94	94	94	94	95	95	95	95	95	95
91	91	91	91	91	91	92	92	92	92	92	92	92	92	92	92	92	93	93	93	93	93	93	93	93	93	93	93	94	94	94	94	94	94	94	94	94	94	94	95	95	95	95	95	95	95	95	95	95	95	96
92	92	92	92	92	92	92	93	93	93	93	93	93	93	93	93	93	93	93	94	94	94	94	94	94	94	94	94	94	94	94	94	95	95	95	95	95	95	95	95	95	95	95	95	96	96	96	96	96	96	96
93	93	93	93	93	93	93	93	94	94	94	94	94	94	94	94	94	94	94	94	94	94	95	95	95	95	95	95	95	95	95	95	95	95	95	95	96	96	96	96	96	96	96	96	96	96	96	96	96	96	97
94	94	94	94	94	94	94	94	94	95	95	95	95	95	95	95	95	95	95	95	95	95	95	95	95	96	96	96	96	96	96	96	96	96	96	96	96	96	96	96	96	96	97	97	97	97	97	97	97	97	97
95	95	95	95	95	95	95	95	95	95	96	96	96	96	96	96	96	96	96	96	96	96	96	96	96	96	96	96	96	96	96	97	97	97	97	97	97	97	97	97	97	97	97	97	97	97	97	97	97	97	98
96	96	96	96	96	96	96	96	96	96	96	96	96	97	97	97	97	97	97	97	97	97	97	97	97	97	97	97	97	97	97	97	97	97	97	97	97	97	98	98	98	98	98	98	98	98	98	98	98	98	98
97	97	97	97	97	97	97	97	97	97	97	97	97	97	97	97	97	98	98	98	98	98	98	98	98	98	98	98	98	98	98	98	98	98	98	98	98	98	98	98	98	98	98	98	98	98	98	98	98	98	99
98	98	98	98	98	98	98	98	98	98	98	98	98	98	98	98	98	98	98	98	98	98	98	98	98	98	99	99	99	99	99	99	99	99	99	99	99	99	99	99	99	99	99	99	99	99	99	99	99	99	99
99	99	99	99	99	99	99	99	99	99	99	99	99	99	99	99	99	99	99	99	99	99	99	99	99	99	99	99	99	99	99	99	99	99	99	99	99	99	99	99	99	99	99	99	99	99	99	99	99	99	100
	1	2	3	4	5	6	7	8	9	10	11	12	13	14	15	16	17	18	19	20	21	22	23	24	25	26	27	28	29	30	31	32	33	34	35	36	37	38	39	40	41	42	43	44	45	46	47	48	49	50

Combined Values Chart (continued)

	51	52	53	54	55	56	57	58	59	60	61	62	63	64	65	66	67	68	69	70	71	72	73	74	75	76	77	78	79	80	81	82	83	84	85	86	87	88	89	90	91	92	93	94	95	96	97	98	99
51	76																																																
52	76	77																																															
53	77	77	78																																														
54	77	78	78	79																																													
55	78	78	79	79	80																																												
56	78	79	79	80	80	81																																											
57	79	79	80	80	81	81	82																																										
58	79	80	80	81	81	82	82	82																																									
59	80	80	81	81	82	82	82	83	83																																							
60	80	81	81	82	82	82	83	83	84	84																																						
61	81	81	82	82	82	83	83	84	84	84	85																																					
62	81	82	82	83	83	83	84	84	84	85	85	86																																				
63	82	82	83	83	83	84	84	84	85	85	86	86	86																																			
64	82	83	83	83	84	84	85	85	85	86	86	86	87	87																																		
65	83	83	84	84	84	85	85	85	86	86	86	87	87	87	88																																	
66	83	84	84	84	85	85	85	86	86	86	87	87	87	88	88	88																																
67	84	84	84	85	85	85	86	86	86	87	87	87	88	88	88	89	89																															
68	84	85	85	85	86	86	86	87	87	87	88	88	88	88	89	89	89	90																														
69	85	85	85	86	86	86	87	87	87	88	88	88	89	89	89	89	90	90	90																													
70	85	86	86	86	87	87	87	87	88	88	88	89	89	89	90	90	90	90	91	91																												
71	86	86	86	87	87	87	88	88	88	88	89	89	89	90	90	90	90	91	91	91	92																											
72	86	87	87	87	87	88	88	88	89	89	89	89	90	90	90	90	91	91	91	92	92	92																										
73	87	87	87	88	88	88	88	89	89	89	89	90	90	90	91	91	91	91	92	92	92	92	93																									
74	87	88	88	88	88	89	89	89	89	90	90	90	90	91	91	91	91	92	92	92	92	93	93	93																								
75	88	88	88	89	89	89	89	90	90	90	90	91	91	91	91	92	92	92	92	93	93	93	93	94	94																							
76	88	88	89	89	89	89	90	90	90	90	91	91	91	91	92	92	92	92	93	93	93	93	94	94	94	94																						
77	89	89	89	89	90	90	90	90	91	91	91	91	91	92	92	92	92	93	93	93	93	94	94	94	94	94	95																				
78	89	89	90	90	90	90	91	91	91	91	91	92	92	92	92	93	93	93	93	93	94	94	94	94	95	95	95	95																			
79	90	90	90	90	91	91	91	91	91	92	92	92	92	92	93	93	93	93	93	94	94	94	94	95	95	95	95	95	96																	
80	90	90	91	91	91	91	91	92	92	92	92	92	93	93	93	93	93	94	94	94	94	94	95	95	95	95	95	96	96	96																
81	91	91	91	91	91	92	92	92	92	92	93	93	93	93	93	94	94	94	94	94	94	95	95	95	95	95	96	96	96	96	96															
82	91	91	92	92	92	92	92	92	93	93	93	93	93	94	94	94	94	94	94	95	95	95	95	95	96	96	96	96	96	96	97	97														
83	92	92	92	92	92	93	93	93	93	93	93	94	94	94	94	94	94	95	95	95	95	95	95	96	96	96	96	96	96	97	97	97	97													
84	92	92	92	93	93	93	93	93	93	94	94	94	94	94	94	95	95	95	95	95	95	96	96	96	96	96	96	96	97	97	97	97	97	97												
85	93	93	93	93	93	93	94	94	94	94	94	94	94	95	95	95	95	95	95	96	96	96	96	96	96	96	97	97	97	97	97	97	97	98	98											
86	93	93	93	94	94	94	94	94	94	94	95	95	95	95	95	95	95	96	96	96	96	96	96	96	97	97	97	97	97	97	97	97	98	98	98	98										
87	94	94	94	94	94	94	94	95	95	95	95	95	95	95	95	96	96	96	96	96	96	96	96	97	97	97	97	97	97	97	98	98	98	98	98	98	98									
88	94	94	94	94	95	95	95	95	95	95	95	95	96	96	96	96	96	96	96	96	97	97	97	97	97	97	97	97	97	98	98	98	98	98	98	98	98	99								
89	95	95	95	95	95	95	95	95	95	96	96	96	96	96	96	96	96	96	97	97	97	97	97	97	97	97	97	98	98	98	98	98	98	98	98	98	99	99	99							
90	95	95	95	95	96	96	96	96	96	96	96	96	96	96	97	97	97	97	97	97	97	97	97	97	98	98	98	98	98	98	98	98	98	98	99	99	99	99	99	99						
91	96	96	96	96	96	96	96	96	96	96	96	97	97	97	97	97	97	97	97	97	97	97	98	98	98	98	98	98	98	98	98	98	98	99	99	99	99	99	99	99	99					
92	96	96	96	96	96	96	97	97	97	97	97	97	97	97	97	97	97	97	98	98	98	98	98	98	98	98	98	98	98	98	98	99	99	99	99	99	99	99	99	99	99	99				
93	97	97	97	97	97	97	97	97	97	97	97	97	97	97	98	98	98	98	98	98	98	98	98	98	98	98	98	98	99	99	99	99	99	99	99	99	99	99	99	99	99	99	99	100			
94	97	97	97	97	97	97	97	97	98	98	98	98	98	98	98	98	98	98	98	98	98	98	98	98	99	99	99	99	99	99	99	99	99	99	99	99	99	99	99	99	99	100	100	100			
95	98	98	98	98	98	98	98	98	98	98	98	98	98	98	98	98	98	98	98	99	99	99	99	99	99	99	99	99	99	99	99	99	99	99	99	99	99	99	99	100	100	100	100	100	100		
96	98	98	98	98	98	98	98	98	98	98	98	98	99	99	99	99	99	99	99	99	99	99	99	99	99	99	99	99	99	99	99	99	99	99	99	99	99	100	100	100	100	100	100	100	100	100	
97	99	99	99	99	99	99	99	99	99	99	99	99	99	99	99	99	99	99	99	99	99	99	99	99	99	99	99	99	99	99	99	99	99	100	100	100	100	100	100	100	100	100	100	100	100	100	100
98	99	99	99	99	99	99	99	99	99	99	99	99	99	99	99	99	99	99	99	99	99	99	99	99	100	100	100	100	100	100	100	100	100	100	100	100	100	100	100	100	100	100	100	100	100	100	100
99	100	100	100	100	100	100	100	100	100	100	100	100	100	100	100	100	100	100	100	100	100	100	100	100	100	100	100	100	100	100	100	100	100	100	100	100	100	100	100	100	100	100	100	100	100	100	100

Index